Ward Rounds in
Obstetrics and Neonatology

Ward Rounds in Obstetrics and Neonatology

Tania Gurdip Singh
MS (Obs and Gyne) Fellowship in Gynecological Endoscopy
Bodyline Trauma and Maternity Center
New Delhi, India

Earl Gaganjot Jaspal
MBBS MD (Ped) PGPN (Boston, USA)
Consultant Pediatrician and Head
Department of Neonatology
Government Hospital
Ambala, Haryana, India

Foreword
Nutan Jain

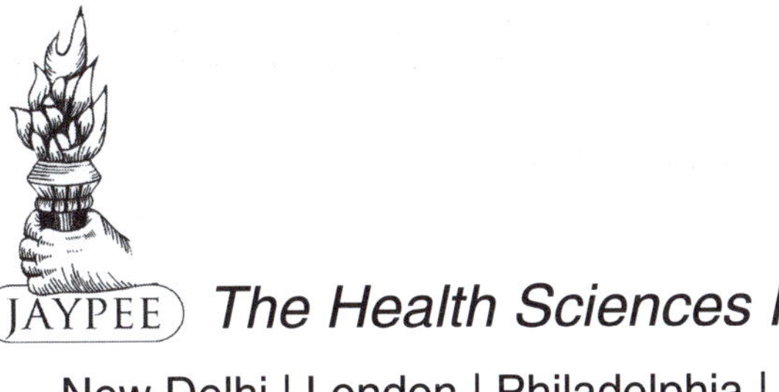

The Health Sciences Publisher
New Delhi | London | Philadelphia | Panama

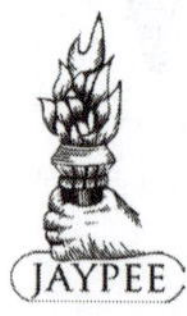 **Jaypee Brothers Medical Publishers (P) Ltd**

Headquarters

Jaypee Brothers Medical Publishers (P) Ltd
4838/24, Ansari Road, Daryaganj
New Delhi 110 002, India
Phone: +91-11-43574357
Fax: +91-11-43574314
Email: jaypee@jaypeebrothers.com

Overseas Offices

J.P. Medical Ltd
83 Victoria Street, London
SW1H 0HW (UK)
Phone: +44 20 3170 8910
Fax: +44 (0)20 3008 6180
Email: info@jpmedpub.com

Jaypee-Highlights Medical Publishers Inc
City of Knowledge, Bld. 237, Clayton
Panama City, Panama
Phone: +1 507-301-0496
Fax: +1 507-301-0499
Email: cservice@jphmedical.com

Jaypee Medical Inc
325 Chestnut Street
Suite 412, Philadelphia, PA 19106, USA
Phone: +1 267-519-9789
Email: support@ jpmedus.com

Jaypee Brothers Medical
Publishers (P) Ltd
17/1-B Babar Road, Block-B, Shaymali
Mohammadpur, Dhaka-1207
Bangladesh
Mobile: +08801912003485
Email: jaypeedhaka@gmail.com

Jaypee Brothers Medical Publishers (P) Ltd
Bhotahity, Kathmandu, Nepal
Phone +977-9741283608
Email: kathmandu@jaypeebrothers.com

Website: www.jaypeebrothers.com
Website: www.jaypeedigital.com

© 2016, Jaypee Brothers Medical Publishers

Inquiries for bulk sales may be solicited at: jaypee@jaypeebrothers.com

Ward Rounds in Obstetrics and Neonatology

First Edition: **2016**

ISBN 978-93-85891-65-6

Printed at Rajkamal Electric Press, Plot No. 2, Phase-IV, Kundli, Haryana.

Dedicated to

*Our daughter Aira, who is the ultimate source of motivation
and is a real boost in whatever we do, including this work*

Foreword

When I got the invitation to write foreword for this book, the first thought in my mind was "to read this book" because of very attractive name of the book. This book makes a solid base for MBBS, postgraduates, interns, and nursing students.

After reading, I was so happy about it as it was more than what I expected. The book goes in a soft flow of rounds, OPD, antenatal ward, labor room and ending up in neonatal unit. In the section of obstetric emergency, I had developed a feeling that I am present at bedside and participating in revival of the patient. Tricky situations demanding blood transfusion and proper fluid management are dictated in such a simple manner which will raise confidence of reader 'yeah, I can also do'. The most appreciable thing of this book is its limited length and simple language. It is amazing how the whole obstetrics and neonatology is covered in around 360 pages so fluently. Students generally struggle with multiple different books, just to find out few details or some special points which they can write down or mumble in their exams.

Dr Tania Singh and Dr Earl Jaspal has reduced all their struggle and tension due in their examinations, by involving all the chapters and details in very concise form in their book. Students can go through a rapid reading and revision of this book.

I must congratulate Dr Tania Singh and Dr Earl Jaspal for this rewarding hard work which will definitely help students and nursing staff who are really in need of such guidance.

It will also have a place of honor in my library.

Nutan Jain MS (Obs and Gyne)
Vardhman Trauma and Laparoscopy Centre Pvt Ltd
Muzaffarnagar, Uttar Pradesh, India

Preface

Ward Rounds in Obstetrics and Neonatology extensively covers all bedside cases which are routinely met in obstetrics and neonatology, wherein main stress is laid only on diagnosis and management in wards. It does not include the time consuming etiology and pathogenesis of any disease.

The book has been presented in two sections.

Section 1: Obstetrics covers all the aspects related to OPD Rounds, Antenatal Cases in High-risk and Low-risk Patients, Labor in High-risk and Low-risk patients, Obstetric Emergencies, Infections in Obstetrics, Blood Transfusion and Fluid Management.

Section 2: Neonatology has been added to cover all current and practical approaches in management of problems encountered in neonatal care including Prematurity and Low Birth Weight, Perinatal Asphyxia, Meconium Aspiration Syndrome, Sepsis, Neonatal Seizures, Hypoglycemia, Hypocalcemia, Fluid and Electrolyte Management, Neonatal Jaundice, Bag and Mask Ventilation and routine procedures in neonatal nursery.

The book will make the ward rounds easy for students as the chapters are very small each consisting of 3–5 pages on an average. Section on OPD rounds will enable a student to counsel any patient attending obstetric OPD. A complete chapter is provided only on HIV counseling.

The basic aim of this book is to provide complete and latest information in a simplified manner with focus on quality rather than quantity.

The information provided in each chapter has been condensed in an easy-to-read format with a point-wise description and important points are highlighted in side boxes to allow quick but at the same time, proficient understanding of the material.

This book has been exclusively designed for medical students, residents, postgraduates, fellows, interns, consultants and nursing staff working in both government and private set-up.

The information provided is up-to-date and include latest protocols and clinical knowledge in fields of obstetrics and neonatology.

We hope this book will provide a better understanding of basic concepts and bedside clinical approach related to all topics in management of obstetrics and neonatology.

Tania Gurdip Singh
Earl Gaganjot Jaspal

Acknowledgments

We take this opportunity to thank all our teachers, friends and well-wishers, that is very much justified at this stage of the completion of our book.

It is our great privilege, though finding words inadequate to express our indebtedness and deep gratitude to Dr Nutan Jain. Her never-ending willingness to render help, loving guidance, coupled with her rich knowledge and keen interest, were a constant source of inspiration for us throughout.

We are deeply grateful to all our revered teachers and shall ever remain obliged to them.

We are very grateful to Shri Jitendar P Vij (Group Chairman) and Mr Ankit Vij (Group President) for showing trust in us and getting this book published. We are sincerely thankful to Mr Tarun Duneja (Director–Publishing), Ms Samina Khan (Executive Assistant to Director–Publishing), Ms Seema Dogra (Cover Designer), Ms Hansika Seth (Copy Editor) Ms Ritu Verma (DTP Operator) of M/s Jaypee Brothers Medical Publishers (P) Ltd, New Delhi, India, who rendered great help in the completion of this project.

We shall be failing in our duty if we do not acknowledge with a deep sense of gratitude, all our patients, from whom we have learnt a lot.

We cannot express in words the indebtedness we owe to our dearest parents, without whose inspiration and blessings, this work could not have been accomplished. Wholeheartedly, we are very thankful to them and entire credit goes to them.

We owe our sincere admiration and thanks to Dr Gagandeep Anand and Dr Nisha Munjal Anand, for their contribution. Their valuable and constructive suggestions were the mainstream to bring this work to the present shape.

And finally, we thank God for everything and pray for His continued blessings and success.

Contents

OBSTETRICS

NEONATOLOGY

Abbreviations

ACE Inhibitors	Angiotensin converting enzyme inhibitors
ADH	Antidiuretic hormone
AED	Antiepileptic drug
AFI	Amniotic fluid index
AFV	Amniotic fluid volume
AIDS	Acquired immunodeficiency syndrome
ALT	Alanine aminotransferase
Anti-TPO	Antithyroid peroxidase
APFS	Antepartum fetal surveillance
aPTT	Activated partial thromboplastin time
ARM	Artificial rupture of membrane
ART	Antiretroviral therapy
AST	Aspartate aminotransferase
BMI	Body mass index
BT	Blood transfusion
CA	Cholic acid
CAD	Coronary artery disease
CBC	Complete blood count
CCT	Controlled cord traction
CDCA	Chenodeoxycholic acid
CFT	Capillary filling time
CHC	Community health center
CHF	Congestive heart failure
CIN	Cervical intraepithelial neoplasia
CMV	Cytomegalovirus
COC	Combined oral contraceptive
CPAP	Continuous positive airway pressure
CPD	Cephalopelvic disproportion
CPR	Cardiopulmonary resuscitation
CTG	Cardiotocography
CVS	Chorionic villus sampling; Cardiovascular system
DBP	Diastolic blood pressure
DCA	Deoxycholic acid
DFKC	Daily fetal kick count
DIC	Disseminated intravascular coagulopathy
DM	Diabetes milletus
DNA	Deoxyribonucleic acid
DV Doppler	Ductus venosus Doppler
DVT	Deep vein thrombosis
ECV	External cephalic version
EDD	Expected date of delivery
EEG	Electroencephalography
EFW	Estimated fetal weight

EPO	Erythropoietin
FHR	Fetal heart rate
g	gauze
G6PD	Glucose 6 phosphate dehydrogenase
GFR	Glomerular filtration rate
GGT	Gamma glutamyl transpeptidase
GI	Gastrointestinal
GIT	Gastrointestinal tract
gm	grams
GTCS	Generalized tonic-clonic seizure
GTN	Gestational trophoblastic neoplasia
Hb	Hemoglobin
HC	Head circumference
hCG	Human chorionic gonadotropin
HDL	High density lipoproteins
ICT	Indirect Coomb's test
IM	Intramuscular
INR	International normalized ratio
IQ	Intelligence quotient
IU	International units
IUD	Intrauterine death; Intrauterine device
IUGR	Intrauterine growth restriction
IV	Intravenous
IVF	In vitro fertilization
IWL	Insensible water loss
JVP	Jugular venous pressure
Kg	Kilogram
KMC	Kangaroo mother care
LCA	Lithocholic acid
LDH	Lactate dehydrogenase
LDL	Low density lipoproteins
LFT	Liver function test
LMP	Last menstrual period
LMWH	Low molecular weight heparin
LNG IUD	Levonorgestrel intrauterine device
LSCS	Lower segment cesarean section
LV	Left ventricle
MAS	Meconium aspiration synrdrome
MCA	Middle cerebral artery
MCDA	Monochorionic diamniotic
mcg	Micrograms
MCH	Mean corpuscular hemoglobin
MCHC	Mean corpuscular hemoglobin concentration
MCMA	Monochorionic monoamniotic
MCV	Mean corpuscular volume
mEq	Milliequalent
mL	Milliliter
MMR	Measles, mumps, rubella
MOA	Mechanism of action
MRI	Magnetic resonance imaging
MUFA	Monounsaturated fatty acids
NICU	Neonatal intensive care unit
NPO	Nil per os
NSAID	Nonsteroidal anti-inflammatory drugs
NST	Nonstress test
NTD	Neural tube defect

NYHA class	New York Heart Association class
OCP	Oral contraceptive pill
OGTT	Oral glucose tolerance test
p.o	per os
PCV	Packed cell volume
PDA	Patent ductus arteriosus
PHC	Primary health center
PI	Pulsatility index
PID	Pelvic inflammatory disease
PPBS	Postprandial blood sugar
PPD	Purified protein derivative
PPH	Postpartum hemorrhage
PPROM	Preterm premature rupture of membranes
PROM	Premature rupture of membranes
PT	Prothrombin time
RBC	Red blood cell
RDS	Respiratory distress syndrome
RFT	Renal function test
RHD	Rheumatic heart disease
RI	Resistance index
RNA	Ribonucleic acid
ROM	Rupture of membranes
RPL	Recurrent pregnancy loss
RUQ	Right upper quadrant
SBP	Systolic blood pressure
SFH	Symphysis-fundal height
SGA	Small for gestational age
SIADH	Syndrome of inappropriate secretion of antidiuretic hormone
SIDS	Sudden infant death syndrome
SLE	Systemic lupus erythematosus
STD	Sexually transmitted diseases
TAS	Transabdominal scan
TBG	Thyroxine-binding globulin
TFT	Thyroid function test
TSH	Thyroid stimulating hormone
TTTS	Twin to twin transfusion syndrome
TVS	Transvaginal scan
UA	Umbilical artery
UPT	Urine pregnancy test
UTI	Urinary tract infection
vWF	Von Willebrand disease
FBS	Fasting blood sugar

PART 1

OBSTETRICS

Section Outline

Section I:

OPD Rounds

Chapter **1**

Preconceptional History and Counseling

Tania G Singh

HISTORY

Genetic History: Risk Factors

Risk Factors for Numerical Chromosomal Abnormalities and New Mutations

- Maternal age
- Paternal age (≥40 years, r/o child having new gene mutations)
- Radiation/chemicals/drugs.

Risk Factors for Inherited Mutations

- Presence of such an illness in either parent, in his or her family or in a previous child
- Couple's ethnic background
- Consanguinity—risk of autosomal recessive disorders increases.

Family History

Construct three-generation pedigree which includes the following:

Genetic Disorders in the Family

- Muscular dystrophy; Hemophilia; Cystic fibrosis; Fragile X syndrome
- Congenital heart disease; Phenylketonuria; Dwarfism
- Sickle-cell anemia; Tay-Sachs disease.

Multifactorial Congenital Malformations

- Spina bifida; Anencephaly; Cleft palate and cleft lip
- Hypospadias; Congenital heart disease.

Familial Diseases with a Major Genetic Component

- Developmental disability; Premature atherosclerosis
- Diabetes mellitus; Psychosis; Epileptic disorders
- Hypertension; Rheumatoid arthritis; Deafness
- Severe refractive disorders of the eye.

Age: Women less than 20 or more than 35 years carry increased risks.

Health History

Chronic Conditions

- Diabetes mellitus; Anemia; Thyroid disorders; Gynecological disorders
- Asthma; STDs; Heart disease; Hypertension
- Deep venous thrombosis; Kidney disease; SLE; Epilepsy

High-risk Ethnic Groups

- Cystic fibrosis in Europe, the Mediterranean region and Middle East
- Sickle-cell anemia and thalassemia (where prevalence of malaria is ↑)
- Tay-Sachs disease and several other rare disorders in Ashkenazi Jewish background
- Neural tube defects

Past Obstetric History Includes

- Early/late miscarriages/stillbirths
- Number of pregnancies and live issues
- Mode of previous deliveries
- Length/course of labor
- Complications (preterm labor or delivery, gestational diabetes milletus, hypertension in pregnancy, postpartum depression)

Lab. Testing
- CBC; Urinalysis; ABO Rh; VDRL; HIV;
- HbsAg; Rubella antibody titer
- FBS/OGTT ; TFT; TORCH – when indicated

No Personal Health Risks and Planned Pregnancy
- Folate-rich foods-fortified grains, spinach, lentils, chick peas, asparagus, broccoli, peas, Brussels sprouts, corn, and oranges
- A multivitamin with folic acid (0.4–1.0 mg) x 2–3 months before conception and throughout pregnancy and postpartum period (4–6 weeks and as long as breastfeeding continues)

Patients with Health Risks or a Family History of Neural Tube Defects or Belonging to a High-risk Ethnic Group (e.g., Sikh)
- Require increased dietary intake of folate-rich foods
- A multivitamin with 5 mg folic acid, beginning at least three months before conception, continuing throughout pregnancy and 4–6 weeks postpartum or as long as breastfeeding continues, supplementation should consist of a multivitamin with folic acid (0.4–1.0 mg)

- Hemoglobinopathies; Cancer; Seizure disorders
- Tuberculosis; Rheumatoid arthritis; Mental health/psychiatric disorders.

Infectious Conditions

- Rubella or varicella susceptible—offer vaccination, if not vaccinated
- Hepatitis B and C—routine preconception testing is not currently recommended
- Routine serologic testing for toxoplasmosis is not recommended
- Evaluate (woman and her partner) for sexually transmitted disease (e.g., Chlamydia, HIV, gonorrhea, syphilis)
- Periodontal screening
- Nonpregnant women immunized with a live or live-attenuated vaccine should be counseled to delay pregnancy by at least four weeks.

Reproductive History

- Menstrual history (regularity, duration and amount of flow, length of cycle, clots, dysmenorrhea)
- Contraceptive; sexual history; infertility; abnormal Pap smears
- In utero exposure to diethylstilbestrol
- Past obstetric history.

Lifestyle Assessment

- BMI; nutrition; physical activity; sufficient sleep; minimum stress
- Prescription and over-the-counter drug use; other substance abuse
- Environmental exposures (current and past).

Counseling

- Ideal BMI—19.6-26.0 kg/mt^2
- Laboratory testing
- Folic acid (vitamin B9) to decrease the incidence of fetal congenital anomalies)
- Vitamin D intake of minimum 5 µg/day for nonpregnant women with limited exposure to sunlight (i.e. those whose hands and face are exposed to the open air for <15 min/day) and 10 µg/day for pregnant women
- Avoid exposure to cat feces, raw/undercooked meats and unpasteurized milk
- Smoking and alcohol cessation
- Consumption of vitamin A to less than 3000 µg/day
- Polytherapy changed to monotherapy in case of epilepsy with prior consultation with aneurologist
- Adequate glycemic control in a patient of pregestational diabetes
- Consultation with cardiologist, if having cardiac disease
- ACE inhibitors should be changed to a different drug.

Chapter **2**

Prepregnancy Counseling in a Cardiac Case

Tania G Singh

- Thorough history of cardiac symptoms including arrhythmias and physical exam
- Explain features of present heart condition/lesion → functional and risk classification
- Should be made aware that deterioration of NYHA class may occur as pregnancy advances
- Obtain records
- Explain the effects of cardiac condition on pregnancy and vice versa
- Adjust medications to avoid adverse fetal effects
- Genetic counseling in cases of heritable lesions
- Need for surgery (valve replacement or repair, if symptomatic prior to pregnancy)/anticoagulation
- Do all baseline investigations (blood tests, exercise tolerance test, ECG, Echocardiography)
- Prenatal visits and need for maternal and fetal testing
- Fetal and neonatal complications (with her specific condition)
- Timing of birth/type of hospital facility required for childbirth
- Pain control and type of anesthesia (during labor and delivery)
- Explain need for cesarean section
- Effective contraception until pregnancy desired

Other important points to be discussed:

- All potential sources of infection to be looked for
- Infection may lie dormant in genital tract
- Dental roots and caries (dangerous source)
- No root filling or capping of teeth in cardiac cases, whether pregnant or not
- UTI has to be looked for
- Anemia → add to complications and failure. Therefore, need to correct it
- ACE inhibitors—contraindicated in pregnancy
- Need for diuretics to be reassessed
- Anticoagulant advice
- Pregnancy best to be avoided (or if conceived) → terminated (maternal mortality → 30–50%) in few situations
- Explain them effects of pregnancy on cardiac disease
- Explain the patient 'Dangerous periods' in pregnancy ("RULE OF 5") in a cardiac patient
  - 5th week—When cardiac output begins to increase (physiological changes start)
  - 5 weeks before term—when all changes reach maximum (mainly cardiac output)
  - 5 minutes after delivery

Side Effects of ACE Inhibitors

- Fetal hypotension
- Anuria
- Oligohydramnios
- IUGR
- Pulmonary hypoplasia
- Renal tubular dysplasia
- Hypocalvaria

Anticoagulants in Cardiac Case

- Oral anticoagulants → to be switched over to heparin at ≈ 6 weeks
- Pregnancy diagnosed → stop warfarin
- Up to 12th week → Inj. Heparin 5000 IU BD s/c
- From 12th week up to 36th week → Tab. Warfarin 3 mg daily (at the same time)
- From 36th week up to Day 7 postpartum → Heparin
- Afterwards → give warfarin

Absolute Contraindications to Pregnancy

- Eisenmenger's syndrome
- 1° pulmonary hypertension
- Corpulmonale
- Single ventricle
- Marfan's syndrome with dilated aortic root
- Terminate in 1st trimester (even for class III and IV patients). They can have permanent sterilization

<table>
<tr><td valign="top" width="30%">

Relative Contraindications to Pregnancy

- Parous women with grade III/IV
- Grade I or II with previous history of cardiac failure in early months or in between pregnancies

During Labor and Immediately after Delivery

- Labor: Every uterine contraction injects 300–500 mL of blood from utero placental circulation into maternal blood stream increasing cardiac output by 15–20%
- Simultaneously during 2nd stage—maternal pushing decreases venous return to heart causing a decrease in cardiac output
- These sudden and frequent variations during 2nd stage may be critical
- When obstructive effect of pregnant uterus upon return circulation to heart disappears → sudden transfusion of blood from lower extremities and utero placental vasculature to systemic circulation → there is ↑ chance of CHF

</td><td valign="top">

- 5 hours after delivery
- 5 days after delivery.
- Mortality lowest with RHD and acyanotic heart disease— less than 1%.

Fetal Prognosis

- Good in RHD (not different from normal patients)
- Cyanotic—increased mortality (45%)
- Causes:
  - Abortion
  - Intrauterine growth restriction (IUGR)
  - Prematurity.
- Fetal congenital malformation increases by 3–10%, if either of parents have congenital lesions, therefore, fetal echo at 20–24 weeks is recommended.

</td></tr>
</table>

Chapter 3

General History Taking

Tania G Singh

CHIEF COMPLAINTS OF THE PATIENT

Past Obstetric History (Gravida Parity Abortions Ectopic Twins Death)

- Married life (years)
- Consanguinity
- Whether ANCs were taken in each previous pregnancy
- Grand multiparity
- Abortions (type, period of gestation, management done)
- Ectopic pregnancy
- Any h/o molar pregnancy
- Any h/o twin gestation (nonidentical twins tend to recur)
- Any perinatal deaths (at what period of gestation, cause, delivery by induction or spontaneous, appearance of the baby: macerated, peeling of skin, any gross congenital anamolies seen, did the baby cry after birth)
- Mode and time of each delivery—vaginal or cesarean section; h/o prolonged labor; home or institutional delivery; any instruments used
- If delivery was by cesarean section—cause, any postoperative complications, any history of blood transfusion
- Was Anti-D taken in cases of Rh negative pregnancy
- Whether any baby was kept in NICU, it's cause and for how long
- Intervals between pregnancies
- Whether all babies are alive and healthy now
- Breastfeeding done and for how long.

Present Pregnancy

- Type of conception (spontaneous or after infertility treatment)
- Any history of fever with or without rash, vaginal bleeding, burning micturition, etc.

Menstrual History

- Last menstrual period
- Periods were regular or irregular
- Whether the patient had any spotting even after LMP
- Any history of oral contraceptives or injectable contraception used just prior to conception

Complications in previous antenatal periods (pre eclampsia, preterm labor, gestational diabetes, antepartum hemorrhage) should be enquired

Previous Ectopic Pregnancy

Ask whether managed medically or surgically; what surgery was done; was the tube saved; any blood transfusions were done; if medically treated, any reaction to the drug used, when was the treatment ended

History of Following Illnesses should be asked

- Hypertension
- Diabetes mellitus
- Rheumatic or other heart disease
- Epilepsy
- Asthma
- Tuberculosis
- Psychiatric illness
- Any other major illness
- Certain drugs can be teratogenic to the fetus. So they need to be changed or stopped at all

<table>
<tr><td valign="top" width="30%">

Social Circumstances of the Patient

- ❧ Occupation (to exclude occupational hazards or occupation as a cause of stress)
- ❧ Unemployment, poor housing (kuccha or pucca house, electricity), overcrowding
- ❧ Daily calories of the patient need to be counted
- ❧ Smoking/alcohol consumption

Abdominal Examination Includes

- ❧ Pigmentation "linea nigra"
- ❧ Striae gravidarum (color, site)
- ❧ Any scar (any previous surgery), its site (horizontal, vertical), its condition
- ❧ Fetal movements; fetal parts; external ballotment; any contractions; fundal height; Symphysis fundal height (with measuring tape)
- ❧ Leopold manoeuvres
- ❧ Fetal heart sound by stethoscope

</td><td valign="top">

Personal and Family History

- History of medications, surgeries or allergies in the past
- Parents and first degree relatives with a condition, such as diabetes, multiple pregnancy, bleeding tendencies or mental retardation increases the risk of these conditions in the patient and the fetus
- Some birth defects are inherited.

Physical Examination

General Appearance

- Built, height, weight, BMI, nutrition, sleep
- Face—any pigmentation
- Systemic examination:
    - Pallor, icterus, cyanosis, clubbing, lymphadenopathy, edema (feet, hands, face)
    - Enlarged thyroid, goitre
    - Breasts: enlargement, warmth, tenderness, any discharge, inverted or flat nipples, Montgomery's follicles "glandular tubercles".
- Spine (lordosis, kyphosis, scoliosis)
- Respiratory system: breath sounds, bilateral air entry, respiratory rate, dyspnea
- Cardiovascular system: BP, PR, functional murmurs
- Abdomen (always warm your hands before abdominal palpation)
- Both external and internal genitalia
    - Any ulcers, purulent or excessive discharge
    - Suspicious looking cervix (cervical smear must be taken) or any growth on the cervix
    - Bimanual examination for condition of the internal os
    - Any tenderness in the fornices.
- Pelvic assessment at 37 weeks.

In the end, calculate period of gestation and write the provisional diagnosis.

</td></tr>
</table>

Chapter 4

Routine Antenatal Checkup and Advice

Tania G Singh

FIRST TRIMESTER (FIRST 12 WEEKS OF PREGNANCY)

Symptoms

- Amenorrhea
- Nausea and vomiting
- Frequency of micturition
- Breast changes—discomfort, enlargement, pain/heaviness
- Fatigue/lassitude
- Change in appetite—craving for certain foods, odors and particular objects
- Sleepiness
- Emotional changes/mood swings.

Signs

Breast Signs

- Appear at 6–8 weeks
- Enlargement with vascular engorgement
- Discomfort—fullness, heaviness and pricking sensation
- Nipple and primary areola become more pigmented
- Montgomery's tubercles appears
- Expression of colostrum as early as 12th week
- More in primigravidae.

Pelvic Signs

Hegar's sign

- Bimanual examination with two fingers in the anterior fornix and the fingers of the other hand on the abdomen behind the uterus
- The internal and external fingers can be approximated due to the fact that the lower segment is soft and empty and upper part of body of uterus is enlarged
- Present from 6 weeks until the 12th week of pregnancy.

Palmer's sign

- Pregnancy should be of at least 8 weeks duration
- Two fingers of gloved right hand are placed into the vagina and left hand palpates the lower abdomen from above, wait for 2–3 minutes
- Uterus becomes firm and then ill-defined as there is contractions and relaxation.

The first antenatal visit should be between 6-10 weeks

Frequency of Micturition

- Due to congestion and pressure on the bladder
- Appears from 8–12 weeks
- Reappears again near the end of pregnancy when the fetal head descends into the maternal pelvis

Placental Sign

- Bleeding at the time of next menstruation

Hartman's Sign

- Implantation bleeding

Ladin's Sign

- Softening in the midline of the uterus anteriorly at the junction of the uterus and cervix
- Occurs at about 6 weeks gestation

Goodell's Sign

- A significant softening of the vaginal portion of the cervix from increased vascularization of uterus in pregnancy
- Can be seen at 6th week

Others

- Placental sign, Hartman's sign, Goodell's sign, Von Braun-Fernwald's sign, Chadwick's sign, Piskacek's sign, Osiander's sign.

SECOND TRIMESTER (13–28 WEEKS)

There should be a minimum of three visits in this trimester.

Symptoms

- Amenorrhea
- Morning sickness and urinary symptoms decrease
- Progressive abdominal enlargement.

Signs

- Breasts become engorged
- Uterus feels soft and elastic, and becomes ovoid shape
- Braxton-Hicks contractions are evident
- Increased softening of the cervix
- Internal ballottement can be elicited between 16th and 28th week.

14–16 Weeks

- Colostrum becomes thick and yellowish by 16th week
- Injection tetanus toxoid 0.5 mL IM (1st dose) should be given
- Prescribe iron and calcium.

18–20 Weeks

- Quickening
- Secondary areola
- Prominent montgomery's tubercles extend to the secondary areola
- Striae (both pink and white)
- Linea nigra
- Palpation of fetal parts
- Active fetal movements
- External ballottement
- Fetal heart sound detected with stethoscope
- Continue iron and calcium
- Injection T.T. 0.5 mL IM (2nd dose).

24–25 Weeks

- Face—chloasma gravidarum may appear at 24th week
- Measure weight and blood pressure
- Plot symphysis–fundal height
- Test urine for proteinuria and rule out asymptomatic bacteriuria
- Oral glucose tolerance test where indicated
- Fetal echocardiography, if mother has heart disease or any fetal cardiac abnormality detected at the time of anamoly scan.

Fundal Height (McDonald's Rule)

- Fundal height, or McDonald's rule, is a measure of the size of the uterus used to assess fetal growth and development during pregnancy

---

Von Braun-Fernwald's Sign

- Irregular softening and enlargement of the uterine fundus at 5–8 weeks gestation

Chadwick's Sign

- Bluish discoloration of the cervix, vagina and labia resulting from increased blood flow
- Observed at 6–8 weeks

Piskacek's Sign

- Can be observed at 7–8 weeks
- One half of uterus - more firm than other half
- Observing a soft palpable bulge at the uterine cornu

Osiander's Sign

- Increased pulsations felt through lateral fornix by 8 weeks

---

- Uterus remains a pelvic organ until 12th week
- From 12–14 weeks, it can be felt as suprapubic bulge

Quickening

- When movements made by the fetus are perceived for the first time by mother
- Occurs at 18–20 weeks in primigravida and 16–18 weeks in multi gravida

- It is measured from the top of the mother's uterus to the top of the mother's pubic bone in centimeter.

THIRD TRIMESTER (29–40 WEEKS)

- As the fetus and uterus grows, patient will complain of more and more discomfort
- Abdomen enlarges further
- There may be physiological edema of the feet
- Frequency of micturition again increases
- Fetal movements are more distinct
- Pigmentation and striae—more dark.

Examination

Lie

- Relationship between the longitudinal axis of fetus and mother
- Longitudinal (resulting in either cephalic or breech presentation)
- Oblique (unstable, will eventually become either longitudinal or transverse)
- Transverse (resulting in shoulder presentation).

Presentation

- Refers to leading anatomical part of the fetus, i.e. is closest to the pelvic inlet of the birth canal
- The various presentations are:
  - Cephalic presentation (96.5%)
  - Breech presentation (3%)
  - Shoulder.

Presenting Part

- The part which is usually felt first on per vaginal examination
- Depending on the degree of flexion, in a cephalic presentation, the presenting part can be
  - Vertex — most common
  - Sinciput
  - Brow
  - Face
  - Chin.

Attitude

- Relationship of fetal head to spine
  - Flexed, (this is the normal situation) where sinciput is higher than the occiput
  - Neutral ("military"), a deflexed state, when both sinciput and occiput are at the same level
  - Extended.

Denominator

It is the bony point on the presenting part which comes in contact with the various quadrants of the maternal pelvis.

Gestational Age	Fundal Height
40 weeks	1–2 finger width below subcostal arch
36 weeks	At costal arch
32 weeks	Between umbilicus and xiphoid process
28 weeks	3 finger widths above umbilicus
24 weeks	At umbilicus
20 weeks	3 finger widths below umbilicus
16 weeks	3 finger widths above symphysis

Two other sounds are confused with FHS:

Uterine Soufflé

- Soft blowing and systolic
- Synchronous with maternal pulse
- Due to increased blood flow though the dilated uterine vessels

Funic or Fetal Soufflé

- Due to rush of blood through the umbilical arteries
- A soft, blowing murmur
- Synchronous with the FHS

Presenting Part	Denominator
Vertex	Occiput
Face	Mentum
Brow	Frontal eminence
Breech	Sacrum
Shoulder	Acromion

LOA is the most common position and lie

Position

- Relationship of presenting part to maternal pelvis
- Based on various presentations, the different positions can be as follows:

Vertex presentation with longitudinal lie

- Left occipitoanterior (LOA)—the occiput is close to the vagina (hence known as vertex presentation) faces anteriorly (forward with mother standing) and towards left
- Right occipitoanterior (ROA)—the occiput faces anteriorly and towards right
- Left occipitoposterior (LOP)—the occiput faces posteriorly (behind) and towards left
- Right occipitoposterior (ROP)—the occiput faces posteriorly and towards right
- Occipitoanterior—the occiput faces anteriorly (absolutely straight without turning to any of the sides)
- Occipitoposterior—the occiput faces posteriorly (absolutely straight without turning to any of the sides).

Face Presentation

Breech presentation with longitudinal lie

Shoulder Presentation with Transverse Lie

Classified into four types, based on the location of the scapula

- Left scapula-anterior (LSA)
- Right scapula-anterior (RSA)
- Left scapula-posterior (LSP)
- Right scapula-posterior (RSP)

- Left sacrum anterior (LSA)—the buttocks, as against the occiput of the vertex presentation, like close to the vagina (hence known as breech presentation), which like anteriorly and towards the left
- Right sacrum anterior (RSA)—the buttocks face anteriorly and towards the right
- Left sacrum posterior (LSP)—the buttocks face posteriorly and towards the left
- Right sacrum posterior (RSP)—the buttocks face posteriorly and towards right
- Sacrum anterior (SA)—the buttocks face anteriorly
- Sacrum posterior (SP)—the buttocks face posteriorly.

Shoulder presentation with transverse lie

Physiological Edema in Pregnancy

- Caused by increased venous pressure of lower extremities by gravid uterus pressing on common iliac veins
- Slight degree (ankle edema) usually confined to 1 leg (right > left)
- Unassociated with increase in BP or proteinuria
- Disappears on rest alone
- Check it over medial malleolus and anterior 1/3rd of tibia
- Press with thumb for 5 seconds

28–30 Weeks

- Measure blood pressure and weight
- Check edema (pedal)
- Check hemoglobin
- Offer anti-D prophylaxis to all rhesus-negative women
- Measure symphysis–fundal height.

32–34 Weeks

- Measure weight, blood pressure and symphysis fundal height
- Ultrasound for fetal wellbeing, liquor, placental localization
- Urine routine to be done
- Repeat ICT at 34–36 weeks
- Some prefer to give anti-D again at 34 weeks (if dual dose regimen was adopted at 28 weeks)
- Confirm the presenting part by Leopold's manoeuvres.

LEOPOLD'S MANOEUVRES

First Manoeuvre: Fundal Grip

- While facing the woman, palpate the woman's upper abdomen with both hands

- Determine the size, consistency, shape, and mobility of the form that is felt
- Fetal head is hard, firm, round, and moves independently of the trunk while the buttocks feel softer, are symmetric, and the shoulders and limbs have small bony processes; unlike the head, they move with the trunk.

Second Manoeuvre: Umbilical Grip or Lateral Grip

- Attempt to determine the location of the fetal back
- Still facing the woman, palpate the abdomen with gentle but also deep pressure using the palm of the hands
- First the right hand remains steady on one side of the abdomen while the left hand explores the right side of the uterus
- This is then repeated using the opposite side and hands
- The fetal back will feel firm and smooth while fetal extremities (arms, legs, etc.) should feel like small irregularities and protrusions
- The fetal back, once determined, should be continuous with the part found at fundus and also to the one in the maternal inlet or lower abdomen.

Third Manoeuvre: First Pelvic Grip

- Face the woman's feet
- The fingers of both hands are moved gently down the sides of the uterus toward the pubis
- The side where the resistance to the descent of the fingers towards the pubis is greatest, is where the brow is located
- If the head of the fetus is well-flexed, it should be on the opposite side from the fetal back
- If the fetal head is extended and the occiput is felt, instead, it is located on the same side as the back.

Fourth Manoeuvre: Pawlick's Grip (Second Pelvic Grip)

- In this manoeuvre, attempt to determine which fetal part is lying above the inlet, or lower abdomen
- First grasp the lower portion of the abdomen just above the pubic symphysis with the thumb and fingers of the right hand
- If it is the head and is not engaged, it may be gently pushed back and forth.

36–38 Weeks

- Measure weight, blood pressure
- Fetal presentation
- 'Lightening'—when the baby has dropped down in the pelvis and the diaphragm is relieved of pressure
- Per vaginal examination is done
- If it is a breech presentation, ECV can be offered after excluding contraindications to it
- Explain the patient about the labor process in brief
- Woman is made aware of signs of onset of true labor pains
- If cesarean section is to be done, indication is discussed with the woman and appropriate gestational age for it is decided
- Women should be made aware about the advantages of breastfeeding.

Prerequisites before Leopold's Manoeuvres

- Difficult to perform on obese women and women who have polyhydramnios
- The maneuvers consist of four distinct actions
- Woman is relaxed and adequately positioned
- Bladder emptied
- The woman should lie on her back with her shoulders raised slightly on a pillow and her knees flexed
- Abdomen uncovered
- Warm the hands by rubbing prior to palpation

Per Vaginal Examination at 36–38 Weeks for:

- Adequacy of pelvis
- Any cervical changes
- And then mode of delivery is discussed with the patient

Woman should Report if She has the Following:

- Pain abdomen which is radiating
- Intermittent and increasing in frequency, duration and intensity
- Per vaginal leak or blood-stained discharge
- Decreased fetal movements

Chapter 5

Blood Pressure Measurement

Tania G Singh

BLOOD PRESSURE RECORDING IN PREGNANCY—IDEAL METHOD

Position

- Rest—5 minutes
- Sitting with feet supported on flat surface (avoid supine position)
- Remove all tight clothing from the arm
- Arm well supported at the level of the heart (different arm positions can alter the BP significantly)
- Measure BP on both arms at first visit (this excludes rare vascular disorders)
- BP of the arm giving higher reading is to be taken
- In labor → left recumbent position.

Cuff

- Length—1.5 times the circumference of the arm
- Wide enough to cover at least 2/3rd of the upper arm
- Arm circumference greater than 33 cm → use larger cuff
- Smaller cuff size will overestimate BP
- Larger cuff will underestimate BP
- Lower edge of the cuff should be 2–3 cm above the point of brachial artery pulsation (easy access to antecubital fossa)
- Application should be firm.

Measurement Apparatus

- Mercury sphygmomanometer is still considered the best for measuring BP (especially in pre eclamptic patients)
- Automated devices may underestimate BP by 10–15 mm Hg.

Measurement

- Do not kink or twist the tube on the cuff
- Inflated and deflated smoothly
- Korotkoff V is taken for diastolic BP
- Korotkoff IV only when sounds are audible as level approaches "0" mm Hg (due to hyperdynamic circulation of pregnancy).

Chapter 6

Weight Gain in Pregnancy

Tania G Singh

Weeks	Weight gain (Pounds)	Weight gain (kg)
0–10 weeks	No weight gain	No weight gain
10–14 weeks	3–4 pounds	1.5 kg
14–20 weeks	4–6 pounds	2.5 kg
20–30 weeks	10–12 pounds	4.5 kg
30–36 weeks	6 pounds	2.7 kg
36–38 weeks	2 pounds	1.0 kg
38–40 weeks	Almost no weight gain	Almost no weight gain
Total	25–30 pounds	12–14 kg

- Underweight: BMI below 18.5
- Normal weight: 18.5 to 24.9
- Overweight: 25.0 to 29.9
- Obese: 30.0 and above

Chapter 7

Symphysis-Fundal Height Measurement

Tania G Singh

Fundal Height (McDonald's Rule)

Fundal height, or McDonald's rule, is a measure of the size of the uterus used to assess fetal growth and development during pregnancy. It is measured from the top of the mother's uterus to the top of the mother's pubic bone in centimeter

Gestational Age	Fundal Height
40 weeks	1–2 finger width below subcostal arch
36 weeks	At costal arch
32 weeks	Between umbilicus and xiphoid process
28 weeks	3 finger widths above umbilicus
24 weeks	At umbilicus
20 weeks	3 finger widths below umbilicus
16 weeks	3 finger widths above symphysis

SYMPHYSIS-FUNDAL HEIGHT MEASUREMENT

Symphysis-fundal measurement is done by using a measurement tape:

- To determine
  - Period of gestation
  - Growth of the fetus
  - Multiple pregnancies
  - Complications of pregnancy, e.g. amniotic fluid disorders
  - Hydatidiform mole and fetal growth disturbances.
- Between 20 and 34 weeks gestation, the height of the uterus correlates closely with measurements in centimeter (except in obesity).

STEPS OF MEASUREMENT

Step I

- Explain the procedure to the mother and gain verbal consent
- Wash hands
- Obtain an on-elastic measuring tape
- Ensure that the mother is comfortable in a supine position and extended legs, with an empty bladder
- Expose enough of the abdomen to allow a thorough examination.

Step II

- Ensure the abdomen is soft (not contracting)
- Perform abdominal palpation to enable accurate identification of the uterine fundus.

Step III

- Use the measuring tape with the centimeter on the underside to reduce bias
- Place the zero mark of the tape measure at the uppermost border of the symphysis pubis
- Measure from the top of symphysis pubis to the top of fundus
- The tape should stay in contact with the skin.

Step IV

- Measure along the longitudinal axis without correcting to the abdominal midline
- Do not hold the tape between the fingers
- Tape should then be turned so that the numbers are visible and the value can be recorded
- Measure only once
- Measurements should be in centimeter only.

Caution:

- If the bladder is full, it can increase the fundal height by 3 cm
- Supine position has the least variations in measurements
- After 34 weeks, not recommended as it may give erroneous readings due to descent of fetus into pelvis
- A discrepancy of >2 cm should be reported

Chapter 8

Gestational Age Calculation (Good Dates/Bad Dates)

Tania G Singh

GESTATIONAL AGE CALCULATION

Calculation of period of gestation is by:
- Last normal menstrual period (if dates are sure)
- Size of the uterus on bimanual (up to 12 weeks) examination
- Abdominal examination from 12–22 weeks, when fundal height is still below the umbilicus, is considered very accurate
- SFH between 24 and 36 weeks
- The size of the fetus (rule out IUGR/SGA or large for date fetus)
- Ultrasound measurements
- If the ultrasound examination is done at less than or equal to 14 weeks, the error in determining the gestational age is only one week
- In patient is more than 24 weeks pregnant, ultrasound cannot be used to determine the gestational age
- If still not clear, look for serial growth after 3 weeks.

Wrong Dates (How to Exclude?)

- Menstrual age = Gestational age
- Fetal age = Conceptional age → begins at conception (e.g. in IVF/Artificial insemination)
- Menstrual age → Conceptional age + 14 days.

Good Dates

Criteria

- Patient is certain of LMP
- Previous regular menses
- No exposure to hormonal contraceptives for more than or equal to 3 regular cycles prior to conception
- No unusual bleeding
- Patient didn't conceive in lactational amenorrhea.

Bad Dates

Criteria

- Uncertain of LMP
- Unusual bleeding/Oligomenorrhea/Abnormal bleeding
- Use of hormonal contraceptives (ovulation may be delayed by 4–6 weeks)
- Became pregnant in 1st ovulatory cycle after a recent delivery
- Ovulation very early (<D11) or very late (>D21)

Uterus Bigger than Dates Suggests

- Error in calculating dates or wrong dates
- Multiple pregnancy
- Polyhydramnios
- Large for the gestational age
- Diabetes mellitus
- Complete molar pregnancy
- Hydrops
- Any mass (fibroid, ovarian tumour, etc.) with pregnancy
- Sometimes fetus in breech presentation looks bigger

Uterus Smaller than Dates Suggests

- Error in calculating dates or wrong dates
- Intrauterine growth restriction
- Oligohydramnios
- Small for gestational age
- Transverse lie
- Fetal descent into the pelvis
- Intrauterine death
- Rupture of membranes

METHODS FOR DETERMINING MENSTRUAL AGE

Add the following to conceptional age:
- IVF ± 1 day
- Ovulation induction ± 3 days
- Artificial insemination ± 3 days
- Single intercourse ± 3 days
- BBT record ± 4 days.

PREDICTION OF GESTATIONAL AGE

Patient's Statement

- Date of fruitful coitus
  - Add 266 days to it (± 7 days)
- Naegele's formula: ± 7 days
  - If interval of cycles is longer, extra days are to be added
  - If interval is shorter, lesser days are to be subtracted to get EDD.
- Date of quickening
  - Add 22 weeks in primigravida and 24 weeks in multi (to it).

Previous Records

Required weeks to be added to make it 40 weeks
- Clinical
  - Size of uterus less than 12 weeks ≈ period of amenorrhea
  - Palpation of fetal parts by 20th week
  - Auscultation of FHR by 18–20 weeks (by stethoscope) and by Doppler by 10th week.
- Investigation record of 1st half of pregnancy
  - UPT +ve at first missed period by earliest
  - USG: visualization of gestational sac at 5th week
  - CRL → 10 mm (at 7 weeks)
              34 mm (at 10 weeks)
    (CRL in cm + 3.5 = week of pregnancy).

Objective Signs

- Height of uterus above symphysis pubis (or SFH)
- Lightening: labor commences approximately at or within 3 weeks
- Size of fetus, change in uterine shape, volume of liquor amnii, hardening of skull and girth of abdomen.

USG

Gestational age (1st and 2nd trimester) should be compared with menstrual age
- When difference in gestational age and menstrual age is less than 7 days → EDD by LMP is taken
- When more than 7 days → EDD by USG age is taken.

Chapter 9

Routine Investigations in Pregnancy

Tania G Singh

LABORATORY TESTS

Immunological Tests for Diagnosis of Pregnancy

Principle

Measurement of human chorionic gonadotrophin (hCG) in maternal urine or serum with antibody, either polyclonal or monoclonal, available commercially.

Tests used are as follows:

Urine pregnancy tests

- Agglutination Test: Latex particles or sheep erythrocyte (tube) coated with anti-hCG
- Agglutination Inhibition Tests
- Dipstick test
- Rapid and simple tests based on enzyme-labelled monoclonal antibodies assay.

Serum pregnancy tests

- Radioimmunoassay of β-subunit of hCG
- Radio receptor assay.

Test using both urine and serum

- Enzyme-linked immunosorbent assay (ELISA).

Progesterone

- Serum progesterone is a reflection of progesterone production by the corpus luteum, which is stimulated by a viable pregnancy
- Measured by radioimmunoassay and fluoroimmunoassay
- Results after 3–4 hours
- A dipstick ELISA that can determine a serum progesterone level of lower than 15 ng/mL is also available.

HOME PREGNANCY TEST

- These tests now use the modern immunometric assay
- Most of these tests claim "99% accuracy"
- These are most commonly used in the week after a missed menstrual period (4th completed gestational week)

---

hCG

- Detectable in the serum in >98% of patients by day 11
- At 4 weeks' gestation (Day 18–22 post conception), the dimer and β subunit of hCG doubling times are ≈ 2.2 days
- Doubling time falls to 3.5 days by 9 weeks' gestation
- Levels peak at 10-12 weeks' gestation and then begin to decline rapidly until another, more gradual rise begins at 22 weeks' gestation, which continues until term

The Pregnancy Test Becomes Negative about

- 1 week after labor
- 2 weeks after abortion
- 4 weeks after evacuation of vesicular mole

Serum Progesterone Levels

- >25 ng/mL → viable intrauterine pregnancy
- < 5ng/mL → a nonviable pregnancy
- 5–25 ng/mL → further testing using ultrasound, additional hormonal assays or serial examinations is warranted

- Urine hCG values are extremely variable at this time and can range from 12 mIU/mL to higher than 2500 mIU/mL
- Therefore, during 4th and 5th week, they may not be highly accurate.

Reading the Test

- 'C' indicates a control (this band must always appear because this is the comparison band)
- 'T' indicates the test sample
- If only one red/pink/purple band appear, in the region marked 'C', it means that the test is negative
- If two red/pink/purple bands appear, one in the 'C' region and the other in the region marked 'T', it means that the test is positive for pregnancy
- In case no bands appear or if a faint line appears in the 'T' region, then the test is invalid
- Repeat the test with a new pack after 72 hours.

OTHER ROUTINE TESTS

- Hemogram
- Screening for hemoglobinopathies
- Complete urine analysis (to detect asymptomatic bacteriuria, if present)
- VDRL, HIV (after pretest counseling and written consent)
- ABO Rh; If Rhesus negative, check husband's blood group
- HbsAg, Anti-HBC Ag
- Rubella susceptibility
- USG to confirm intrauterine gestation, cardiac activity, measure gestational age using CRL, to rule out multiple gestation and ectopic pregnancy
- Cervical cytology, if indicated
- A wet smear of any symptomatic vaginal discharge (i.e. itching, burning or offensive)
- Down's syndrome screening.

Nuchal Translucency (NT)

- Single most powerful marker for Down's syndrome
- Refers to normal subcutaneous fluid-filled space between back of fetal neck and overlying skin
- Seen in all normal fetuses
- Called a 'translucency' because on ultrasound this appears as a black space beneath the fetal skin
- Normally less than 2.5 mm
- More than and equal to 2.5 mm may indicate Down's syndrome or another chromosomal abnormality
- Best time to measure: 10–14 weeks
- Increased in Trisomy 21; Trisomy 18; Pregnancy loss less than 24 weeks; congenital heart defect.

Nasal Bone (NB)

- Clear association between absence of fetal nasal bone and Down's but absent NB is not related to NT
- It is an independent marker.

Collection of Urine for Home Pregnancy Test

- ❧ Try to perform first thing in the morning, though this is not mandatory
- ❧ Collect urine in a clean, dry, plastic container
- ❧ Wash only with water and not with any detergent
- ❧ Take out the strip from the pack and keep it on a flat surface
- ❧ Put about 2–3 drops of urine on it with a dropper (provided in the kit)
- ❧ Do not spill urine on the reading strip
- ❧ Wait for 3–5 minutes and then read the test results
- ❧ Trying to read the results before the stipulated time or waiting too long, can both lead to inaccurate readings

Recommendations for Noninvasive Tests

- ❧ 1st trimester: Combined screening (NT + PAPP A + hCG at 10-13^{+6})
- ❧ 2nd trimester:
  - Quadruple (hCG + Inhibin A + MSAFP + uE3 at 15-20^{+6}) OR
  - Triple test (MSAFP + uE3 + hCG at 15-20 weeks)
  - Level II (anamoly scan) ultrasound at 18–22 weeks

Hemogram

- If hemoglobin level is lower than 10 g/100 mL, investigate and consider additional iron supplementation
- If MCH is lower than 27 picograms, offer HPLC (high-performance liquid chromatography)
- If woman is found to be carrier of a clinically significant hemoglobinopathy, father should also be screened without delay.

Rhesus Negative Blood Group

- If Rh negative blood group with husband's rhesus positive, offer indirect coomb's test
- If ICT is negative, repeat at 28 weeks and then at 34 weeks
- If positive, send for anti-D antibodies titer.

VDRL Positive

- If either the VDRL (Venereal Disease Research Laboratory) or RPR (Rapid Plasmin Reagin) test is negative, then the patient does not have syphilis and no further tests for syphilis are needed
- If the titre is higher than or equal to 1:16, patient has syphilis and must be treated
- If the titre is lower than or equal to 1:8, the laboratory should test the same blood sample by means of the TPHA (Treponema Pallidum Hemagglutin Assay) or FTA (Fluorescent Treponemal Antibody) test.

HIV Positive

- Confirm by western blot or repeat ELISA.

AMNIOTIC FLUID

Appearance

- During the first two trimesters: clear and yellow
- During the third trimester: becomes colorless
- Approximately from the 33–34 week onwards: cloudiness and flocculation occur
- At term: moderately cloudy and contains a moderate number of flakes of vernix.

Constituents

- 1st trimester: water and electrolytes only
- 2nd trimester
  - Water and electrolytes (99%)
  - Glucose
  - Lipids from the fetal lungs
  - Proteins with bactericide properties
  - Flaked-off fetal epithelium cells
  - Normally has a pH of 7.0 to 7.5.

Functions of Amniotic Fluid

- Amniotic fluid is "inhaled" and "exhaled" by the fetus—essential for the development of lungs

- Swallowed amniotic fluid also forms urine and contributes to the formation of meconium
- Amniotic fluid protects the developing fetus by cushioning against blows to the mother's abdomen
- Allowing for easier fetal movements
- Promotes muscular and skeletal development.

Placental Grading

- Refers to an ultrasound grading system of the placenta depending upon it's maturity
- This primarily portrays the extent of calcifications.

Grade '0'

- At less than 18 weeks
- Features: uniform echogenicity; smooth chorionic plate.

Grade 'I'

- At 18–29 weeks
- Features: occasional parenchymal calcification/hyperechoic areas.

Grade 'II'

- At more than 30 weeks
- Occasional basal calcification/hyperechoic areas
- May also have comma type densities at the chorionic plate.

Grade 'III'

- At more than 39 weeks
- Significant basal calcification
- Chorionic plate interrupted by indentations
- An early progression to grade III is a matter of concern and is sometimes associated with placental insufficiency.

Chapter 10

Tetanus Toxoid in Pregnancy

Tania G Singh

WHO TETANUS TOXOID IMMUNIZATION SCHEDULE

Dose	When to give	Protection%	Duration of protection
TT-1	At first contact or as early as possible in pregnancy	Nil	None
TT-2	At least 4 weeks after TT-1	80	3 years
TT-3	At least 6 months after TT-2 or during subsequent pregnancy	95	5 years
TT-4	At least 1 year after TT-3 or during subsequent pregnancy	99	10 years
TT-5	At least 1 year after TT-4 or during subsequent pregnancy	99	Throughout childbearing

Chapter 11

Diet in Pregnancy

Tania G Singh

GENERAL PRINCIPLES

- Pregnant women need between 2,200 and 2,900 calories a day which should be gradually increased with the growth of the fetus
    - 1st trimester → does not require any extra calories
    - 2nd trimester → an additional 340 calories a day is recommended
    - 3rd trimester → recommendation is 450 calories more, a day.
- Add variety to your food
- Choose foods high in starch and fiber, such as whole-grain breads, cereals, pasta, rice, fruits, and vegetables
- Eat and drink at least four servings of calcium-rich foods a day to help ensure that you are getting 1200 mg of calcium in your daily diet
- Vitamin D which will helps the body absorb calcium
- Eat at least three servings of iron-rich foods per day to ensure getting 27 mg of iron in the daily diet
- Choose at least one source of vitamin C every day
- Choose at least one source of folic acid every day
- Choose at least one source of vitamin A every other day
- Choose at least one source of vitamin B_{12} a day
- Avoid:
    - Left over food
    - Frozen and deep-frozen food
    - Cold drinks
    - Tobacco
    - Alcohol/Smoking.
- Liver and liver products may also contain high levels of vitamin A, and therefore, consumption of these products should also be avoided
- Tea, coffee, chocolates and ice cream can be taken only in moderation (only 2 cups of either tea or coffee permitted/day)
- Those who suffer from constipation, gas, bloating must avoid peas and other 'heavy to digest' cereals, and potato, they must take green gram as it is easy to digest and gives protein
- Butter, clarified butter, milk, honey, fennel seeds, sweets made from jaggery rather than white sugar can be taken in small quantity
- Items, such as sandwich, bakery bread, bun, dhokla, pizza, khandvi, pancake, khaman, steamed rice cake, curd, tomato, tamarind, kadhi usually increase the swellings and acidity.
- Most important, water intake should, by no means be less than 2.5 litres/day
- Limit fats and cholesterol
- Do not diet or try to lose weight during pregnancy.

Protein Sources:

- *For vegans:* nuts, peanut butter, legumes, soy products, quinoa, and tofu
- *For nonvegans:* meat, poultry, fish, eggs, or dairy products

Sources of Calcium include dairy products, seafood, leafy green vegetables, dried beans or peas, and tofu

Adequate amounts of **vitamin D** can be obtained through exposure to the sun and in fortified milk, eggs, and fish. Vegans should receive 10–15 minutes of direct sunlight to the hands, face, or arms three times per week or take a supplement

Sources of Iron Source of iron include enriched grain products (rice), eggs, leafy green vegetables, broccoli, brussels sprouts, sweet potatoes, dried beans and peas, raisins, prunes, and peanuts

Vitamin B_{12} is found in animal products including fish and shellfish, eggs, and dairy products

CALORIE CHART FOR BASIC FOOD ITEMS

Fruits Per 100 Grams

- Apple—56
- Avocado Pear—190
- Banana—95
- Chickoo—94
- Cherries—70
- Dates—281
- Grapes Black—45
- Guava—66
- Kiwi Fruit—45
- Lychies—61
- Mangoes—70
- Orange—53
- Orange juice 100 mL—47
- Papaya—32
- Peach—50
- Pears—51
- Pineapple—46
- Plums—56
- Strawberries—77
- Watermelon—26
- Pomegranate—77.

Vegetables Per 100 Grams

- Broccoli—25
- Brinjal—24
- Cabbage—45
- Carrot—48
- Cauliflower—30
- Fenugreek (Methi)—49
- French beans—26
- Lettuce—21
- Mushroom—18
- Onion—50
- Peas—93
- Potato—97
- Spinach—23
- Tomato—21
- Tomato juice 100 mL—22.

Cereals Per 100 Grams

- Bajra—360
- Maize flour—355
- Rice—325
- Wheat flour—341

Milk and Milk Products Per Cup

- Butter 100 gms—750
- Buttermilk—19
- Cheese—315
- Cream 100 gms—210
- Ghee 100 gms—910
- Milk Buffalo—115
- Milk Cow—100
- Milk Skimmed—45.

Chapter 12

Advice on General Ailments in Pregnancy

Tania G Singh

NAUSEA AND VOMITING IN EARLY PREGNANCY

- Women should be informed that most cases of nausea and vomiting in pregnancy will resolve spontaneously within 16–20 weeks and that nausea and vomiting are not usually associated with a poor pregnancy outcome
- The following interventions appear to be effective in reducing symptoms:
  - Nonpharmacological: ginger, P6 (wrist) acupressure
  - Pharmacological: antihistamines.

HEARTBURN

- Lifestyle and diet modification
- Antacids may be offered to women whose heartburn remains troublesome despite lifestyle and diet modification.

CONSTIPATION

- Diet modification, such as bran or wheat fibre supplementation
- Increase water intake.

HEMORRHOIDS

- Diet modification
  - Intake of fibre-rich diet
  - Isabgol husk.
- If clinical symptoms remain troublesome, standard hemorrhoid creams should be considered.

VARICOSE VEINS

- A common symptom of pregnancy that will not cause harm
- Avoid long standing hours (relax in between)
- Elevation of legs using pillows, etc. while lying down
- While sitting on chair, keep a step under your feet
- Compression stockings can improve the symptoms but will not prevent varicose veins from emerging.

LEG CRAMPS

- Administration of adequate calcium and vitamin D_3
- Gentle massage of the legs
- Local application of topical analgesics.

Backache

- Women should be informed that exercising in water, massage therapy and group or individual back care classes might help to ease backache during pregnancy

Breast Care

- Maintain cleanliness
- Massaging the breasts
- Try to express the discharge (colostrum)

INCREASED VAGINAL DISCHARGE

- A common physiological change in pregnancy
- If it is associated with itch, soreness, offensive smell or pain on passing urine, there may be an infective cause and investigated
- A 1-week course of a topical imidazole is an effective treatment and should be considered for vaginal candidiasis infections
- The effectiveness and safety of oral treatments for vaginal candidiasis in pregnancy are uncertain and these treatments should not be offered routinely.

Chapter 13

HIV Counseling

Tania G Singh

> * HIV leads to decline in the CD4 cell count
> * ART may lead to preterm labor, gestational diabetes and pre eclampsia in some

PREPREGNANCY

- Assess viral load
- If not possible → clinical staging and CD4 count
- Start 1st line preferred therapy (triple line regimen) to all women of childbearing age, irrespective of CD4 count and clinical staging and this therapy is to be continued throughout pregnancy starting from the 1st day
- Adequate and balanced diet with folic acid should be started
- Screening for:
  - Syphilis; Rubella; Hepatitis B and C
  - Opportunistic infections (*P. carinii pneumonia*).
- Other routine blood tests
  - Hemogram; Urine analysis
  - Blood group and type; FBS/PPBS.
- HIV testing of sex partners is to be encouraged
- Counseling for cessation of smoking and illicit drug use is necessary
- Explain the effects of pregnancy on the disease and vice versa
- Counseling regarding the risk of vertical transmission, measures available to decrease it and infant feeding options, the benefits to infants of early diagnosis of HIV
- Advice barrier contraceptives to those who choose to continue sexual contact
- Where the female partner is HIV negative but husband is positive, assisted reproduction with either donor sperms should be advised
- Try to delay conception until plasma viral load comes down
- All women who are HIV positive are recommended to have annual cervical cytology.

> **Routes of Transmission**
> * Heterosexual 87.4%
> * Parent to child 5.4%
> * Injecting drug use 1.6%
> * Homosexual/bisexual 1.3%
> * Blood and blood products 1.0%
> * Unknown causes 3.3%

PERINATAL TRANSMISSION

- Vertical transmission accounts for most pediatric HIV infections
- Intrapartum transmission can occur
  - During labor → through maternofetal exchange of blood
  - Delivery → by contact of infant's skin or mucous membrane with infected blood or other maternal secretions.

FACTORS WHICH INCREASE RISK OF MOTHER-TO-CHILD TRANSMISSION

Clinical Factors

- Immunologically or clinically advanced HIV disease in mother

- High plasma viral load
- Maternal injectable drug use during pregnancy
- Preterm delivery
- Failure to receive antiretroviral therapy
- Breastfeeding (risk increases if breast abscesses, nipple fissures, mastitis, oral disease in infant, e.g. thrush/sores).

Obstetric Factors

- Increases with every hour after membrane rupture → delivery more than 4 hours after rupture of membranes can double the risk of HIV transmission
- Maternal infection with another STD during pregnancy and certain obstetric procedures like
  - CVS
  - Amniocentesis
  - Invasive fetal intrapartum monitoring.
- Chorioamnionitis.

HIV TESTING IN PREGNANCY (WHO 2013)

- Counseling and testing is recommended for women as a routine component of the package of care in all antenatal, childbirth, postpartum and pediatric care settings
- Testing should be done at the booking antenatal visit
- Retesting is recommended in all mothers in the 3rd trimester, or during labor, or shortly after delivery because of the high-risk of acquiring HIV infection during pregnancy
- Testing is usually done by HIV serology and if confirmed by other tests, clinical assessment, viral load and CD4 count should be done
- If feasible, other tests to be done are:
  - HBV serology
  - HCV serology
  - Screening for STDs
  - Assessment for major noncommunicable chronic diseases and comorbidities.
- Cryptococcus antigen, if CD4 count less than or equal to 100 cells/mm^3
- Treatment failure is defined by a persistently detectable viral load more than 1000 copies/mL after at least six months of using ARV drugs
- Viral load
  - Less than or equal to 1000 copies/mL → maintain 1st line preferred therapy
  - 1000 copies/mL → switch to 1st line alternative therapy or 2nd line therapy.
- If viral load is not routinely available, CD4 count and clinical monitoring should be used to diagnose treatment failure
- If a woman declines an HIV test, this should be clearly documented in her antenatal card, her reasons should be sensitively explored and screening offered again in the 3rd trimester
- Rapid HIV testing at the time of labor is recommended, if HIV infection status has not previously been documented during the index pregnancy.

COUNSELING

Counseling plays a very vital role in a disease like HIV/AIDS.

"At Risk" Women
- Exchanging sex for money or drugs
- With a history of STD
- A new or multiple sex partners during pregnancy
- Use of illicit drugs
- Sex partners known to be HIV positive or at high-risk
- Who have signs and symptoms of seroconversion
- Injection drug users
- High prevalence geographic areas or healthcare facilities

Viral load is recommended as the preferred monitoring approach to diagnose and confirm ARV treatment failure in comparison to CD4 count or clinical staging. Why?
- It provides an early and more accurate indication of treatment failure and the need to switch to second-line drugs, reducing the accumulation of drug-resistance mutations and improving clinical outcomes
- Measuring viral load can also help to discriminate between treatment failure and nonadherence
- Many people who are identified with immunological failure (decreasing CD4 count inspite of ARV therapy) in fact have adequate virological suppression and they are misclassified as having treatment failure and are switched, unnecessarily to 2nd line therapy

Pretest Counseling

- Informed consent
- Emphasize confidentiality
- Explore high-risk behavior
  - Unsafe sex practices
  - IV drug use
  - Blood/blood products received.
- Explore HIV/AIDS knowledge
  - Explain
  - Clarify misconceptions.
- Explore test implication
  - Meaning of negative or positive test result.
- Reason for testing
  - Removes uncertainty.
- Arousing hope: advice and empowerment
  - Focus on quality of life
  - No cure yet but let us hope
  - Express your availability when needed.
- Right to decline testing as it is a voluntary test
- Causative agent, modes of transmission, methods of testing should be explained to the patient
- Done on one to one basis or as lectures with slide shows, posters, charts and video clips
- HIV testing should not be imposed as a precondition for employment or providing healthcare facilities.

Post-test: Test Negative

- Renew relationship
- Explain negative results
- Explain about window period
- Clarify doubts/misconceptions
- Evaluate need for retest
- Repeat preventive education.

Post-test: Test Positive

- Renew relationship
- Follow patients lead when to disclose
- State result clearly
- Wait, give time, listen
- If positive
  - Make adaptive change in lifestyle
  - Plan for future.
- Assess strategies for coping
  - Evaluate past handling to stressful situations
  - Evaluate patient's social support network.
- Preventive education.

Chapter 14

Pelvic Assessment

Tania G Singh

ASSESSMENT OF PELVIC

In vertex presentation: Assessment is done at any time beyond 37th week but better at beginning of labor because of softening of tissues, assessment can be done effectively during this time.

Sacral Promontory

- Attempt should be made to tip the sacral promontory
- Try to establish the length of the diagonal conjugate
- Method
  - Fingers are to follow anterior sacral curvature
  - In normal pelvis, it is difficult to feel sacral promontory (or felt with difficulty)
  - To reach it, elbow and wrist are to be depressed sufficiently and fingers are mobilized in an upward direction
  - Point at which bone recedes from fingers is sacral promontory
  - Fingers are then mobilized under symphysis pubis and a marking is placed over gloved index finger by index finger of the left hand
  - Internal fingers are removed
  - Distance between marking and tip of middle finger gives measurement of diagonal conjugate
  - Practically, if middle finger fails to reach promontory or touches it with difficulty → conjugate is adequate for average size head to pass through.
- If it is easily tipped, it should alert one to the possibility of a contracted pelvis.

Curvature of the Sacral Curve

- It is next assessed to see if it is flat or well-curved
- A well-curved sacrum allows for internal rotation of the fetal head.

Pelvic Side Walls

- Assessed next to see if they are parallel or convergent
- Normally not easily palpable.

Ischial Spines

- These are palpated to see if they are prominent and sticking in (that is decreasing the space in mid pelvis)
- Normally, these are everted.

Features of a Gynecoid Pelvis Include:

- A wide diagonal conjugate
- A well-curved sacrum
- Parallel side walls
- Ischial spines that are not prominent
- A wide subpubic angle and lastly
- A wide intertuberous diameter

Sacrosciatic Notch

- Sufficiently wide to place two fingers over sacrospinous ligament covering the notch
- Gives information of the capacity of posterior segment and side walls of lower pelvis.

Posterior Surface of Symphysis Pubis

- Smooth-rounded curve
- Angulation/beaking → abnormal.

Pubic Arch

- Normally rounded
- Should accommodate palmar aspect of two fingers
- Configuration more important than pubic angle.

Subpubic Angle

- Before the fingers are removed from the vagina, the subpubic angle is assessed to see if it is acute or obtuse.

Now take out your fingers

Intertuberous Diameter

Having removed the fingers, the intertuberous diameter is assessed to see if it accommodates more than four knuckles → if it does, it is adequate.

CONCLUSION

The most suitable pelvis for vaginal delivery is that of a gynaecoid pelvis that has adequate dimensions.

Chapter **15**

Twin Gestation Assessment

Tania G Singh

DIAGNOSIS

History

- ART—ovulation induction drugs (esp. gonadotropins)
- Family history of twins (maternal >> paternal, especially for dizygous twins)
- If mother herself is a member of pair of dizygous twins, she has 2% chances of conceiving with twins as compared to dizygous husband whose wife has only 1% chance of giving birth to twins
- Increased age and parity
- Increased maternal body weight (not clear, may be because of increased circulating levels of pituitary gonadotropins)
- Race (highest—Nigeria and lowest in Japan).

Symptoms

- Hyperemesis or increased nausea in early months
- Pressure symptoms:
  - Edema of legs [vulva/abdominal wall (may be)]
  - Shortness of breath
  - Palpitations
  - Varicose veins
  - Hemorrhoids
  - Digestive discomfort.
- Undue uterine enlargement because of polyhydramnios
- Excessive fetal movements.

GPE

- Anemia
- Unusual weight gain, not explained by pre eclampsia/obesity
- Gestational hypertension/pre eclampsia.

Per Abdomen

- Shape—Elongated shape of normal pregnant uterus changed to barrel shape
- Abdomen—unduly enlarged.

Palpation

- Height of uterus more than period of gestation (SFH)
- ↑↑ Abdominal girth (at term)

Ultrasound Parameters

- Determination of chorionicity and amnionicity
- Confirmation of gestational age
- Diagnosis of anomalies and complications
- Measurement of cervical length
- Assessment of growth and amniotic fluid
- Placental localization
- Fetal position for intra-partum management

Dichorionic Pregnancy

- 2 layers of amnion
- 2 layers of chorion
- Membrane thicker and more reflective than the monochorionic diamniotic membrane
- Membrane thickness of >2 mm

Monochorionic Pregnancy

- Membrane thickness ≤2 mm

DZ Twins (Binovular)

- They can be same sex or opposite sex twin pairs
- Number of placenta – 2 (except in cases where they are fused to form 1)
- Number of intervening membranes – 4
- They are always dichorionic diamniotic (DCDA)
- Constitute 70% of all the twin pregnancies
- There is no vessel communication
- Blood type will be different
- Usually discordant for chromosomal anomalies

- Fetal bulk—disproportionately more in relation to fetal size
- Palpation of at least 3 poles or 2 fetal heads (too many fetal parts).

Auscultation

Two separate FHS (heard simultaneously by 2 different observers) separated by a silent area with a discrepancy of at least 10 beats per minute—this may not be that easily heard because of presence of hydramnios (very commonly associated).

Determination of Chorionicity and Amnionicity

- Chorionicity relates to placentation and is more accurate before 14 weeks
- Amnionicity: Before 8–10 weeks, separate and distinct amnions may be visible on USG as they have not enlarged sufficiently to contact each other and create intertwin membrane (they are extremely thin and delicate)
- Before 10 weeks gestation
  Number of gestational sacs: Each gestational sac forms its own placenta and chorion
  - 2 gestational sacs → dichorionic
  - 1 gestational sac with 2 identified heartbeats → monochorionic.

  Number of amniotic sacs within the chorionic cavity
  - 2 amnionic cavities → diamniotic
  - 1 amnionic cavity → monoamniotic (only criteria for MCMA).

  Embryos per sac
  - 1 embryo per sac in diamniotic diamniotic
  - 2 embryos per sac in monochorionic diamniotic
  - 2 embryos per sac in monochorionic monoamniotic.

  Number of yolk sacs
  - This may help diagnose the amnionicity
  - 2 yolk sacs → diamniotic
  - A single yolk sac → in most cases indicate monoamniotic twins but a single yolk sac seen with dual embryos → a follow-up first trimester scan to definitively assign amnionicity.

MZ Twins (Uniovular)

- Constitute 30%
- Arise when an embryo splits soon after fertilization
- These can be:
  - DCDA (33%)
  - MCDA (66%)
  - MCMA (<1%)
- Carry essentially identical genetic instructions (share 100% of their genes)
- Are always of the same sex (boy–boy or girl–girl)
- Number of intervening membranes depends upon the time of fertilization
- High incidence in humans

- After 10 weeks gestation
  Fetal genitalia (should not be done routinely)
  Placental number
  - Single placenta → mostly monochorionic (except where 2 placentas are fused to form one)
  - Two distinct placentas → dichorionic
  - Ability of USG to identify 2 discrete placental masses depends on proximity of implantation of 2 blastocysts.

  Chorionicity
  - Twin peak or Lambda sign → Dichorionic diamniotic (100% dichorionic placenta)
  - Absence of the twin peak sign → monochorionic
  - T-sign (Monochorionic diamniotic): There is a 90° relationship between membrane and placenta with no apparent extension of dividing membrane.

ZYGOSITY

- Genetic identity of each twin in the pregnancy
- Zygosity cannot always be inferred from the determination of chorionicity
- There are two types of twins, dizygotic (DZ) and monozygotic (MZ) twins.

Recurrent Pregnancy Loss Assessment

Tania G Singh

FIRST LINE

- Pelvic ultrasound (to exclude uterine abnormalities)
- Complete blood count
- Thyroid profile
- Antithyroid antibodies
- Anticardiolipin antibodies
- Lupus anticoagulant
- Fasting insulin, glucose, homocysteine
- Activated protein C resistance
- Karyotype of both partners.

SECOND LINE

- Hysterosalpingogram, sonohysterogram or hysteroscopy
- Methylenetetrahydrofolate reductase mutation
- Factor V Leiden, prothrombin gene mutation, protein C, protein S
- Antithrombin III
- Anti-Müllerian hormone.

THIRD LINE

- Male karyotype deletion
- Sperm DNA fragmentation
- Peripheral blood natural killer cells
- Uterine natural killer cells
- Embryo quality (IVF).

Chapter 17

Rh Negative Pregnancy

Tania G Singh and Nisha M Anand

UNDERSTANDING THE DISEASE

- Rh antigen is identified in the red cell membrane as early as 38 days after conception
- If fetomaternal hemorrhage occurs in 1st pregnancy of a mother who is Rh -ve (i.e. she lacks the red blood cell antigen) carrying Rh +ve fetus, during pregnancy or during labor, she gets exposed to RhD +ve fetal erythrocytes into her circulation (i.e. she is 'sensitized', a process called "alloimmunization" or "isoimmunization")
- The initial response of mother to this D antigen is slow (sometimes taking as long as 6 months to develop), that's why 1st pregnancy is usually not affected
- But re-exposure to this antigen (in subsequent pregnancies) produces a rapid immunological response (i.e. formation of IgG anti–D antibodies) which usually can be measured in days
- These IgG anti-D antibodies cross the placenta → coat D-positive fetal red cells → which are then destroyed and removed from circulation in the fetal spleen (hemolysis)
- Once sensitization has occurred, it is irreversible.

RESULTS OF HEMOLYSIS

Before Birth

- Mild to moderate hemolysis: manifest as increased indirect bilirubin (of the fetus) which appears in the amniotic fluid → it is cleared by placenta and is not harmful
- Severe hemolysis → severe anemia → ↑RBC production by the spleen and liver of the fetus
- Subsequently:
  - Hepatic circulatory obstruction (portal hypertension)
  - Placental edema, leading to ascites in fetus
  - Hepatomegaly, increased placental thickness and polyhydramnios
  - Progressive liver damage
  - Decreased albumin production results in the development of hydrops fetalis
  - Fetal heart failure.

After Birth

- Hemolytic disease of the newborn
- If not treated in time, damage of specific areas of the neonatal brain

- Kernicterus
- Cerebral palsy, deafness, motor and speech delay.

ANTEPARTUM MANAGEMENT OF RH NEGATIVE PREGNANCY

First Pregnancy (Unaffected with no Previous Sensitizing Events)

- Check father's blood group
- If Rh –ve: nothing to be done
- If father's Rh +ve: ICT (at 28 weeks)
- Give Anti-D 300 µg at 28 weeks
- After delivery, determine baby's blood group
- If baby's blood group negative: nothing is to be done
- If positive: consider anti-D within 72 hours of delivery.

First Affected Pregnancy (Sensitized due to Previous Event but no Severely Affected Pregnancy)

- Check maternal titers (method used should be stated by the lab.)
- An albumin titer of 1:16 is equal to an indirect antiglobulin test (IAT) titer of 1:32 to 1:128
- Titer of higher than 1:4 → considered sensitized
- If titer is lower than or equal to 1:32, repeat antibody titers every 4 weekly till 24 weeks and then every 2 weeks thereafter
- If titer is higher than or equal to 1:64 (critical titer, for each lab it is different) → amniocentesis → fetal RhD status (if facility for fetal genotyping from maternal plasma is not available)
- If fetus RhD positive → serial fetal MCA Doppler OR serial amniocentesis for Δ OD450 every 1–2 weeks starting at 24 weeks and continued till 35 weeks
- When peak MCA velocity is higher than 1.5 MoM: cordocentesis, to determine fetal hematocrit
- If fetal hematocrit is less than 30% → intrauterine transfusions.

First Sensitized Pregnancy/Previously Affected Pregnancy

- The initial procedure is usually performed at least 4–8 weeks earlier than the prior gestational age at which significant morbidity occurred in previous pregnancy
- Usually amniocentesis is started at 15 weeks (determine fetal genotype) or if MCA Doppler is opted, testing should be started at 18 weeks
- Rest managed as mentioned above.

Anti-D is not required after complete spontaneous abortion <12 weeks gestation, provided there is no instrumentation of the uterus

If pregnancy is followed only with Doppler assessments and values remain normal till 35 weeks, amniocentesis need to be done at 35 weeks for fetal lung maturity and Δ OD450 values and further pregnancy managed accordingly

Where the titers are extremely high (≥256) at <28 weeks and the fetus does not demonstrate hydrops, but there is a documented history of IUD due to hydrops in the previous pregnancy, IV immune serum globulin might be offered

- Dose = 400 mg/kg/day × 5 days
- Repeat infusions every 15–21 days
- Contraindications to its use
  - A previous episode of intravenous immunoglobulin-induced anaphylaxis (rare)
  - Selective IgA deficiency

Chapter 18

Hypothyroidism in Pregnancy

Tania G Singh

ASSESSMENT BEFORE CONCEPTION

- If known hypothyroid on treatment → achieve TSH levels lower than 2.5 mIU/L (adjust dose)
- If known autoimmune thyroid disease → do TSH prior to or in early pregnancy
- If known other autoimmune disease (Type 1 DM): do TSH prior to or in early pregnancy.

ANTENATAL MANAGEMENT

If Hypothyroid (known case)

- Levothyroxine is the treatment of choice for maternal hypothyroidism, if the iodine nutrition status is adequate
- Better to achieve a target TSH level of lower than 2.5 mIU/L before pregnancy
- Adjust the dose as early as 4–6 weeks of gestation → ↑ it by 30–50%, then titrate according to TSH levels.

Why Should Dose be Increased?

- There is a rapid rise in TBG levels resulting from the physiological rise in estrogen
- There is increased distribution volume of thyroid hormones (vascular, hepatic, fetal-placental unit)
- There is an increased placental transport and metabolism of maternal T4
- ↓ to prepregnancy dose immediately after delivery.

Detected for 1st Time

Start Levothyroxine

- 1.8–2.0 µg/kg/day (T4 → synthetic) in cases of overt disease
- 100 µg thyroxine daily in mild cases (TSH <10 mIU/L).

Increment in Thyroxine Dose can be Based on the Initial Degree of TSH Elevation

- Serum TSH between 5 and 10 mIU/L → average increment in thyroxine dosage is 25–50 µg/d
- Serum TSH between 10 and 20 mIU/L → increase up to 50–75 µg/d
- Serum TSH higher than 20 mIU/L → 75–100 µg/d
- Serum TSH and TT4 should always be evaluated 3–4 weeks after every change of dosage

- There should be a 4 hour delay between LT4 and iron and calcium supplements usually prescribed in pregnancy as these interfere with levothyroxine absorption.

Frequency of Testing

- Do TSH after 4 weeks and titrate
- Then do every 6–8 weeks throughout pregnancy
- If patient is noncompliant → check TSH and TT_4 minimum 3 times (once in each trimester)
- Check TFT immediately after delivery and decrease the dose accordingly
- Recheck TSH 4–6 weeks postpartum.

Women with Thyroid Autoimmunity (TAI)

- Euthyroid antibody positive women: check TFT every 4 weeks
- In the case of recurrent miscarriage: treat with low dose thyroxine with judicious monitoring of thyroid function.

If Previous Thyroidectomy or ^{131}I Ablation Done (No Native Thyroid Function)

- ↑↑ dosage required.

Subclinical Hypothyroidism

- TSH ↑ but normal free T_4
- Even mild form (delayed mental and motor function) has:
  - Increased risk of abruptio
  - Increased cases of preterm birth (< 34 weeks)
  - Central congenital hypothyroidism in newborns (requiring thyroxine): in infants of female with undiagnosed or inadequately treated Graves' disease during pregnancy
- Long-term neurodevelopment of offspring is adversely affected
- Thyroxine treatment improves obstetrical outcome but does not modify long-term neurological development in the offspring
- Still prudent to give thyroxine.

COMPLICATIONS OF HYPOTHYROIDISM IN PREGNANCY

Maternal

- Pre eclampsia/Gestational hypertension
- Eclampsia
- Anemia
- Abruptio
- Preterm delivery
- Antepartum depression
- ↑ risk of cesarean section (Indication—fetal distress)
- PPH/Postpartum hypertension
- Lactation problems.

Fetal

- Miscarriage
- IUGR/Low birth weight
- Increased perinatal mortality
- Lower IQ and poorer cognitive function in infants.

Screening Recommendations

- Thyroid function: TSH and Total T4
- Presence of autoimmune thyroid disease: anti TPO antibodies and anti Thyroglobulin antibodies
- Ultrasound: Only when nodular disease is suggested by examination

Central Hypothyroidism

- Free T4 ↓ and TSH normal or ↓

Overt Hypothyroidism

- ↑ serum TSH concentration and ↓ free T4 concentration

Section II:

High-risk Antenatal Ward Rounds

Chapter 19

Iron Deficiency Anemia in Pregnancy

Tania G Singh

CONCEPT OF PHYSIOLOGICAL ANEMIA IN PREGNANCY

- RBC increases by (350 mL) 20–30%
- Plasma volume increases by (250 mL) 40–50%
- Erythrocyte dilution by 5–15%
- Decrease in hemoglobin concentration by ≈ 2g/dL
- Total blood volume, increases by (1500 mL) 30–40%
- Because of hemodilution → physiological anemia occurs → hemoglobin is brought down to 11 gm%
- Blood picture of physiological anemia in pregnancy: normocytic, normochromic.

FACTORS LEADING TO ANEMIA DURING PREGNANCY

- Increased demand
  - Multiparity (increased iron demand by 2-folds)
  - Women with rapidly occurring pregnancy within 2 years following last delivery
  - Teenage pregnancy (e.g. at the age of 17, additional demand is ≈ 270 mg during pregnancy) → becomes nil by age 21
  - Parturition
  - Lactation.
- Diminished intake of iron
  - Low socioeconomic status
  - Vegetarian diet
  - Lack of balanced diet or poor intake (e.g. diet rich only in carbohydrates)
  - Alcoholism
  - High-risk ethnic groups
  - Increased absorption by presence of HCl in stomach
  - Drugs—alphadopa/levodopa/ciprofloxacin/cimetidine: interfere with iron absorption
  - Achlorhydria and copious intake of antacids decreases it
  - Loss of appetite and vomiting.
- Disturbed metabolism: presence of infection
  - Asymptomatic bacteriuria
  - Chronic and latent pyelonephritis
  - UTI.

Therefore, antibacterial therapy is necessary before response to hematinics is expected.

Physiological Anemia of Pregnancy

Benefits

- Decreases blood viscosity: decreases load on heart
- Facilitates blood flow through placenta
- Increases blood volume : acts as protective barrier against blood loss in third stage of labor

Harmful effects

- In case of cardiac disease, the increased circulatory burden can be dangerous, especially in presence of anemia and fetus may be less efficiently oxygenated because of decreased oxygen carrying capacity of diluted blood

During lactation, absorption rate increases by 20%, therefore, demand hardly fulfilled

According to Indian tradition—housewife eats last, after all male members and children have eaten and in many families, the women eat only the leftovers. Hence, even though the food prepared for the family is the same, women are more prone to develop iron deficiency anemia than other members of the family

It requires ≈ 2 years to replenish ≈ 1000 mg of iron lost during delivery and lactation

Each worm extracts up to 0.05 mL of blood/day, i.e. 0.5–2 mg of iron daily
A hookworm burden of 40–160 worms (depending on the iron status of the host) is associated with iron deficiency anemia

Why iron is not prescribed in first trimester?
- Absorption of exogenous iron is regulated by state of body store
- Females generally have adequate iron stores when they enter pregnancy, leading to it's little absorption in 1st trimester
- Later in gestation, there is increased demands → depletion of stores and accordingly iron absorption is increased from 7% in 1st trimester to 66% in 3rd trimester

Risk Periods for Anemic Mother
- At approximately 30–32 weeks of pregnancy
- During labor
- Immediately following delivery
- Any time in puerperium especially first 7–10 days after delivery due to pulmonary embolism

- Decreased absorption
  - Dietary factors (tannins, phytates in fibre, calcium in milk, tea, coffee, carbonated drinks)
  - Upper GI pathology: chronic gastritis; chronic diarrhea; gastric lymphoma; celiac disease; Crohn's disease
  - Medications that decrease gastric acidity or bind iron
  - Gastrectomy or intestinal bypass
  - Duodenal pathology
  - Chronic renal failure patients.
- Iron loss
  - Loss by sweat ≈ 15 mg/month
  - Repeated pregnancy at short intervals (along with prolonged lactation)
  - Increased blood loss during menstruation
  - Hookworm infestation
  - Malaria (falciparum and vivax), chronic blood loss due to bleeding piles/dysentery
  - Sickle-cell anemia and thalassemia
  - GI bleeding
  - Regular blood donors
  - Hematuria
  - Intravascular hemolysis: hemoglobinuria
  - Extreme physical exercise (endurance athletes)
  - Pathological (hemolytic).
- Prepregnancy health status: anemic or inadequate state of stored iron
- Polymorphism of anemia in pregnancy: Pregnancy interferes with maternal erythropoiesis by competing for available raw materials.

EFFECTS OF ANEMIA ON MOTHER AND FETUS

Mother

During Pregnancy

- Abortions
- Pre-eclampsia because of malnutrition and hypoproteinemia
- Intercurrent infection; heart failure at 30–32 weeks
- Preterm labor; IUD (24% at term).

During Labor

- Uterine inertia; Postpartum hemorrhage
- Cardiac failure; Shock.

Puerperium

- Puerperal sepsis; subinvolution; failing lactation
- Puerperal venous thrombosis; pulmonary embolism.

Fetus

- Preterm birth; IUGR; IUD.

Baby

- Low Apgar score; developmental delay; iron deficiency in infancy.

TREATMENT PROPER

The points to be remembered before starting therapy are as follows:
- Oral route is the first choice to replenish iron stores unless indicated otherwise
- Oral therapy takes about 6–10 weeks for Hb to return to normal level
- In iron deficiency anemia, stores are exhausted and need to be replenished which begins only after Hb returns to normal
- Therefore, stopping iron soon after Hb is normal means inadequate therapy and predisposes to recurrence
- Absorption of iron diminishes after Hb has returned to normal and therefore, replenishment of stores is a very slow process, taking about 3–4 months
  - Thus, iron therapy should be continued for 5–6 months
  - The best absorption occurs during the first few weeks of treatment
  - A positive response to treatment can be defined as a daily increase in hemoglobin concentration of 0.1g/dL from the 4th day onwards.
- Start iron tablet with 1 tablet/day, increase gradually till full dose is reached and well-tolerated
- If patient complains of side effects, try a low dose preparation with an iron enhancer like ascorbic acid or try alternative salts with less gastric intolerance
- More than 2 tablets/day → not recommended and not favored
- Side effects are directly related to amount of elemental iron and the actual compound and not to the brand used
- Ferrous salts → 3 times readily absorbed than ferric forms
- Ideally, iron should be taken on an empty stomach but it ↑ side effects, therefore, can be taken in between meals. If taken after meals, absorption is ↓ to 5%
- Tea, coffee, antacids, calcium salts (other than calcium carbonate and citrate) should be avoided for atleast 2–3 hours after iron intake
- Vitamin C is an enhancer so can be taken with iron
- Liquid preparations are expensive, deteriorate on storage, has metallic taste, make feces black, cause temporary discoloration of teeth (due to formation of iron sulphide), therefore, taken with straw or mix with water or fruit juice. Use a dropper to the back of the mouth and then rinse the mouth thoroughly
- There is no significant difference in absorption when a ferrous salt is given in form of sulphate, gluconate, lactate, fumarate or succinate but absorption is poor
  - When given as carbonate, citrate and pyrophosphate
  - In ferric forms
  - Colloidal iron preparations
  - Iron carbohydrate complexes.
- Cheapest and well-absorbed form—ferrous sulphate
- Most commonly used salt in commercial preparations—ferrous fumarate
- Side effects:
  - Upper GIT: nausea, gastric discomfort, loss of appetite, staining of teeth with liquid preparations
  - Lower GIT: constipation, diarrhea, flatulence.
- Enteric-coated or sustained release oral iron preparations are generally not recommended as majority of the iron is carried past the duodenum resulting in poor absorption

---

Iron Requirements/Day in Different Trimesters

Normal iron requirement in pregnancy is roughly 4.0 mg/day, i.e. ≈ 120–150 mg/month

In pregnancy
- Early: 2.5 mg/day
- 20–32 weeks: 5.5 mg/day (1.9 mg/1000 kcal in 2nd trimester)
- >32 weeks: 6–8 mg/day (2.7 mg/1000 kcal in 3rd trimester)

Lactation
- 2.4 mg/day

Response to Oral Therapy
- Usually begins 1 week after starting treatment and thereafter hemoglobin increases at the rate of 0.8 g/dL/week
- Retic count ↑ by 7–10 days

Daily Versus Weekly Iron Supplementations

Studies have shown that weekly supplementation is simple, economical, with less side effects and equally efficacious when compared to daily doses

Fetus usually remains unaffected even if mother suffers from iron deficiency anemia

Various Oral Iron Preparations

Preparation	Iron compound (mg/tab)	Elemental iron (mg/tab) (%)
Ferrous sulphate (hydrous)	300	60 (20%)
Ferrous sulphate (dried)	200	65 (325%)
Ferrous gluconate	300	36 (12%)
Ferrous fumarate	200	66 (33%)
Ferrous succinate	100	35 (35%)
Ferric ammonium citrate	125	25 (17–22%)
Carbonyl iron	100	90 (90%)
Iron polymaltose complex	100 mg /50 mg	-
Ferrous ascorbate	100	
Ferrous fructose	25%	
Ferrous lactate	19%	
Ferrous carbonate	16%	
Ferrous glycine citrate	23%	
Iron choline	12%	

- Colloidal ferric hydroxide has high elemental iron (52.26%) → gets reduced to ferrous state easily by action of gastric juices → assuring its greatest and better absorption with minimal gastric irritation.

NEWER ORAL IRON PREPARATIONS

Iron III Hydroxide Polymaltose Complex (Mumfer)

Advantages

- Less side effects (nonionic)
- Can be used by people who cannot tolerate other oral preparations
- Does not stain teeth
- Can be taken at any time irrespective of meals
- No metallic taste.

Disadvantages

- Recently, therapeutic efficacy of IPC is questioned
- Comparatively costlier as compared to other preparations
- Ferric iron preparation
- Very poor bioavailability.

Iron Bisglycinate

- Glycine (smallest of all amino acids) on reacting with ferrous iron, forms a more stable compound, bisglycinate chelate with least GI symptoms
- It protects the iron from harmful chemical reaction in stomach and duodenum, therefore, phytates will not reduce its absorption
- Disadvantage: high-cost.

Carbonyl Iron

- "Carbonyl" refers to a manufacturing process
- Iron is obtained by controlled heating of vaporized iron pentacarbonyl → leading to the deposition of unchanged elemental iron (purity >98%) as microscopic spheres of diameter less than 5μ → which then becomes soluble in gastric juices
- The gastric juices solubilizes this iron, consuming H^+ ions → increasing its pH → for much slower but complete absorption
- ↓↓ toxicity (no risk of iron poisoning even if taken by children by mistake)
- Has high bioavailability and less side effects than other preparations.

Na- Feredetate

- Newer formulation, chelate form of iron
- Does not dissociate in stomach thereby producing minimal gastric irritation
- Bioavailability is 2.5 to 10 times of ferrous sulphate and carbonyl iron respectively
- Produces faster rise in hemoglobin as compared to conventional and carbonyl iron
- Absorption → unaffected by phytates and oxalates
- Available as tabs and solution
- Tablet provides:
    - 231 mg of sodium feredetate equivalent to 33 mg of elemental iron
    - 1.5 mg of folic acid
    - 15 mcg of vitamin B_{12}.

- Each 5 mL of solution contains
  - 231 mg of sodium feredetate equivalent to 33 mg of elemental iron
  - Available in lemon orange flavor.

Gastric Delivery Systems

- Bioadhesive polymer (cross-linked polyacrylic acid)
- It adheres to the gastric mucosa or epithelium and floats there
- Releases iron slowly (over 5–12 hours) but continuously in stomach, reducing the dosage to once daily
- Eliminates GI side effects
- Absorption ↑↑
- Very costly.

Short Gun Therapy of Anemia

- Contain different vitamins and trace elements, an added advantage
- High-cost
- Technical advisory board (India) has recommended that B complex, other vitamins and zinc should not be included in iron and folic acid containing hematinics.

PARENTERAL ADMINISTRATION

- Caution before use: Iron deficiency should be confirmed by ferritin levels before use of parenteral preparations as free iron may lead to the production of hydroxyl radicals with potential toxicity to tissues
- Rate of response → same as oral therapy
- Oral iron to be discontinued when IM or IV iron is given, otherwise receptor sites get chocked → ↑ toxicity from free circulating iron (especially 48 hours before in case of iron sorbitol) who would otherwise receive transfusion.

ROUTES

Intramuscular

- Technique: Test dose 0.5 mL (at same site where full dose is to be given)
- After 1 hour, give full dose
- Give only into muscle mass of upper outer quadrant of buttock in a Z track technique (before injection, skin is laterally displaced so as to avoid staining in case it leaks into subcutaneous tissues)
- Do not rub the injection site
- Recommended dosage—1.5 mg/kg/day or on alternate days
- Formula—[(normal Hb – patient's Hb) × wt (kg) × 2.21] + 1000
- It takes ≈ 200 mg of elemental iron to raise Hb by 1gm/dL of blood
- Anaphylaxis is less with IM than IV preparations
- Side effects: pain, discoloration at injection site, injection abscess, sarcomatous change (rare).

Intravenous

- Advantages over IM therapy
  - Less painful
  - Better compliance—complete treatment ensured
  - Less hospital stay.

Indications for Parenteral Therapy

- Demonstrated intolerance to oral iron
- Disorder of GIT (Inflammatory bowel disease) – poor absorption
- Along with erythropoietin
- Non compliance / Non adherence → patient is not taking it at all (color of stools to be asked)
- Late in pregnancy
- Poor response to oral therapy (≈ after 4 weeks in a confirmed case of iron deficiency anemia)
- Chronic uncorrectable bleeding
- Hemoglobin <6 g /dL (60 g per L) with signs of poor perfusion, in patients

Contraindications to Parenteral Therapy

- History of anaphylaxis or reactions to parenteral iron therapy
- 1st trimester of pregnancy
- Active acute or chronic infection
- Chronic liver disease

Parenteral Preparations

Iron carbohydrate complexes

- Iron dextran (Imferon)
- Iron sorbitol (Iron sorbitol citric acid complex- Jectofer)
- Iron sucrose (Orofer S)

Iron dextran	Iron sorbitol citric acid complex
IM and IV preparation both	IM only
High molecular weight	Low molecular weight and high transferrin saturation capacity, therefore, cannot be given as high IV bolus or infusion
Available as 2 mL (IM) and	Available as 1.5 mL ampule 10 mL (IV)
Elemental iron – 50 mg/mL	Elemental iron – 50 mg/mL
50–90% absorbed	Absorbed completely
Slow absorption	Absorption rapid
Not excreted in urine	30% excreted in urine, therefore, treatment comparatively costlier
Molecule – large as compared to sorbitol	Small molecule as compared to dextran
Takes 3–4 weeks for complete absorption	≈ 2/3rd of the dose is absorbed from local site in 3 hours and little or no residue remains at injection site after 10 days
Side effects: Joint pain in 20%	Side effects: pain at injection site, fever in 5% of cases

- Dose calculation:

$$\frac{\text{Hb deficit (g/dL)} \times \text{blood vol (65 mL/kg body wt)} \times 3.4}{100}$$

  - Where $3.4 \rightarrow$ mg iron/gm Hb
  - Total dose is diluted in 0.9% NS
  - 5% dextrose $\rightarrow\uparrow$ incidence of local pain and phlebitis
  - Test dose: 0.5 mL (25 mg) diluted in 50 mL IV over 10–15 min
  - After 1 hour—give total dose (to be completed within 30 minutes).

Iron Sucrose

- Polynuclear ferric hydroxide
- Molecular weight 34,000–60,000 daltons
- Can be given only by intravenous route
- Each 2.5 mL/5 mL ampule contains 50 mg and 100 mg elemental iron, respectively, i.e. each mL contains 20 mg of iron
- Plasma $t_{1/2} \approx 6$ hours
- After IV administration, it dissociates into iron and sucrose
- Peak levels reach in 10 minutes
- Does not oversaturate transferrin
- Dose calculation—The cumulative dose depends on total iron deficit
- Total iron (mg) = [2.4 × wt.(kg) × Hb deficit (gm)] + 1000 mg (for pregnancy)
- Administration: as slow IV injection or infusion
  - Slow IV injection: 100 mg injected IV over 2–5 minutes
  - IV Infusion: 5 mL Iron sucrose is usually diluted in 100 mL of 0.9% NaCl, immediately prior to infusion and infused IV at the rate of 100 mg of iron over a period of at least 15 minutes
  - Unused diluted solution must be discarded
  - Each dose of 100 mg IV may be repeated up to 3 times per week $\rightarrow$ maximum of 200 mg/sitting.
- Advantages
  - More safe
  - Effective
  - Well-tolerated
  - Very rare anaphylactic reaction.
- Disadvantage: high-cost
- Contraindications
  - In patients with evidence of iron overload
  - In patients with known hypersensitivity to formulation
  - In patients with anemia not caused by iron deficiency.
- Side-effects (though uncommon)—keep patient in hospital for minimum 2 hours for observation
  - Hypotension, chest pain, hypertension, hypervolemia
  - CHF, cramps, musculoskeletal pain
  - Diarrhea, nausea/vomiting, abdominal pain
  - Elevated liver enzymes, skin irritation, pruritus
  - Application site reaction, dizziness, dyspnea
  - Headache, fever, asthenia/malaise
- Absence of response—complete investigation including bone marrow biopsy.

SEVERE ANEMIA IN LATE PREGNANCY

Late Pregnancy

- Blood transfusion—life saving in last 4 weeks of pregnancy
- Packed cells are to be transfused slowly instead of whole blood
- Diuretics (Frusemide)—simultaneously administered
- Propped-up position
- O_2 inhalation
- Vitals charting
- Intermittent chest auscultation
- Keep a check on uterine contractions (may go into preterm labor).

ROLE OF ERYTHROPOEITIN IN ANEMIA

Indications

- Pregnancy with renal insufficiency
- Refractory anemia
- Severe anemia in late pregnancy
- Member of Jehovah's witnesses.

Product Detail (in India)

Available as

- Vials containing 1000, 2000 and 4000IU
- Prefilled erythropoietin syringe for subcutaneous use.

Safety

- Seems to be safe for the fetus: it does not cross the placental barrier and, therefore, lacks any direct fetal effect
- Also safe for the mother.

Prerequisite for Successful Treatment

- Adequate iron supplementation.

Contraindications

- Uncontrolled hypertension
- Hypersensitivity to the drug.

Side Effects (uncommon)

- High blood pressure
- Muscle and joint pain
- Flu-like syndrome (headache, dizziness, insomnia, pyrexia, cough, URTI)
- Pruritis, rashes, urticaria
- Nausea, vomiting, stomatitis, dysphagia
- Injection site pain and irritation.

Route

- For subcutaneous or IV administration only
- Not for intradermal, intramuscular or intra-arterial administration
- IV route recommended for patients on hemodialysis.

Caution in Giving Iron Sucrose

- The whole infusion should get over in 20–30 minutes (and not 4–5 hours)
- Most cases of anaphylactoid reaction (recently observed) occurs in the last half hour of the slow infusions, due to the release of free iron radicals with DELAYED INFUSIONS and NOT due to compound

Response to Iron Sucrose Treatment

- Reticulocyte count >12%
- Rate of rise in Hb in pregnancy is 0.8 gm/dL/week and in nonpregnant women 1.0–1.2 gm/dL/week
- Maximum Hb response does not appear till 4–9 weeks, therefore, if Rx is not started until last month of pregnancy → insufficient time to increase Hb till delivery

Causes of Treatment Failure in Iron Deficiency Anemia

- Noncompliance
- Continuous blood loss through hookworm infestation or bleeding piles
- Coexisting infection
- Faulty iron absorption
- Folic acid deficiency
- Noniron deficiency microcytic anemia
  - Thalassemia; Pyridoxine deficiency; Lead poisoning

Place of Blood Transfusion in Case of Iron Deficiency Anemia
- Hemoglobin<5 gm/dL– at any gestational age
- After 36 weeks of pregnancy
- Nonresponders to oral or parenteral therapy
- PPH

Place of Exchange Transfusion
- Rare
- Indicated in very severe cases in cardiac failure

Precautions before using Erythropoeitin
- Do not shake or vigorously agitate vial → prolonged, vigorous shaking may denature the glycoprotein, rendering it biologically inactive
- Rotate subcutaneous injection site
- Single-dose vials contain no preservative
- Use only 1 dose/vial
- Do not reenter the vial
- Discard any unused portion
- Do not combine unused portions or save unused portions for later use
- Do not administer in conjunction with other drug solutions. However, at the time of subcutaneous administration, single-use vials may be admixed in a syringe with bacteriostatic sodium chloride 0.9% and benzyl alcohol 0.9% in a 1:1 ratio
- Multidose vials contain benzyl alcohol and admixing is not necessary
- Individualize dosing and use the lowest dose sufficient to reduce the need for blood transfusions

Drug Administration

Two methods exist:

Method 1: Erythropoietin + iron sucrose in same sitting

200 mg iron sucrose diluted in 100 mL 0.9% NS infused over 15–20 minutes → flush cannula with 5 mL saline solution→ inject erythropoietin (1 mL) bolus

Method 2: Erythropoietin s/c with oral iron therapy

150 IU/kg × 3 times/week for a total of 4 weeks
- When adjusting therapy, consider hemoglobin rate of rise, rate of decline and hemoglobin variability
- A single hemoglobin excursion may not require a dosing change
- Evaluate the iron status in all patients before and during treatment and maintain iron repletion.

NRHM (NATIONAL RURAL HEALTH MISSION) RECOMMENDATIONS 2013

As anemia is very common among pregnant females in India and majority of anemia related complications occur at low resource settings, utmost importance should be given to treatment of anemia at subcentre/outreach/PHC/CHC levels. Screening by Sahli's hemoglobinometer or by Standard Hemoglobin Color scale is done.

ANTEPARTUM

Hb between 9 and 11 gm/dL
- 2 IFA tablets /day × min 100 days
- Reassess Hb after a month → if normal → stop treatment
- If not → refer to higher centre.

Hb between 8 and 9 gm/dL
- Investigate for the cause
- Rest same as above.

Hb between 7 and 8 gm/dL
- Investigate for the cause
- If iron deficiency → IM iron therapy in divided doses + folic acid (if no other obstetric or systemic complications)
- Repeat Hb after 8 weeks
- If she is in her 3rd trimester → refer to higher centre
- Multiple dose regimen
  - Intramuscular (IM)—Test dose of 0.5 mL given deep IM and woman observed for 1 hour
  - Iron dextran or iron sorbitol citrate complex given as 100 mg (2 mL) deep IM in gluteal region daily
  - Recommended dose is 1500–2000 mg (IM in divided doses) depending upon the body weight and Hb level.

Hb between 5 and 7 gm/dL
- Refer to higher centre.

Hb lower than 5 gm/dL
- Immediate hospitalization in tertiary care.

Postpartum
- Hemoglobin checked within first 48 hours after delivery

- If woman is nonanemic, prophylactic regime should be given (1 tab daily × 100 days)
- If Hb lower than 10 gm/dL (WHO) → treat.

Features Pointing Towards Aetiology of Anemia
- Presence of jaundice – Hemolytic anemia
- Leg ulcer—Sickle-cell anemia
- Spotted nails and koilonychia—Iron deficiency anemia
- Neurological deficit—Megaloblastic anemia
- Cold intolerance, reduced resistance to infection—Iron deficiency anemia
- Hepatosplenomegaly—Hemolytic anemia
- Malignancy and parasitic infestation—Thalassemia
- Frontal bossing—Thalassemia
- Lymphadenopathy or sternal tenderness—Blood dyscrasias and metastasis
- Scleral icterus—Hemolytic anemia
- Restless leg syndrome—Iron deficiency anemia
- Glossitis—Pernicious anemia/folic acid/vit B_{12} deficiency
- Tongue fiery red—Vitamin B deficiency
- Pale tongue—Pernicious anemia
- Fatigue, leg cramps on climbing stairs, craving ice or cold vegetables—Iron deficiency anemia
- Petechiae—Thrombocytopenia from a bone marrow disorder
- Glossy tongue, with atrophy of the lingual papillae—Iron deficiency anemia
- Ecchymosis, purpura, lymphadenopathy, splenomegaly—Hemolytic malignancy
- Melena, hematochezia, hematuria, hematemesis—Iron deficiency anemia secondary to bleeding
- Chelitis, glossitis, decreased proprioception and vibratory sensation—Vitamin B_{12} deficiency
- Dermatitis herpetiformis (DH) or Duhring's Disease—Iron deficiency anemia secondary to malabsorption
- Dysphagia with solid foods together with esophageal web (dysphagia results from weakened esophageal muscle contractions)—Plummer-Vinson syndrome
- Pseudotumour cerebri—Iron deficiency anemia (a rare finding in severe cases)

Chapter 20

Thalassemia in Pregnancy

Tania G Singh and Nisha M Anand

STEPS IN DIAGNOSIS OF THALASSEMIA

Step I: RBC Indices
- MCV and MCH → low
- MCHC → Normal
- Serum iron and TIBC → normal or ↑.

Step II: Confirm by electrophoresis
- ↑HbA$_2$ ($\alpha_2\delta_2$) → >3.5% with or without ↑ HbF.

Step III: Investigations of the partner
- Send Hb electrophoresis: if normal, nothing is to be done
- If both have trait: offer prenatal diagnosis (there is 25% chance that the fetus will have thalassemia major)
- If yes, terminate pregnancy.

HB ELECTROPHORESIS

- For routine Hb analysis
- Quantification and identification of various hemoglobins
- Best technique for diagnosis of Thalassemia syndromes
- Thalassemia syndromes
  - Are a heterogenous group of inherited anemias characterized by reduced or absent synthesis of either α or β globin chains of HbA
  - Most common single gene disorder.

POSSIBLE CHAINS OF GLOBIN

HbA ($\alpha_2\beta_2$)

- A pair of alpha and a pair of beta chain
- It is higher than 95% in normal adult blood.

HbA$_2$ ($\alpha_2\delta_2$)

- Approximately 1–3%.

HbF ($\alpha_2\gamma_2$)

- Fetal hemoglobin
- 80% of Hb in cord blood at term
- Falls to 25% by 1st month of life
- Almost completely changed to HbA in 1st year of life
- Constitutes less than 1% of adult blood.

Classification

- When synthesis of alpha chain is suppressed
  - Level of all three is reduced, i.e. HbA $(\alpha_2\beta_2)$; HbA$_2$ $(\alpha_2\delta_2)$ and HbF $(\alpha_2\gamma_2)$ leading to Alpha thalassemia
- When synthesis of beta chain is suppressed, adult Hb is reduced $\rightarrow$ leading to Beta thalassemia
- Inheritance: autosomal recessive.

BETA THALASSEMIA

- Results from point mutations of the two genes responsible for beta chain that are located on chromosome 11
- Characterized by total or near total absence of beta chains resulting in marked decrease in HbA
- Results in compensatory increase in other chains
  - γ chain synthesis persists in adult life ($\uparrow$ HbF)
  - δ chain synthesis is also increased ($\uparrow$ HbA$_2$)
  - Excess of α chains precipitate in cytoplasm of affected RBC $\rightarrow$ destruction of RBC $\rightarrow$ Anemia

Classification of Beta Thalassemia

Classification	β globin genes	HbA	HbA$_2$	HbF
Normal	Homozygous β	97–99%	1–3%	<1%
Thal major	Homozygous $\beta°$	0%	4–10%	90–96%
Thal major	Heterozygous β^+	0–10%	4–10%	90–96%
Thal intermedia	Homozygous β^+	0–30%	0–10%	60–100%
Thal minor	Heterozygous $\beta°$	80–95%	4–8%	1–5%
Thal minor	Heterozygous β^+	80–95%	4–8%	1–5%

ALPHA THALASSEMIA

- Results from gene deletions of the four genes responsible for alpha chains that are located on chromosome 16
- Mutation of one gene
  - "Silent" carrier
  - No clinical or laboratory abnormality.
- Mutation of two genes
  - Alpha thalassemia "Minor"
  - Goes unrecognized
  - Pregnancy well-tolerated.
- Mutation of three genes
  - "Hb H disease" (Hb H Ds) or "Intermediate"
  - Hb Bart (4 γ chains) $\rightarrow$ present at birth
  - Gradually replaced by HbH (4 β chains) $\rightarrow$ 5–30%
  - These women suffer from hemolytic anemia
  - During pregnancy $\rightarrow$ anemia worsens.
- Mutation of four genes (Bart's Hydrops Fetalis Syndrome)
  - Most severe form $\rightarrow$ "α Thalassemia major"
  - Incompatible with life
  - Have no functioning alpha chain genes (--/--)
  - Mother may develop Mirror Syndrome

β^+thal $\rightarrow$ reduced synthesis of β globin chain; Heterozygous $\beta°$thal $\rightarrow$ absent synthesis of β globin chain; Homozygous

Pathophysiology of the Disease

Lack of adequate HbA$\rightarrow$ anemia$\rightarrow\uparrow$ tissue hypoxia$\rightarrow\uparrow$ EPO production$\rightarrow\uparrow$ erythropoiesis in the marrow and at times extramedullary also $\rightarrow$ expansion of medullary cavities of various bones Liver/spleen enlarges$\rightarrow$ extramedullary hematopoiesis

Mirror Syndrome

- Hydramnios
- Edema
- Pre eclampsia

- Neonate born with hydrops fetalis
- Hepatosplenomegaly and cardiomegaly present
- Predominant hemoglobin is hemoglobin bart, along with hemoglobin portland and traces of hemoglobin H
- Bart's hemoglobin has high oxygen affinity so cannot carry oxygen to tissues
- Fetus dies in utero or shortly after birth
- At birth, has severe hypochromic, microcytic anemia
- Pregnancy → dangerous to mother
- Increased risk of severe pre eclampsia and postpartum hemorrhage.

MANIFESTATIONS

Marrow Expansion

- Hemolytic facies with frontoparietal, occipital bossing
- Malar prominence; malocclusion of teeth
- Distortion of ribs and vertebrae
- Pathological fractures of long bones due to cortical thinning
- Sinus and middle ear infection due to ineffective drainage
- Folate deficiency
- Increased absorption of iron from intestine
- Hypermetabolic state → fever, wastage, leg ulcers.

Hepatomegaly

- Iron released from breakdown of endogenous or transfused RBCs cannot be utilized for hemoglobin synthesis→ hemosiderosis
- Hemochromatosis
- Infections (transfusion related) → Hepatitis B, C, HIV
- Chronic hepatitis; Jaundice—obstructive (due to gall stones).

Splenomegaly

- Work atrophy due to constant hemolysis
- Hypersplenism
- Jaundice—unconjugated hyperbilirubinemia.

Clinical Spectrum of β Thalassemia

Thalassemia Major

- Serious homozygous form
- Severe microcytic hypochromic anemia
- Detected early in childhood
- Present in early infancy with progressive pallor, hepatosplenomegaly, bony changes
- Fatal during first few years of life, if left untreated
- Hemoglobin level between 4 and 8 gm/dL
- Peripheral blood shows:
  - Markedly hypochromic, microcytic erythrocytes
  - Extreme poikilocytosis, target cells, teardrop cells and elliptocytes
  - Marked basophilic stippling.
- Repeated blood transfusions required
- Physical growth and development delayed.

Which is more common of the two?

Beta thalassemia (COOLEY'S ANEMIA) is more common of the two. Alpha thalassemia is rare

Thalassemia Minor

- Heterozygous form
- Presents late and patient can lead a normal life except for persistent mild hemolytic anemia
- Compatible with normal life
- Have one normal beta gene and one mutated beta gene
- Hemoglobin level in 10–13 g/dL range, with normal or slightly elevated RBC count
- Anemia usually hypochromic and microcytic
- Rarely see hepatomegaly or splenomegaly
- Make sure that these are not diagnosed with iron deficiency anemia.

Thalassemia Intermedia

- Patients are able to maintain minimum hemoglobin (7 g/dL or greater) without transfusions
- They are also homozygous
- Patient presents somewhere between two extremes with variable clinical manifestations—
  - Progressive pallor hepatosplenomegaly
  - Bony changes, have significant increase in bilirubin.
- Life is fairly comfortable
- Not dependent on blood transfusions
- Anemia usually becomes worse with infections, pregnancy, or folic acid deficiencies
- Tend to develop iron overloads as a result of increased gastrointestinal absorption.

Management of β Thalassemia Major in Pregnancy

These patients have iron overload. Iron deposition in various organs

- Brain (hypothalamus and pituitary) → Endocrine abnormalities → Hypogonadotrophic hypogonadism. Manifests as:
  - Primary or secondary amenorrhea
  - Chronic anovulation
  - Decreased estradiol levels.
- Hypothyroidism; Diabetes Milletus
- Direct ovarian damage due to iron deposition and redox-active iron in follicular fluid.

Preconception Period (Very Important)

- Need to investigate the mother as well as the partner
- Chelation therapy
  - With desferrioxamine + vitamin C
  - Aim → serum ferritin level of 1000–2000 ng/mL.
- Start folic acid.

Antenatal Management

- Investigations mentioned above
- Discontinue desferrioxamine
  - Harmful effects on fetus
  - Risk of iron deficiency in neonates.

Mother's Investigations in Preconceptional Period

- Maternal cardiac status
- Thyroid function tests
- FBS/PPBS/HbA$_1$C
- Serum ferritin
- Blood group and type
- Screening for blood group antibodies (anti-Kell and Duffy) should be performed→ If not available→ ICT
- Hepatitis B, C, HIV
- Partner: Hb electrophoresis

These Fetuses are at Increased Risk of:

- Anemia →↑ blood transfusions (continue folic acid throughout pregnancy)
- Increased risk of IUGR (frequent fetal growth monitoring and biophysical profile)
- Increased risk of pregnancy loss
- Cardiac failure due to overload of pregnancy
- Increased chances of undergoing cesarean section

- Discontinue vitamin C
  - It increases dietary absorption of iron.
- Iron supplements should not be given.

Management of α Thalassemia

Diagnosis by CVS or Amniocentesis

When There is Mutation of 1 or 2 Genes

- Iron and folate therapy
- Never to be given parenteral therapy
- Pregnancy → well-tolerated.

HbH disease

- 5 mg folate/day
- Offspring will either be a silent carrier or will carry "trait".

α Thalassemia Major

- Incompatible with life and pregnancy
- Vaginal delivery is complicated due to large placenta and fetus.

Chapter 21

Megaloblastic Anemia

Tania G Singh

Deficiency of folic acid and/or vitamin B_{12}
- Deficiency of folic acid → very common
- Deficiency of vitamin B_{12} → rare.

Why there is Impaired DNA Synthesis or Abnormal Maturation?
- For maturation, the following are required:
  - Vitamin B_{12} → In synthesis of RNA
  - Folic acid → In synthesis of DNA
  - Vitamin C → For conversion of folic acid to folinic acid.
- Therefore, if there is inadequate vitamin B_{12} → Defective synthesis of DNA and RNA
- If folic acid is not adequate → Defective synthesis of DNA only
- Folic acid is required for conversion of uridine to thymidine in nucleic acid synthesis.

FOLIC ACID (AN OVERVIEW)

- Also known as folate, vitamin M, vitamin B_9, etc.
- Folic acid is itself not biologically active, but it's biological importance is due to tetrahydrofolate and other derivatives after it's conversion to dihydrofolic acid in the liver
- Humans cannot synthesize folate de novo; therefore, folate has to be supplied through the diet to meet their daily requirements
- Derived it's name from the Latin word 'folium' (which means "leaf"), therefore, leafy vegetables are principal sources of folic acid
- Folate in body stores: 500–20,000 µg
- A complete lack of dietary folate takes months before deficiency develops
- Folate requirement of newborn → 20–50 µ/day

Vitamin B_{12} Deficiency is Rare-Why?
- Very long storage life
- Stores usually not depleted by pregnancy
- Absorption usually normal in pregnancy
- Vitamin B_{12} binds to intrinsic factor (secreted by gastric parietal cells) → absorbed in distal ileum
- Pre-existing vitamin B_{12} deficiency is often associated with infertility
- Intake (animal products)
  - In nonpregnant females → 2 µg/day
  - In pregnancy → 3 µg/day.
- Only strict vegans have a problem→ may require supplementation in pregnancy.

Mechanism

- Vitamin B_{12} deficiency alone will not cause the syndrome in the presence of sufficient folate
- The actual mechanism is loss of B_{12} dependent folate recycling, followed by folate-deficiency → which in turn will affect the nucleic acid synthesis (specifically thymine) → leading to defects in DNA synthesis
- Folic acid supplementation in the absence of vitamin B_{12} prevents this type of anemia (although other vitamin B_{12}-specific pathologies continue)

Functions of Folic Acid

- To synthesize DNA
- Repair DNA
- Methylate DNA
- To act as a cofactor in certain biological reactions
- Aids in rapid cell division and growth

Causes of Megaloblastic Anemia in Pregnancy

It is mainly because of folic acid deficiency and the other causes are as follows:

- Deficient supply (poor nutrition)
- Decreased intake because of hyperemesis
- Defective absorption (e.g. in tropical sprue)
- Alcohol consumption (interferes with folate metabolism)
- Smoking ($\downarrow$ availability)
- Frequent child birth and multiple gestation (increased demands)
- Hemolytic factors
  - Congenital $\rightarrow$ sickle cell disease
  - Parasitic $\rightarrow$ e.g. malaria
  - Peptic ulcer; hookworms; hemorrhoids.
- Infection decreases life span of RBCs $\rightarrow$ folic acid is required to make more RBCs
- Increased demand (in pregnancy $\rightarrow$ minimum 400 µg/day)
- Female on anticonvulsant drugs (in epilepsy) $\rightarrow$ rapid decrease in RBC folate
- Intestinal malabsorption syndrome $\rightarrow$ recurrence in subsequent pregnancies
- Woman on OCPs have reduced cobalamin levels, which may exaggerate a pre-existing cobalamin deficiency
- Hepatic disorders ($\downarrow$ storage)
- Vitamin C deficiency
- Excessive cooking destroys much of folate.

Investigations which can Confirm Diagnosis of Megaloblastic Anemia

Hemogram

- Hb lower than or equal to 10 gm%
- MCV higher than 100 µm^3
- MCH higher than 33 pg
- MCHC normal
- The reticulocyte count is decreased due to destruction of fragile and abnormal megaloblastic erythroid precursor
- Leucopenia/Thrombocytopenia
- Serum iron $\rightarrow$ normal or $\uparrow$
- Total iron binding capacity $\rightarrow \downarrow$.

Peripheral Smear

Presence of any two of the following:

- Hyper/multisegmented neutrophils ($\geq$5 lobes) $\rightarrow$ "Senile neutrophil"
  - This is thought to be due to decreased production and a compensatory prolonged lifespan for circulating neutrophils, which increase numbers of nuclear segments with age.
- Anisocytosis (increased variation in RBC size) and poikilocytosis (abnormally-shaped RBCs)
- Macrocytosis (larger than normal RBCs) and Giant polymorphs
- Megaloblasts
- Ovalocytes present
- Howell-Jolly bodies (chromosomal remnant).

Management

- Deworm the patient
- Iron supplementation → is a must with folic acid
- Folic acid 5 mg starting at least 3 months before conception → throughout pregnancy → up to 4 weeks postpartum
- Injection Vitamin B_{12} 100 μg daily or on alternate days OR Inj. Methyl-cobalamin
    - Methylcobalamin → It is a kind of endogenous coenzyme B_{12}
    - It has an important role in transmethylation as a coenzyme in synthesis of methionine from homocysteine
    - Promotes nucleic acid and protein synthesis
    - 1 mL of injection contains 500 μg vitamin B_{12}.
- Vitamin C 100 mg three times a day should be included
- Transfusion → Antepartum hemorrhage is the main indication (but before that take blood sample for peripheral smear) → it will unmask folate deficiency
- Established anemia: Start an additional tablet of 5 mg folic acid especially in last month of pregnancy, along with
    - Parenteral iron (while waiting for investigations)
    - In multiple gestation (risk of preterm labor).

Once megaloblastic hemopoiesis is established → treatment of folic acid deficiency becomes more difficult, due to megaloblastic changes in GIT resulting in impaired absorption → becomes normal in 5 weeks with oral treatment → if ineffective → parenteral treatment.

Diagnostic (Definitive)

- Serum folate (fasting) <3 ng/mL (6.68 mmol/L) → Diagnostic
- Erythrocyte folate activity <20 ng/mL (50 mmol/L) → indicates folic acid deficiency
- Serum B_{12} <90 pg/mL

Maternal and Fetal Complications

- Abortion
- Dysmaturity
- Prematurity (fetus at risk of megaloblastic anemia because preterm infant in folate deficient mother is in severe negative folate balance because of high-growth rate)
- Abruptio
- Fetal malformation (cleft palate, NTDs)

Chapter 22

Sickle Cell Disease (SCD)

Tania G Singh

UNDERSTANDING THE DISEASE

- Normal hemoglobin cells are smooth, round, flexible and quiet elastic, like the letter "O," which enables them to deform to pass through the vasculature easily
- Sickle-cell hemoglobin cells are stiff, rigid, sticky, lose their elasticity and form into the shape of a sickle, or the letter "C," promoted by low oxygen tension
- They fail to return to normal shape when normal oxygen tension is restored
- They are unable to deform as they pass through narrow capillaries, leading to vessel occlusion and ischemia. Therefore, a person with sickle cell disease is chronically anemic
- Sickle cells only survive 10–20 days and are destroyed by spleen
- In this process, spleen is also damaged → ischemia and infarction occurs → hyposplenism → auto splenectomy.

Clinical Manifestations

Chronic Manifestation

- Sickle red cells
  - ↑ mechanical fragility
  - ↑ blood viscosity - 'seeding in microvasculature'
  - Hemolysis: Anemia; Icterus; Gallstones.
- Chronic pain
- Chronic renal failure due to Sickle cell nephropathy—hypertension, proteinuria, hematuria and worsened anemia.

Acute Manifestation

- Infarctive or painful crisis: Severe skeletal pain but no change in Hb%
- Sequestration crisis:
  - Sudden massive pooling of red cells in spleen with an acute fall in Hb concentration with the potential for hypovolemic shock
  - Because of its narrow vessels and function in clearing defective red blood cells, the spleen is frequently affected → infarction of spleen
  - This autosplenectomy increases the risk of infection from encapsulated organisms.
- Hemolytic crisis: Uncommon
  - Acute accelerated ↓ in Hb concentration with ↑↑ in jaundice
  - This is particularly common in patients with coexistent G6PD deficiency.
- Vaso-occlusive crisis: ↑ blood viscosity → ischemia, pain and infarction

---

Also known as: "HbSS"; "SS disease"; "Hemoglobin S"; Drepanocytosis

Caused by a point mutation in the β-globin chain of hemoglobin, causing the hydrophilic amino acid glutamic acid to be replaced with the hydrophobic amino acid valine at the sixth position

Affected newborn seldom exhibits clinical features of sickle cell disease. Anemia develops over the first 2–4 months paralleling replacement of much of fetal Hb by HbS. Clinical manifestations are uncommon before 5–6 months of age

- HbA is $\alpha_2\beta_2$: It thus needs to have both α and β chains.
- β chains are defective in sickle cell disease such that:
  - In heterozygotes or sickle cell trait: 40% chains are defective
  - In homozygotes or sickle cell disease: 100% chains are defective
- HbA$_2$ is $\alpha_2\delta_2$ and HbF is $\alpha_2\gamma_2$
- There is no underlying defect in δ chains or γ chains in sickle cell disease and hence HbF and HbA$_2$ may well be seen

- Lung–Pulmonary hypertension due to vaso-occlusive disease in lung vessels—leading to strain on the right ventricle and a risk of heart failure; typical symptoms are shortness of breath, decreased exercise tolerance and episodes of syncope
- Bone—Osteomyelitis

  The most common cause of osteomyelitis in sickle cell disease is Salmonella (especially the nontypical serotypes, *Salmonella typhimurium*, *Salmonella enteritidis*, *Salmonella choleraesuis and Salmonella paratyphi B*), followed by *Staphylococcus aureus* and Gram-negative enteric bacilli perhaps because intravascular sickling of the bowel leads to patchy ischemic infarction
- Avascular necrosis (aseptic bone necrosis) of the hip and other major joints, which may occur as a result of ischemia
- Spleen—hyposplenism; autosplenectomy
- Priaprism
- Kidney—Acute papillary necrosis
- Eye—Background retinopathy, proliferative retinopathy, vitreous hemorrhages and retinal detachments, resulting in blindness
- Stroke, which can result from a progressive narrowing of blood vessels, preventing oxygen from reaching the brain. Cerebral infarction and cerebral hemorrhage in adults
- Silent stroke is a stroke that causes no immediate symptoms but is associated with damage to the brain. Silent stroke is probably five times as common as symptomatic stroke, predominating in the younger patient.
- Aplastic crisis
  - This is an acute worsening of the patient's baseline anemia, producing pallor, tachycardia, and fatigue
  - This crisis is normally triggered by parvovirus B19, directly affecting erythropoiesis by invading the red cell precursors and eventually leading to their destruction
  - Parvovirus infection nearly completely prevents red blood cell production for two to three days, which in normal individuals, is of little consequence, but the shortened red-cell life of sickle-cell patients results in an abrupt, life-threatening situation
  - Reticulocyte counts drop dramatically during the disease, and the rapid turnover of red cells leads to the drop in hemoglobin
  - This crisis takes 4 days to one week to disappear
  - Overwhelming post-(auto) splenectomy infection (OPSI), which is due to functional asplenia, caused by encapsulated organisms, such as *Streptococcus pneumoniae and Haemophilus influenzae.*

Most episodes of sickle-cell crises last between five and seven days.

Management

Preconceptional Counseling

- These women should ideally be reviewed annually from adolescence
- Patient should be made aware of the factors favoring sickling/polymerization
  - Hypoxia: (2,3 diphosphoglycerate $\uparrow$ polymerization)
  - Dehydration
  - Stress/overexertion
  - Acidosis: ($\downarrow$ pH enhances polymerization)

Consequences of Anemia

- Cardiomegaly: Heart failure
- Hepatomegaly
- Reactive bone marrow hyperplasia
  - Stunted growth; Bossing skull; Fish mouth vertebra
- Chronic leg ulcers
- Most common acute presentation of sickle-cell anemia is: Bone pain (recurrent episodes) → produced as a result of intermittent episodes of vaso-occlusion in connective tissue and musculoskeletal structures → painful ischemia

- Hb concentration: Higher concentration →↑ polymerization
- Combination of HbS with other Hbs→ It depends upon extent of homology with other Hbs.
- Any urinary infection, if present should be treated before pregnancy
- Patient should be made aware of the increased risk of:
  - Worsening anemia
  - Sickling crises and acute chest syndrome
  - Urinary tract infection during pregnancy.
- Recommend pregnancy keeping in mind any previous damage due to serious complications and their screening in advance
  - Echocardiography to screen for pulmonary hypertension
  - Blood pressure and Urine analysis to rule out hypertension and/or proteinuria
  - RFT/ LFT
  - Ophthalmic examination
  - Screening for iron overload (if undergone multiple transfusions or who have high ferritin levels)
  - Screening for red cell antibodies.
- Partner's Hb electrophoresis
- Prenatal diagnosis
- Folic acid 5 mg daily
- Patients taking hydroxyurea (to decrease the incidence of crisis and acute chest syndrome) should be counseled regarding the associated congenital defects in the fetus and the drug should be stopped at least 3 months prior to conception
- Angiotensin-converting enzyme inhibitors and angiotensin receptor blockers should be stopped before conception
- Penicillin prophylaxis and vaccinations (Hep B, influenza, pneumococcal vaccine, etc.) should be considered especially in those who are hyposplenic
- Effects of pregnancy on the disease and how the disease affects pregnancy, should be discussed in detail.

EFFECT OF SICKLE CELL DISEASE ON PREGNANCY

Mother

Sickle-cell Trait

- Not much affected
- There is an increased incidence of:
  - Painful crises during pregnancy
  - IUGR; Antepartum hospital admission
  - Postpartum infection; UTI.

Sickle Cell Disease

- Encounter frequent urinary tract infections
- Lung infection
- They can have iron deficient anemia while pregnant, requiring iron supplementation
- Gallstones; Acute painful crisis
- Antenatal hospitalization
- Maternal mortality
- Delivery by cesarean section

Effect of Pregnancy on Sickle Cell Disease

- In some pregnancy may go uneventful
- In others there may be worsening of the disease
- Sickle-cell crises may still occur in pregnancy and can be managed conservatively
- Pre-existing kidney disease and congestive heart failure may worsen during pregnancy, even with proper treatment and care

- Infection; Thromboembolic events
- Antepartum hemorrhage
- Hypertensive disorders of pregnancy
- Cardiac enlargement and heart failure from anemia.

Fetus

- Miscarriage; Intrauterine growth restriction
- Preterm birth; Low birth weight
- Stillbirth and neonatal death.

Antepartum Management

Sickle-cell Trait

- Folic acid 5 mg daily
- Mother not at higher risk
- But baby may be affected, if the father also carries the trait
- Investigate the husband at the 1st visit, if not done preconceptionally
- If the baby's father has sickle cell trait, amniocentesis or other methods of prenatal diagnosis may be offered to help determine if the fetus has the trait or the disease.

Sickle Cell Disease

Care of the mother

- Should see both obstetrician and the hematologist
- Early and regular prenatal care is very important
- Folic acid 5 mg daily
- Avoid excessive nausea and vomiting to prevent dehydration
- More frequent prenatal visits allow for close monitoring of the disease and for fetal well-being
- Healthy diet, prenatal vitamins, folic acid, prevent exertion and extreme temperatures
- Blood pressure (often have a low BP) and urine analysis at each visit
- Urine culture—performed monthly
- Serial ultrasounds and Doppler studies (in case of IUGR fetus)
- Though pregnancy is not contraindicated while patient is on hydroxyurea, but stop the drug as soon as pregnancy is diagnosed and ultrasound should be done to rule out any defects
- Live attenuated vaccines should be deferred in pregnancy
- Iron supplementation only, if there is documented iron deficiency
- Low dose aspirin 75 mg daily from 2nd trimester onwards, to minimize the risk of preeclampsia is advisable
- If admitted to hospital, LMWH should be considered
- No recommendation for prophylactic blood transfusions
- Blood transfusions to replace the sickled cells, if acute emergency arises. This is to be continued several times in pregnancy
- There is no recommendation as when to start the transfusion but Hb lower than 6 gm% or a fall in Hb of higher than or equal to 2 gm% any time in pregnancy is an indication for blood transfusion
- Such women are to be screened for antibodies that may be transferred from transfused blood
- The most common antibodies are to the Rh factor
- Exchange transfusion in case of acute chest syndrome or acute stroke.

Place of Blood Transfusion

- Only when there are concomitant serious complications
- From 26 weeks onwards
- Exchange transfusion (2 units removed for every 3–4 units transfused)

Investigations

- CBC; Blood group and type
- Antibody screen
- HIV; HbsAg; Anti-HCV
- LFT/KFT; Viral screen
- Urine routine and culture; Partner screening (as soon as pregnancy is diagnosed).

Care of the fetus

- Started in the 2nd trimester
- TAS (level II scan)
- Nonstress test (after 32 weeks)
- Biophysical profile
- Doppler flow studies (if IUGR).

Complications

Painful Crisis

- Most frequent complication during pregnancy
- Incidence ranges from 27–50%
- Most frequent cause of hospital admission
- Avoidance of precipitants, such as a cold environment, excessive exercise, dehydration and stress is important
- Pain management
  - Mild pain—paracetamol
  - Mild to moderate pain—NSAIDs (only in 2nd trimester)
  - Moderate pain—Weak opioids
  - Severe pain—Stronger opiates (morphine) by oral, subcutaneous, IM or IV route
  - Pethidine to be avoided.

Prognosis

- About 90% of patients survive to age 20, and close to 50% survive beyond the fifth decade
- Acute splenic sequestration has a peak incidence between 6 months and 3 years and can be rapid in onset → death
- Most common cause of mortality → sepsis and acute chest syndrome
- Chronic transfusion therapy (repeated B.T.) required in severely ill-patients

Acute Chest Syndrome

- 2nd most common complication
- Reported in 7–20% of pregnancies
- Respiratory symptoms—tachypnea, chest pain, cough, dyspnea
- Management:
  - IV antibiotics; Hydration; Oxygen
  - Blood transfusion
  - Ventilatory support—if severe hypoxia.

Acute Stroke

- Is an emergency
- Urgent exchange transfusion.

Acute Anemia

- Isolate the woman (may be attributed to erythrovirus)
- It may be due to malaria or splenic sequestration
- Reticulocyte count
- Blood transfusion
- With erythrovirus, there is a risk of vertical transmission to the fetus, leading to hydrops. Therefore, careful fetal monitoring is necessary.

Medical Management of Tubal Ectopic Pregnancy

Tania G Singh

PRESENTATION

- Most common gestational age → 6–10 weeks
- Classic triad of ectopic
  - Abdominal pain; Vaginal bleeding; Adnexal mass.

PHYSICAL EXAMINATION

- Abdominal tenderness (97.3%)
- Adnexal tenderness (98%)
- Amenorrhea with vaginal spotting/bleeding (60–80%)
- Tachycardia or orthostatic changes
- Cervical motion tenderness → in 3/4th of patients but may be present prior to rupture
- Uterine tenderness (from blood irritating the peritoneal surfaces)
- A palpable mass
- Rebound tenderness or peritoneal signs
- Pallor; Abdominal distension
- Enlarged uterus; Shock/collapse.

DIAGNOSIS

Ultrasonography

Transabdominal Scan

- Identification of products of conception in fallopian tubes is difficult
- Intrauterine pregnancy not recognized until 5-6 menstrual weeks or 28 days after timed ovulation
- Corpus luteum cysts and matted bowel can mimic tubal pregnancy
- Indeterminate sac
  - Less than 1cm → TAS
  - 0.6 cm → TVS (sensitivity 20–80%).

Transvaginal

Look for the following:
- 1st USG sign of intrauterine pregnancy → gestation sac "double decidual sign" (double echogenic rings around the sac → eccentrically placed in uterus more than or equal to 1–3 mm in size) at 4.5–5 weeks

---

- 25–30% patients will not have vaginal bleeding
- 10% will have palpable adnexal mass
- ≈ 10% have negative pelvic examination
- Profuse vaginal bleeding is suggestive of incomplete abortion rather than ectopic
- Abdominal pain + vaginal bleeding → 39%
- Abdominal pain + vaginal bleeding + other risk factors → 54%

Even if the classic triad is present, still rule out the following possibilities:
- Implantation bleeding
- Acute appendicitis
- Miscarriage
- Ovarian torsion
- PID
- Ruptured corpus luteal cyst or follicle or chocolate cyst
- Tubo-ovarian abscess
- Urinary calculi

Other reported symptoms:
- ❧ Breast tenderness
- ❧ Gastrointestinal symptoms
- ❧ Dizziness, fainting or syncope
- ❧ Shoulder tip pain (secondary to diaphragmatic irritation)
- ❧ Urinary symptoms
- ❧ Passage of tissue
- ❧ Rectal pressure or pain on defecation

- ❧ β hCG is a glycoprotein hormone that contains both an alpha and a beta subunit
- ❧ Levels begin to ascend in a curvilinear fashion early in pregnancy and continue until they reach plateau at ≈ 9–11 weeks
- ❧ The plateau lasts for only a few days and thereafter β-hCG levels begin to decline at 20 weeks
- ❧ In the absence of a reliable LMP, hCG level is instrumental
- ❧ Ideally, β-hCG levels should increase by 53–63% within 48 hours in normal pregnancy
- ❧ If β-hCG levels increase by <53% during a 48-hour period, there is almost always a nonviable pregnancy associated, be it intra- or extrauterine

Discriminatory zone is defined as the level of β hCG at which an intrauterine pregnancy should be visualized
- ❧ With TAS → 6500 mIU/ mL
- ❧ With TVS → 1500 – 2500 mIU/mL
- ❧ Above these levels, if it is not visualized, it is either an ectopic or an intrauterine nonviable pregnancy

- Intrauterine gestation at 5.5 menstrual weeks → 1 week after missed periods → 100% accuracy
- Yolk sac → at 5–6 weeks and remain until about 10 weeks
- Embryo (fetal pole) and cardiac activity → 5.5–6 weeks
- Look for tubes and adnexa (separate from ovary) to evaluate for heterotopic pregnancy as it is common after IVF
- Fluid in cul-de-sac
- Adnexal masses cannot be seen when they are small or when obscured by bowel.

β-hCG (Human Chorionic Gonadotropin)

Following possible situations:
- β-hCG level has reached DZ and no intrauterine pregnancy
  - Highly suspicious of ectopic → (exception: multiple gestation).
- β-hCG> DZ and no definite USG diagnosis
  - It can be either dead fetus or ectopic
  - Do D and C—if chorionic villi are absent, treat as ectopic
  - Chorionic villi present—No further Rx.
- β-hCG< DZ (patient stable)
  - Serial β-hCG + repeat TVS (at 2–3 days interval).

Medical Management

Methotrexate (MTX)
- Medical treatment of choice currently
- It destroys the ectopic pregnancy tissue and allows the body to reabsorb the latter
- Immunosuppressive drug (folinic acid antagonist)
- Metabolism—binds to the catalytic site of enzyme dihydrofolate reductase; inhibits synthesis of purines and pyramidines (thymidylate, serine and methionine), disrupting synthesis of DNA, RNA and cell replication eventually leading to cell death
- Most widely used → single dose ($50 \, mg/m^2$)
- Can be given as outpatient therapy → cost saving
- Failure:
  - When β-hCG levels plateaus OR
  - Level increases OR
  - There is tubal rupture (which can even occur in face of declining β-hCG levels).

Contraindications

Absolute
- Active intra-abdominal hemorrhage
- Breastfeeding; immunodeficiency
- Liver/renal/severe pulmonary disease
- Alcoholism; pre-existing blood dyscrasias
- Peptic ulcer disease; known sensitivity to methotrexate.

Relative
- Gestational sac lower than 3.5–4 cm
- High initial hCG more than 5000 mIU/mL
- Presence of cardiac activity.

Indications

Absolute

- Hemodynamically stable without active bleeding or signs of hemoperitoneum
- Patient desires future fertility
- Nonlaparoscopic diagnosis
- Patient compliant/reliable
- Administration of general anesthesia poses risk
- Patient has no contraindication to methotrexate.

Relative

- Period of gestation less than 6 weeks
- Unruptured mass smaller than or equal to 3.5 cm at greatest dimension
- No fetal cardiac activity
- β-hCG limit does not exceed a predetermined value, i.e. β-hCG less than 5,000 mIU/mL and only in very few cases upto 15,000 mIU/mL.

METHOTREXATE THERAPY

Protocols

Single Dose (without Folinic Acid)

- The term 'single dose' is actually a misnomer. While the term single describes the number of MTX injections, the regimen includes provision for additional doses when response is inadequate
- Candidates
    - Women with serum β-hCG concentrations less than 1500 mIU/mL, a single-dose MTX regimen ($50 \, mg/m^2$ or 1 mg/kg IM) can be considered.
- Dose
    - 50 mg/sq. mt of body surface methotrexate IM on Day 1.
- Lab values:
    - LFT/CBC/RFT (mainly creatinine) on Day 0
    - β-hCG on Day 0, 1, 4 and 7.
- Repeat dose on Day 7, if β hCG does not decrease by 15% between day 4 and 7
- Follow-up:
    - β-hCG level weekly and continue regimen until no longer detected
    - If difference between day 4 and 7 more than 15% → repeat weekly until undetectable
    - If difference less than 15% → repeat methotrexate dose and begin new Day 1
    - If cardiac activity is present by Day 7 → repeat methotrexate dose, begin new Day 1
    - If β-hCG levels are not decreased and fetal cardiac activity persists after 3 doses of methotrexate → surgical management.

Fixed Multiple Dose (Alternated with Folinic Acid – Leucovorin)

- Candidates
    - Hemodynamically stable; Unruptured tubal ectopic
    - No signs of active bleeding
    - Serum β-hCG concentrations less than 3000 mIU/mL.
- Dose: Alternate every other day, 1 mg/kg methotrexate IM (Day 1, 3, 5, 7) and 0.1 mg/kg leucovorin IM (Day 2, 4, 6 and 8)

'Phantom hCG' is a positive blood pregnancy test without being pregnant but a negative urine test. Following steps are recommended when phantom hCG is found:

- Measure urinary hCG
- Remeasure the hCG concentration using a different method
- Add normal mouse serum or other animal serum to the assay, test for anti-hCG antibodies
- Measure hCG concentrations after several days or weeks

Patient Selection

- No significant pain
- Unruptured ectopic with no cardiac activity
- Adnexal mass <35 mm
- β-hCG levels <1500 mIU/mL (even women up to 5000 IU/lit can be offered MTX therapy, if all other criterias are fulfilled)
- No intrauterine pregnancy (confirmed on ultrasound)
- Candidate reliable and willing for follow-up
- ABO Rh should be checked

Candidates not for MTX

- Liver disease: transaminase level >2 times normal
- Renal disease: creatinine >1.5 gm/dL (133 µmol/l)
- Immune compromise:
    - WBCs <1500/mm³ (1.5 x 10⁹ /lit)
    - Platelets <1 lakh/ mm³
- Significant pulmonary disease (CXR should be done because of the risk of interstitial pneumonitis in these patients)

> ✎ Leucovorin is an antagonist to MTX that can help reduce other prohibitive side effects, particularly when higher doses of MTX are used

> ✎ In both treatment protocols, once hCG levels have met the criteria for initial decline, hCG levels are followed serially at weekly intervals to ensure that concentrations decline steadily and become undetectable
> ✎ hCG levels should decline to <5 mIU/mL before stopping treatment

Predictors of MTX Treatment Failure

> ✎ Presence of fetal cardiac activity
> ✎ Gestational mass >4 cm
> ✎ hCG >5000 mIU/mL
> ✎ Free blood in peritoneal cavity
> ✎ Rapidly increasing hCG concentrations before initiation of MTX treatment (>50% rise in 48 hours)
> ✎ Continued rapid increase in hCG levels during treatment

Congenital Anamolies Associated with MTX

CNS abnormalities
> ✎ Spina bifida; Hydrocephaly; Anencephaly; Mental retardation

Skeletal abnormalities
> ✎ Synostosis of lambdoid sutures
> ✎ Partial or absent ossification of bones
> ✎ Micrognathia; Cleft lip or palate
> ✎ Broad depressed nasal bone; Hypertelorism
> ✎ Short limbs; Syndactyly; Absent digits; Clubfoot

Dextrocardia and IUGR

- Lab values:
  - LFT/CBC/RFT on Day 0
  - β-hCG on Day 0,1, 3, 5 and 7 (i.e. every 48 hours) until levels decrease by 15%.
- Repeat regimen (for up to 4 doses of each), if β-hCG level does not decrease by 15% with each measurement (in 48 hours)
- Follow-up
  - β-hCG level weekly and continue regimen until no longer detected
  - Mean time to resolution of ectopic pregnancy is 2–3 weeks after MTX therapy but can take 6–8 weeks, especially if pretreatment levels were high.

Effects Related to Drug

- Liver involvement (12%); Nausea, vomiting
- Conjunctivitis; Stomatitis; Gastric distress (gastroenteritis 1%)
- Dizziness/fever; Pneumonitis (drug-induced)
- Reversible alopecia (rare); Severe neutropenia (rare)
- Photosensitivity; Bone marrow depression
- A proportion of women need to be admitted for observation and assessment by TVS while on Methotraxate treatment – Why?
  - To differentiate so called 'separation pain' due to tubal abortion from pain due to tubal rupture
  - Separation pain usually develops between day 3 and 7 after treatment begins and subsides within 4–12 hours after onset
  - In 65-75% cases, increasing pain begins several days after therapy
  - Relieved by non narcotic analgesics
  - If not relieved→ check vitals and hematocrit and if ruptured, surgery becomes mandatory.

Effects Related to Treatment

- Increased abdominal pain
- Increase in β-hCG levels from day 1 to day 4
- Increase in abdominal girth
- Vaginal bleeding or spotting (rare, due to thrombocytopenia, occurring within 2 weeks of injection).

Advice to Patients on Methotrexate Therapy

- Prohibition during treatment
  - Sexual intercourse; alcohol
  - NSAIDs lethal interactions; Aspirin
- Maintain ample fluid intake
- Limit sun exposure during treatment, as methotrexate can cause sensitivity to sunlight and sunburn or dermatitis may occur
- Reliable contraception for 3–6 months after MTX because of possible teratogenic risk (minimum 3 months)
- Avoid gas forming foods as they may cause pain

- Avoid pelvic examinations and ultrasound during surveillance of MTX therapy
- Pregnancy occurring before 3 months is not an indication for termination unless USG indicates birth defects
- Although half-life of MTX is 8–15 hours, it's presence in the liver has been reported to last up to 116 days after exposure
- Rh negative woman with confirmed or suspected ectopic should receive anti-D.

Future Fertility and Risk of Recurrence

- $\approx$ 30% will have difficulty conceiving
- $\approx$ 77% $\rightarrow$ overall conception rate REGARDLESS of mode of management
- 5–20% $\rightarrow$ risk of recurrence
- 32% $\rightarrow$ risk with 2 consecutive ectopic pregnancies

Chapter 24

Abortions

Tania G Singh

Expulsion of the fetus from uterus either spontaneously or by induction before the period of viability, i.e. 22 weeks.

TYPES

- Missed abortion; Threatened abortion; Inevitable abortion
- Incomplete abortion and complete abortion.

Missed Abortion

- Embryonic or fetal demise
- Products of conception are dead and retained inside uterine cavity
- Also called 'silent miscarriage'
- No signs and symptoms of abortion
- Regressing symptoms of pregnancy (breast changes, nausea/vomiting).

History

- Amenorrhea and brownish vaginal discharge.

Diagnosis

- Vitals stable
- There is a decrease in uterine size, after considerable time has elapsed (minimum 2 weeks)
- FHS absent when supposed to be heard
- Cervix—uneffaced, os closed; feels firm
- No bleeding
- UPT becomes absent.

Complications (Though Rare)

- DIC → they are autolyzed→ thromboplastin released → initiate the coagulation mechanism
- Infection → any dead tissue is a nidus for infection → sepsis.

Management

- Admission
- Investigations: Hemoglobin; Urine routine; Blood group; Coagulation profile
- Termination:
  - 1st trimester
    - Surgical (suction evacuation or D and C)

Threatened abortion, Inevitable abortion, Incomplete abortion and Complete abortion are spectrum of the same process

Sometimes in 1st trimester, missed abortion proceeds to form a blood mole where the fetus and placenta are surrounded by clotted blood within the capsular decidua. If a blood mole is retained in the uterus for some months, the fluid becomes absorbed and the fleshy hard mass which remains is called a 'Carneous mole'

USG Features of Missed Abortion

- Embryonic pole ≥5 mm without fetal cardiac activity OR
- Embryonic pole <5 mm and no interval growth over one week

Whatever be the measurements on ultrasonography, it is preferable to do a repeat scan before labeling it as missed abortion

- – Medical—800 mcg misoprostol single dose per vaginally preferably
- – Can be given orally, if patient hesitant for vaginal route
- – If bleeding does not start after 24 hours—report back
- – Do not give mifepristone.
- 2nd trimester → medical, using prostaglandins
- Investigate the cause of abortion.

Threatened Abortion

- 'Warning signal'
- History of amenorrhea (<20 weeks)
- Vaginal bleeding → minimal/moderate
- Pain abdomen/backache → mild pain/cramping.

Diagnosis

- Vitals stable
- Per speculum: minimal bleeding/spotting through os present
- Uterine size corresponds to period of gestation
- Cervix uneffaced; Internal os closed.

Management

- Admission/ambulatory care
- Investigations: Hemoglobin; Urine routine; Blood group.

Advice on Discharge

- Bed rest; Coitus contraindicated
- Progesterone supplements → natural micronized progesterone
- Investigate and treat the cause
- May or may not miscarry.

Inevitable Abortion

- History of amenorrhea
- Vaginal bleeding—moderate → becomes severe at the time of expulsion
- Pain abdomen—moderate/severe.

Diagnosis

- Vitals stable
- General condition proportionate to visible blood loss
- P/S: Bleeding through os present
- P/V:
  - – Uterine size corresponds to period of gestation
  - – Uterus tender, firm
  - – Cervix effaced
  - – Internal os open
  - – Products of conception → felt at os.
- Miscarriage unavoidable.

Management

- Admission
- Investigations: Hemoglobin, Urine routine, Blood group and type
- Expedite the process of abortion

USG Features of Threatened Abortion

- Cardiac activity present
- Subchorionic hemorrhage may be present

Urine routine is a very important investigation in Threatened abortion

Threatened abortion is the only abortion which has expectant line of management

USG Features of Inevitable Abortion

- Products of conception visible
- Fetal cardiac activity may or may not be present

- 1st trimester: surgical
- 2nd trimester: medical.
- Investigate the cause.

Incomplete Abortion

Incomplete abortion is very important for here we can even lose the mother

- Most common
- History of amenorrhea
- Vaginal bleeding—moderate/severe
- Pain abdomen—moderate/severe
- History of having passed products of conception but not complete.

Diagnosis

USG Features of Incomplete Abortion

Irregular, heterogeneous and/or echogenic material along endometrial stripe or in cervical canal suggestive of retained products

- Vitals may be stable or patient is in hypovolemic shock
- P/S: Profuse bleeding through os present
- P/V:
  - Uterine size < period of gestation
  - Uterus tender, firm
  - Cervix—effaced; internal os partly closed
  - Products of conception felt at os
- Most likely to occur in 2nd trimester.

Management

- Admission
- Investigations: Hemoglobin, Blood group and type
- Resuscitation
- Investigate the cause
- Complete the process of abortion as fast as possible

USG Features of Complete Abortion

- Uterus empty
- Endometrial lining may be thickened
- Rule out any remaining bits (rare)

- Can be managed surgically or medically
- Medical: 600 μg misoprostol per vaginally (single dose)
- Repeat UPT after 3 weeks, if positive, report to exclude molar pregnancy or ectopic
- Surgical: If gestational age less than or equal to 13 weeks, vacuum aspiration (misoprostol 400 μg sublingually or 600 μg orally can be given before evacuation to speed up the process).

Complete Abortion

- History
- Amenorrhea (usually within first 8 weeks)
- Vaginal bleeding (moderate/severe)
- Pain abdomen (cramps)
- Expulsion of a fleshy mass/products of conception
- On examination:
  - Patient stable
  - Abdominal pain absent
  - Minimal spotting or no bleeding
  - Uterine size smaller than period of gestation
  - Feel of uterus—firm
  - Internal os closed.

Note: Anti-D to be given in all cases where deemed necessary

Management

- No further treatment required.

MEDICAL TERMINATION OF PREGNANCY

Regimen I

First 7 Weeks (49 days)

- Mifepristone 200 mg orally
- After 24–48 hours: Misoprostol (400 µg orally OR 800 µg sublingually OR 800 µg vaginally OR 800 µg by buccal route).

From 7 to 9 Weeks (49–63 days)

- Same as above except that oral route of misoprostol is CONTRAINDICATED

From 9 to 12 Weeks (63–84 days)

- Mifepristone 200 mg orally
- After 36–48 hours—Misoprostol (800 µg vaginally) followed by 200 µg misoprostol either vaginally or sublingually every 3 hours (a total of 4 doses).

From 12 to 24 Weeks

- Mifepristone 200 mg orally
- After 36–48 hours: Misoprostol (800 µg vaginally OR 400 µg orally) followed by 400 µg misoprostol either vaginally or sublingually every 3 hours (a total of 4 doses).

From 24 Weeks Onwards

- Dose of misoprostol should be reduced as the gestation advances, as the uterus becomes more and more responsive even to minor doses.

Regimen II

Till 12 Weeks

- 800 µg misoprostol vaginally OR sublingually followed by
- 800 µg misoprostol every 3 hourly (a total of 4 doses, i.e. for a total duration of 12 hours).

From 12 to 24 Weeks

- Misoprostol 400 µg vaginally OR sublingually every 3 hourly (a total of 5 doses).

From 24 Weeks Onwards

- Same as above.

Surgical Termination of Pregnancy

Up to 12 Weeks

- Vacuum aspiration
- Should not be followed by sharp curettage or D and C
- No need for cervical preparation but can be done as per situation.

From 12–24 Weeks

- Dilatation and evacuation—safest and most effective
- Cervical preparation becomes obligatory: misoprostol 400 µg
- Sublingually or vaginally 2–3 hours prior to the procedure.

Anembryonic Gestation

Pregnancy in which a gestational sac develops without development of any embryonic structures; previously referred to as an "empty sac" or "blighted ovum"

USG

- Gestational sac >13 mm without yolk sac OR
- 18 mm without embryonic pole OR
- Empty sac beyond 38 days' gestation and no interval growth over one week

Placenta Previa

Tania G Singh

JAUNIAUX AND CAMPBELL CLASSIFICATION

- Type I (Low lying): Lower margin within 5 cm of the cervical os
- Type II (Marginal placenta previa): Reaches up to the margin of os but does not cover it
- Type III (Incomplete or partial placenta previa): Placenta partially covers the os
- Type IV (Central or Total): Placenta covers the os completely.

On the basis of placental localization on the anterior or posterior wall:
- *Type A:* When placenta lies on the anterior wall
- *Type B:* When placenta lies on the posterior wall.

BLEEDING IS RECURRENT, CAUSELESS AND PAINLESS IN PLACENTA PREVIA. WHY?

Recurrent

- As lower uterine segment continues to grow in 3rd trimester, bleeding can occur again and again during it's growth. Now, this bleeding is controlled by
  - Thrombosis of open sinuses
  - Mechanical pressure by presenting part
  - Placental infarction.

Causeless

- As this is a natural phenomenon (i.e. growth of lower uterine segment in 3rd trimester) and placenta is inelastic with slower growth in later months whereas lower segment progressively dilates, the inelastic placenta is sheared off the wall of lower segment → opening up of uteroplacental vessels → bleeding episode.

Painless

- Because it is a physiological phenomenon
- Bleeding is almost always because of maternal bleed but trauma may become the cause of fetal bleed.

Clinical Suspicion

- The two classical presentations of placenta previa are:
  - As Antepartum hemorrhage OR
  - As fetal malpresentation in late pregnancy

- Of late, a third important presentation is added to this → diagnosis of asymptomatic placenta previa by routine ultrasound examination
- Bleeding after 20 weeks of gestation and usually before term
- There is often repeated episodes of bleeding
- Maternal vitals corresponds to the amount of bleed
- Uterus relaxed, soft, nontender
- FHS → almost always present
- High presenting part
- Head cannot be pushed down in pelvis, it's persistent displacement is highly indicative of placenta previa
- An abnormal lie
- Painless or provoked bleeding by sexual intercourse, irrespective of previous imaging results
- Painful only when labor accompanies
- Bleeding is bright red (indicative of fresh bleed) → because it occurs from separated uteroplacental sinuses close to cervical opening and escapes out immediately
- *Stallworthy's sign:* Drop the fetal head in the pelvic brim → FHS decreases → release the head → FHS normalizes.

> ✒ Women with a large placenta from twins or erythroblastosis are at higher risk
> ✒ Placental pathology (Velamentous insertion, succenturiate lobes, bipartite, i.e. bilobed placenta)

Warning Hemorrhage
> ✒ Occurs somewhere in mid pregnancy
> ✒ Mild fresh bleed
> ✒ Little amount
> ✒ Lasting for 4–5 days, stopping in a weeks' time
> ✒ Not causing damage to mother or fetus indicative of recurring bouts to come

Definitive Diagnosis

Transvaginal Scan (TVS)

- Considered gold standard
- Imaging is better
- Even safe in presence of bleeding
- Woman does not need a full bladder → avoids both maternal discomfort and distortion of the anatomy of lower uterine segment and cervix
- Though some argue that probe insertion could provoke bleeding but an answer to this is the insertion of probe to no more than 3 cms into the vagina will not come in contact with the cervix or lower uterine segment
- It is helpful in detection and confirmation, follow-up and planning route of delivery.

> **TVS** has a:
> ✒ Sensitivity of 87.5%
> ✒ Specificity of 98.8%
> ✒ Positive predictive value of 93.3%
> ✒ Negative predictive value of 97.6%

Detection and Confirmation of Placenta Previa

- If anamoly scan (at 18–22 weeks) shows low lying placenta → confirm by repeat scan
- In case of asymptomatic suspected minor previa—TVS at 36 weeks
- If placenta is posterior or a case of previous LSCS—repeat scan in 3rd trimester
- In case of asymptomatic suspected major previa—TVS at 32 weeks (for confirmation and planning of management).

Transabdominal Scan (TAS)
Associated with high false positives. What leads to it?
> ✒ Presence of myometrial contraction: contraction may mimic a placenta in appearance or may displace the placental edge low down
> ✒ Overdistended bladder: approximates anterior and posterior uterine walls, giving false impression of previa
> ✒ Poor visualization of posterior placenta
> ✒ Fetal head can interfere with visualization of lower segment

Follow-up

- When placental edge overlaps or exactly reaches the internal os (between 18–24 weeks) → repeat TVS in the 3rd trimester
- If it is between 20 mm away from internal os and 20 mm overlap after 26 weeks → repeat USG at regular intervals
- If more than 20 mm at any time in 3rd trimester → there are ↑chances of cesarean section.

Planning Route of Delivery (After 35 Weeks)

- Depends upon the distance of placental edge from internal os

- Obesity also interferes with accuracy
- Phenomenon of placental migration: development of lower uterine segment in later part of pregnancy (10 fold growth of lower uterine segment compared to placenta)

USG Terminology

- When placental edge does not reach internal os→ designated as "mms" away from internal os
- When placental edge overlaps internal os→ distance is given as "mms of overlap"
- When placental edge exactly reaches internal os→ measurement given as "0 mms"

Cases in which Placenta is Less Likely to Migrate

- When it is posterior
- When it is thicker
- Lower edge is <2 cm from os
- When there is a history of previous cesarean section

- If more than 20 mm away from internal os—vaginal route opted (success rate 63–100%)
- If between 0 and 20 mm away from internal os—vaginal delivery may occur (40–90% chances of C. section)
- If between 0 and <20 mm degree of overlap—Indication of cesarean section
- It is recommended to defer elective cesarean section to 38 weeks to decrease neonatal morbidity
- If placental edge is between 20–35 mm away from os → Anticipate PPH.

Chapter 26

Placental Invasion (Accreta, Increta, Percreta)

Tania G Singh

RISK FACTORS

- Placenta previa with or without previous uterine surgery
- Rising cesarean section rates
- Previous myomectomy
- Previous uterine curettage
- Evacuations associated with trauma or infection
- Asherman's syndrome
- Submucous fibroids
- Maternal age more than 35 years
- Previous trophoblastic disease.

Imaging Modalities in Placenta Accreta, Increta or Percreta

Grayscale Ultrasound

- Diagnostic criteria: When more than or equal to 1 of the following situations is present
  - Placental lacunae
  - Obliteration of clear space
  - Interruption of bladder border
  - Myometrium of less than 1 mm.

2D Color Doppler

- Sensitivity → 82–100%
- Specificity → 92–97%
- Grayscale imaging is found to be equally good.

3D Power Doppler

- Additional information provided by power Doppler
  - Exact site; Extent of involvement
  - Depth of invasion by aberrant vessels over the uterine serosa-bladder junctional region.

MRI

- MRI is performed when the results of ultrasound are inconclusive
- The most common site for placenta accreta is anterior at the lower uterine segment
- When the abnormality is located in the posterior wall or in cases of fundal accreta or when the patient is obese, the resolution will be poor. It is here MRI proves to be a better modality

Definition

- Placenta accreta is typified by chorionic villi on the myometrial surface
- Placenta increta by villus infiltration into the myometrium
- Percreta by infiltration through the entire myometrium to breach the serosa and beyond

Complications of Placenta Percreta

- High maternal mortality ($\approx 10\%$)
- Massive hemorrhage
- Disseminated intravascular coagulation
- Hysterectomy
- Bladder and ureteric trauma
- Acute respiratory distress syndrome
- Acute tubular necrosis
- They may present as acute abdomen and shock from
  - Ruptured uterus
  - Antepartum hemorrhage
  - Hematuria, if bladder is involved
  - As a complication in the third stage of labor

- Disadvantage: Very high cost of the machine and as a result testing is costlier, making it nearly-impossible to use it in all the cases.

RISKS

Massive and/or Repeated Hemorrhage (Discussed Elsewhere)

Preterm Delivery

Hospitalization:
- Not recommended for placenta previa
- Safety precautions should be taken at home (someone should be available to get the patient to hospital in case of emergency – bleeding, contractions, even minor suprapubic pain)
- Not to stay too far from the hospital
- Cervical cerclage: No recommendations
- Tocolysis
  - For prophylaxis: No use
  - When presents with bleeding: Though studies have shown a positive response when 10 mg of ritodrine every 6 hours by intramuscular injections for 7 days was used. There was a prolongation of pregnancy by 2–3 weeks with an increase in birth weight but side effects have to be kept in mind. Each case needs to be individualized.

Thromboembolism

For patients admitted to hospital for a longer time, following precautions should be taken:
- Ambulation
- Adequate hydration
- Thromboembolic stockings
- Anticoagulants—not recommended.

Uterine Perforation

Chapter 27

Previous LSCS

Tania G Singh

Vaginal Birth after Cesarean section can be offered to the following:

- Gestational age: 37–40 weeks
- Adequate pelvis
- Previous C.S. for nonreassuring induction
  - Breech; fetal distress; maternal hemorrhage
- Prior lower segment cesarean section (transverse)
- Vertex presentation
- Patient's consent
- Facility to carry out immediate LSCS
- Women with two previous low transverse scars, who wish to attempt VBAC can also be considered if they had a vaginal delivery in the past
- Blood transfusion facilities are available.

Predictors for VBAC Success or Failure

Increased Chance of Success

- Maternal age less than 40 years
- Adequate pelvis
- Prior vaginal delivery
- Prior VBAC
- Spontaneous labor
- Nonrecurrent indication
- Favorable cervix (Bishop's score >6).

Reduced Chances of Success

- Gestational age more than 40 weeks
- Increased number of cesarean sections
- Estimated fetal weight more than 4 kg
- Previous C.S. requiring induction/augmentation of labor
- Previous postpartum wound infection
- Maternal obesity (BMI >30)
- Diabetes milletus
- Multiple gestation
- Induction of labor
- Recurring indication (CPD/failed 2nd stage)
- Short maternal stature
- Interval less than 19 months after last delivery
- No previous VBAC
- Previous preterm C.S.
- No epidural anesthesia

Success rate of planned VBAC: 60–82%

Success rate of VBAC, if patient has had a vaginal delivery before: 87–90%

Hospital Facilities While Conducting VBAC

- Access to an emergency CS
- Continuous intrapartum monitoring
- Advanced neonatal resuscitation
- On site blood transfusion
- Staff experienced in advanced analgesic techniques

Contraindications to VBAC

- Previous classical or inverted T-shaped or J-shaped uterine incisions
- Previous uterine surgery (myomectomy) or prior low vertical incision
- Previous extensive transfundal uterine surgery
- Previous history of uterine rupture
- Contracted pelvis
- Medical or obstetric complications that precludes vaginal birth
  - Placenta previa
  - Elderly patient

Contd...

Contd...

- – Long standing secondary infertility
- – Previous perinatal deaths
- Two prior uterine scars with no vaginal delivery
- Inability to perform emergency LSCS
- Previous significant sepsis post cesarean section

Placental localization over the site of previous scar is one of the major causes making the scar weak resulting in uterine rupture

If placenta is low lying and anterior → placenta accreta should be sought on USG with color Doppler

Trial of labor → not indicated in these patients

Role of Induction of Labor in Trial of VBAC

- Induction of labor is not a contraindication but chances of success are less
- Oxytocin is safer than prostaglandins
- Risk of uterine rupture ↑↑ when prostaglandins were followed by oxytocin (sequential use)
- Misoprostol should NOT be used [even dinoprostone (E$_2$) is not recommended] in 3rd trimester inductions in such cases

- Advanced maternal age
- Female child.

Benefits of Vaginal Delivery over Repeat Cesarean Section

- Shorter hospital stay
- Early ambulation and resumption to work
- Economical
- Less chance of bleeding
- No contamination of peritoneal cavity
- No pulmonary/wound complications
- Less infection
- Damage to internal organs and major vessels avoided
- Scar-related remote complications are avoided:
    - Keloid; Hypertrophy; Incisional hernia
    - Adhesions; Scar endometriosis.
- Successful VBAC → subsequent obstetric career improves.

Risks of Failed VBAC

- Uterine rupture with increased perinatal mortality
- Hysterectomy
- Operative injury
- Postoperative infection
- Need for blood transfusion
- Hypoxic ischemic encephalopathy in newborn.

Risks for Infant in Elective Repeat Cesarean Section

- Transient tachypnea
- RDS
- Hyperbilirubinemia
- Increased neonatal lacerations
- Iatrogenic prematurity (if dates not reliable).

Risks for Infant in VBAC

- Cord blood gas pH lower than 7
- 5-minute apgar score lower than 7
- Sepsis
- Hypoxic ischemic encephalopathy.

Unknown Scar (No Previous Records Available)

- Always elicit the history
- Under which circumstances, cesarean section was done
- Majority of unknown scars will be lower segment transverse incisions (92%)
- Trial of induction of labor is not contraindicated in patients with an unknown scar, unless there is a high clinical suspicion of a previous classical incision.

Antenatal Management in Women Attempting VBAC

- It is a high-risk pregnancy, requiring special ANCs

- Obtain records or information regarding previous cesarean, it's indication, previous uterine scar
- Correct dating of pregnancy is essential, from
    - History; clinical examination; USG.
- Early detection of other obstetric (esp. placenta previa, PIH, etc.) and medical complications (anemia, etc.)
- All routine investigations to be done
- If VBAC is to be considered, rule out the following:
    - Malpresentations
    - Multiple pregnancy
    - Macrosomia.
- Ultrasound for
    - Fetal maturity especially when LMP is not certain
    - Fetal weight
    - Placental localization
    - Scar integrity assessment.
- In 3rd trimester—at every visit, enquire about:
    - Fetal movements
    - Suprapubic pain
    - Palpate for scar tenderness
    - Vaginal bleeding.
- Pelvic assessment at 37 weeks and again in early labor
- Proper counseling for risks and benefits
    - Patients staying far→ admit at 38 weeks
    - Spontaneous labor has high success rates
    - Trial of labor, should not be attempted if hemoglobin is lower than or equal to 9 gm% or blood is not arranged (correction of anemia is very important)
    - Induction of labor (IOL) → not a contraindication but the risks should be explained
    - Risk of uterine rupture is increased 2–3 folds
    - Likelihood of repeat cesarean section with IOL—1.5-fold
    - Misoprostol should not be used in 3rd trimester for cervical ripening or labor induction in cases of previous LSCS.
- Written and informed consent (explaining all risks and benefits)
- Proper counseling and consent for sterilization (if appropriate at that time).

Assessment of Scar Integrity Antenatally

- TVS is better than TAS
- A scar 'defect' or 'niche' is defined by the presence of a wedge-shaped cystic or hypoechogenic area in the anterior wall within the myometrium of the LUS, at the site of a previous CS
    - In cases of previous elective CS, the scar will appear halfway between the uterovesical fold and the internal cervical os
    - In cases following emergency CS → the scar could well be below, or at the level of the os.
- Various studies have concluded that myometrial scar tissue takes at least 3 months to form and that complete involution and recovery of the zonal anatomy is not achieved until 6 months later
- No ideal cut-off value can yet be recommended which can describe a strong or a weak scar.

Risks to be Included in Consent

- Uterine rupture
- Shock
- Need for blood transfusion
- Operative delivery →↑ chances of surgical injury
- In adverse circumstances, hysterectomy
- Increased fetal morbidity and in few cases mortality
- Increased rate of admission to NICU
- Long separation of mother and baby
- Delayed resumption of breastfeeding
- Risk of postoperative infection
- Longer hospital stay

Benefits to be Included in Consent

- Overall success rates are high
- Shorter hospital stay
- Less postpartum pain
- Less postpartum infections
- Fewer chances of blood transfusions
- Early initiation of breastfeeding
- Reduced chances of respiratory problems requiring admission to NICU
- Less chances of placenta previa accreta in subsequent pregnancy

Chapter 28

Twin Pregnancy (Antenatal Management)

Tania G Singh

Superfetation

- Separate ovulation
- By separate act of coitus
- During different menstrual periods
- Unproven in humans
- Fetuses with markedly different gestational ages

Superfecundation

- Fertilization during same menstrual cycle
- By different act of coitus
- Not necessarily by sperms from same male

PREPREGNANCY (FOR ANY WOMAN TRYING CONCEPTION)

- Counseling of women undergoing ART
- Ideal BMI—19.6–26.0 kg/mt^2
- Laboratory testing:
  - CBC; Urinalysis; ABO Rh
  - VDRL; HIV; HbsAg
  - Rubella antibody titer
  - FBS; Thyroid profile.
- Folate-rich foods—fortified grains, spinach, lentils, chick peas, asparagus, broccoli, peas, Brusselssprouts, corn, and oranges
- A multivitamin with folic acid (0.4–1.0 mg) × 2–3 months before conception
- Vitamin D intake of minimum 5 µg/day for nonpregnant women with limited exposure to sunlight (i.e. those whose hands and face are exposed to the open air for less than 15 min/day) and 10 µg/day for pregnant women
- Avoid exposure to cat feces, raw/undercooked meats and unpasteurized milk
- Smoking and alcohol cessation
- Consumption of vitamin A to less than 3000 µg/day.

ANTENATAL

First Trimester

- Documentation of chorionicity and amnionicity
- Nuchal translucency
- Treatment of exaggerated symptoms
- Folic acid—1 mg/day (1000 mcg/day)
- Diet—300 kcal more than in singletons
- Increased proteins/vitamins/minerals/fiber-rich diet
- Routine investigations (mentioned above)
- Multifetal pregnancy reduction—if required.

Second Trimester

- Iron and calcium supplementation (iron 100 mg/day) in early 2nd trimester
- Triple screen test at 16 weeks
- Tetanus toxoid injection (2 doses)
- Anamoly scan at 18–22 weeks
- If fetal cardiac abnormality is detected, fetal echocardiography at 24 weeks

- Rule out conjoined twins
- OGTT at 24 weeks
- Increased antenatal visits from mid-pregnancy (every 2 weeks) for early detection of the following:
    - Anemia (check hemoglobin minimum 4 times, once in each trimester and then before labor)
    - Pre eclampsia (BP, weight measurement and urine analysis at each visit after mid-pregnancy)
    - Preterm labor.
- Bed rest
- In case of Rh negative pregnancy, consider anti-D at 28 weeks followed by serial ICT measurements
- Careful monitoring throughout antenatal period
- In cases of one fetal death, check well-being of second twin and look for coagulopathy (in case of monochorionic twins)
- If hydramnios develops—therapeutic amniocentesis.

Third Trimester

- Serial USG (every 3–4 weeks but not more than 5 weeks) for growth discordance, to assess liquor, to exclude placenta previa
- Administration of 2 doses of betamethasone 12 mg IM, 24 hours apart in cases of threatened preterm or if delivery is planned before 34 weeks
- Surveillance for hypertensive disorders
- Fetal surveillance
- Discuss with the couple, the mode of delivery and methods of analgesia present.

Fetal Complications

- Vanishing twin syndrome
    - Arrest of development
    - Subsequent resorption of fetus in 1st trimester.
- Malformations—structural defects
- Chromosomal anamolies
- Complications based on chorionicity
- Preterm labor
    - More frequent ANCs (very high-risk)
    - Serial evaluation of cervix
    - Less than 34 weeks → (steroids and tocolytics together to be used with caution as these woman are at increased risk of pulmonary edema).
- PPROM
    - Rupture occurs in presenting sac
    - Per speculum → swab taken for C/S
    - Per vaginum → avoided
    - Look for—infection, abruption, fetal death
    - Give antibiotics and steroids
    - Conservative treatment till 34 weeks → approach individualized.
- IUGR
    - Rate of growth in twins = same as singleton (till 32 weeks) followed by decrease in growth velocity
    - Rate of growth in triplets = same as singleton till 28 weeks
    - In last few weeks → competition for nutrients among fetuses.

Bed Rest

In left lateral position for minimum of 2 hours in morning or afternoon and minimum 10 hours at night, starting at 22 weeks gestation until 34 weeks

Maternal Complications

- Anemia (iron deficiency and folic acid deficiency)
- Pressure symptoms:
    - Edema of legs
    - Shortness of breath
    - Increased varicose veins
- Hyperemesis
- Gestational hypertension and pre eclampsia
- HELLP syndrome/ placental abruption
- Placenta previa
- Polyhydramnios

COMPLICATIONS BASED ON CHORIONICITY

Dichorionic Diamniotic

There are two main complications:

- Discordant growth
- Intrauterine fetal death.

Discordant Growth

- Different definitions/criteria for discordance have been provided:
    - $\dfrac{\text{EFW larger twin} - \text{EFW smaller twin}}{\text{EFW largest twin}} \times 100\%$
        - Intertwin birth weight discordance of more than 20% with reference to weight of larger twin
        - EFW is based on BPD and AC or AC and FL.
    - Difference in AC >20 mm OR
    - Difference in BPD >8 mm
    - Mean intertwin birth weight difference ≈ 10%.
- Causes
    - Twin to twin transfusion syndrome (most common → placental vascular anastomosis)
    - IUGR
    - Structural anamolies occurring in one fetus only
    - Due to different genetic growth potential
    - One placenta with suboptimal implantation.

Intrauterine Death of One Fetus

- When the demise occurs early in pregnancy, the prognosis for the surviving fetus is excellent
- Determining factors: Cause of IUD and gestational age
- As placentas are separate, there is no worry of damage to surviving twin due to hypotensive or embolic phenomena, as in case of monochorionic pregnancy
- Risk is related to preterm labor
- Maternal DIC—rare
- Offer uncomplicated dichorionic twin pregnancies elective birth from 37 weeks onwards
- Risk → negligible in DC twins
- Perform: NST; BPP; give corticosteroids (between 24–34 weeks, if delivery anticipated in 7 days).

MONOCHORIONIC DIAMNIOTIC

Twin to Twin Transfusion Syndrome (TTTS)

- Affects approximately 15% of these pregnancies
- Perinatal mortality is up to 80% if the syndrome is left untreated
- Results from abnormal shunting of blood between the circulations of the unborn twins through anastomoses of the vessels of the shared placenta
- USG diagnosis.

Features of Recipient Twin

- Excessive fluid (hydramnios)
- Normal structure

Superficial Anastomosis
- Bidirectional
- Artery to artery anastomosis
- Vein to vein anastomosis

Deep Anastomosis
- Unidirectional
- Artery to vein anastomosis
- Arterial blood of 1 twin drains into venous system of the other

- Usually, appropriately grown for gestational age
- Has a large distended bladder, visceromegaly
- May, if severely compromised, show tricuspid regurgitation or hydrops fetalis or heart failure
- Polycythemic
- Becomes plethoric
- Neurological sequelae
- Deepest vertical pocket less than 2 mm.

Features of Donor Twin

- Little or no fluid (oligohydramnios) or anhydramnios (the donor twin gets stuck against the wall of the uterus)
- This may lead to renal failure
- Separating membrane completely covering this fetus
- Normal structure
- Frequently, severely growth restricted as it transfuses blood to the recipient twin → pulmonary hypoplasia
- Shows abnormal umbilical artery Doppler waveforms
- The bladder becomes nonvisible
- Anemic, becomes pale
- Neurological sequelae.

Intrauterine Fetal Death

- 25% risk of death
- 25% risk of neurological handicap and multiorgan injury
- Multiple foci of encephalomalacia and ischemic changes in
    - Spleen; Kidney; GIT; Skin; Brain.
- (May be) Because of embolization of thromboplastin material released from dead fetus, which goes to surviving twin through placental anastomosis
             OR
- (May be) That acute bleeding from surviving to dead fetus occurs due to decreased pressure in dead twin which leads to transient severe hypotension and ischemic damage in vital organs of surviving fetus
- Supported by occurrence of sudden anemia in surviving twin with normal coagulation profile after death of one fetus.

Treatment

- Depends on gestational age, chorionicity and condition of surviving fetus
- If it is 1st trimester loss → no harm to surviving fetus
- If it is 2nd or 3rd trimester loss → outcome depends on chorionicity
    - Previable: Termination
    - Viable: Immediate delivery doesn't appear to change the outcome as injury could have occurred at time of demise
- There may be transient increase in FDPs with hypofibrinogenemia, risk of clinically significant maternal coagulopathy → almost nil
- Baseline maternal coagulation profile recommended.

Twin Reversed Arterial Perfusion Syndrome (TRAP)

- Also known as acardiac twinning
- Have a 90% risk of preterm birth and a 30% risk of congestive heart failure in the normal twin (also called pump twin)

Diagnosis of TRAP
- As early as 10 weeks
- Arterial blood flows towards rather than away from affected fetus (reversal of blood flow within the abnormal fetus) on color Doppler → definitive diagnosis
- Serial USG:
  - Grossly malformed fetus with amorphous cephalic pole
  - Poor definition of trunk and extremities (due to severe hypoxia)
  - Absence of cardiac pulsations
- Fetal hemodynamic function should be assessed by fetal echocardiography; hydrops in the pump twin being a poor prognostic feature

Management of TRAP
Interruption of vascular communication
- Ultrasound-guided
- Needle used: 14 gauge radio ablation needle
- Cauterization of umbilical vessels and termination of blood flow to the recipient twin at the site of cord insertion into umbilicus
- Period of gestation at which performed: 18–24 weeks

- Large artery to artery placental shunt can be seen in early 1st trimester
- Imbalance in interfetal circulation and reversal of blood flow in umbilical vessels
- Perfusion pressure of donor twin overpowers that in recipient twin
- "Used" arterial blood reaching recipient twin preferentially goes to iliac vessels and thus perfuses only the lower part of body → disruption and deterioration of growth and development of upper body
- High cardiac output in pump twin → decompensation.

Monochorionic Monoamniotic

- Conjoined Twins
- Intrauterine fetal death in 60%
- Those born alive → die of anomalies
- Diagnosis can be made by ultrasound examination, even at less than 10 weeks period of gestation but again confirmation is required at 11–14 weeks
- Of all conjoined twins, only those who are omphalopagus have a reasonable chance of survival
- Most frequent types:
  - Thoracopagus (anterior)—most common
  - Pygopagus (posterior)
  - Craniopagus (cranial)
  - Ischiopagus (caudal)
- Management:
  - If termination between 18–24 weeks → hysterotomy may be required
  - Close antenatal surveillance from 24 weeks onwards
  - Elective cesarean section at 32–34 weeks
  - Vaginal delivery carries risks of dystocia, trauma to uterus and cervix, cord entanglement and sudden IUD.

Chapter 29

Hypertensive Disorders in Pregnancy

Tania G Singh and Nisha M Anand

GESTATIONAL HYPERTENSION

- New onset of hypertension arising after 20 weeks gestation
- No additional features of pre eclampsia
- Resolves within 3 months postpartum.

Maternal Monitoring

Mild Hypertension (140/90 to 149/99 mm Hg)

- Do not admit
- No treatment required
- Measure BP once a week
- Measure proteinuria at each visit (using automated reagent-strip reading device) or urinary protein:creatinine ratio (taking midstream urine sample)
- Only routine investigations.

Moderate Hypertension (150/100 to 159/109 mm Hg)

- Do not admit
- Treat with oral labetelol (1st line drug) to keep DBP between 80–100 mm Hg and SBP lower than 150 mm Hg
- Measure BP twice a week
- Measure proteinuria at each visit
- Blood tests: KFT with electrolytes, CBC, LFT—only transaminases and bilirubin
- Do not carry out further blood tests, if no proteinuria at subsequent visits.

Severe Hypertension (≥160/110 mm Hg)

- Recheck BP after 15 minutes of rest before making diagnosis
- Admit (until BP is ≤159/109 mm Hg)
- Manage with oral labetelol (1st line drug) to keep DBP between 80–100 mm Hg and SBP lower than 150 mm Hg
- Measure BP at least 4 times/week
- Measure proteinuria daily
- Investigate at presentation and then monitor weekly: KFT with electrolytes, CBC, LFT—only transaminases and bilirubin.

Fetal Monitoring

Mild and Moderate Hypertension

- If less than 34 weeks—USG for growth, AFI, Umbilical artery Doppler

---

Risk Factors Requiring Additional Assessment and Follow-up:

- Nulliparity
- Age ≥40 years
- Pregnancy interval of >10 years
- Family history of pre eclampsia
- Multiple pregnancy
- BMI of ≥35 kg/m^2
- Gestational age at presentation
- Previous history of pre eclampsia or gestational hypertension
- Pre-existing vascular disease
- Pre-existing kidney disease

Severe Hypertension

2nd line management: Methyldopa, nifedepine
Follow-up: BP and proteinuria twice weekly; Blood tests weekly

- If more than 34 weeks—above not required
- NST only if DFKC not adequate.

Severe Hypertension

- NST at diagnosis and weekly
- USG for growth, AFI and Umbilical artery doppler at diagnosis and every 2 weekly.

Time of Delivery

- For mild and moderate hypertension → at 37 completed weeks
- In refractory cases → at 34 weeks after a course of steroids.

Pre Eclampsia

Onset at more than 20 weeks' gestational age of:

- 24-hour proteinuria more than or equal to 300 mg/day or, if not available, a protein concentration more than and equal to 30 mg ($\geq$1+ on dipstick) in a minimum of two random urine samples collected at least 4–6 hours but no more than 7 days apart
- A systolic blood pressure more than 140 mm Hg or diastolic blood pressure higher than or equal to 90 mm Hg as measured twice, using an appropriate cuff, 4–6 hours and less than 7 days apart and
- Disappearance of all these abnormalities before the end of the 6th week postpartum, in a woman who was normotensive prior to pregnancy.

Diagnosis can also be made when:

Hypertension arises after 20 weeks gestation (confirmed on 2 or more occasions) accompanied by one or more of the following:

- Significant proteinuria
- Renal involvement
  - Serum or plasma creatinine more than or equal to 90 micromol/L or
  - Oliguria (<500 mL/24 hours)
- Hematological involvement:
  - Thrombocytopenia (platelets <1 lakh/mm^3)
  - Hemolysis; DIC.
- Liver involvement:
  - Raised transaminases; Severe epigastric or right upper quadrant pain
- Neurological involvement
- Pulmonary edema
- Intrauterine fetal growth restriction (IUGR)
- Placental abruption.

Risk Factors for Pre Eclampsia

- Pre eclampsia in a previous pregnancy
- Family history of pre eclampsia
- Poor outcome in a prior pregnancy (placental abruption, IUGR, fetal death in utero)
- Interdelivery interval more than 10 years
- Nulliparity
- Pre-existing medical conditions
- Maternal age more than or equal to 40 years
- BMI more than 35 kg/m^2

Raised BP is commonly but not always the first manifestation
Proteinuria is also common but should not be considered mandatory to make the clinical diagnosis

Significant Proteinuria
Random urine protein/creatinine ratio $\geq$ 30 mg/mmol OR
A validated 24-hour urine collection shows > 300 mg protein OR
$\geq$ 3+ in dipstick test

Neurological Involvement
- Severe headache
- Persistent visual disturbances (photopsia, scotomata, cortical blindness, retinal vasospasm)
- Hyper reflexia with sustained clonus
- Convulsions (eclampsia)
- Stroke

Pre-existing Medical Conditions
- Chronic hypertension
- Diabetes (pre-existing or gestational)
- Renal disease
- Thrombophilias: Antiphospholipid syndrome, Protein C and S deficiency, Antithrombin III deficiency and Factor V Leiden

- Multiple pregnancy
- Raised BP at booking
- Gestational trophoblastic disease
- No midtrimester fall in BP
- Finger and facial edema
- Fetal triploidy.

Management

Mild PE (140/90 to 149/99 mm Hg)

- Admit in hospital
- No treatment required
- Measure BP at least 4 times/day
- Measure proteinuria everyday (midstream urine sample)
- Investigations: twice/week
    - KFT with electrolytes; CBC
    - LFT: transaminases and bilirubin
- Delivery at 37 completed weeks
- At 34–37 weeks, deliver if—In labor; nonreassuring NST; other obstetric indication.

Moderate PE (150/100 to 159/109 mm Hg)

- Rx with oral labetelol (1st line drug) to keep DBP between 80–100 mm Hg and SBP lower than 150 mm Hg
- Rest management in hospital is the same as for Mild PE mentioned above
- Once BP stabilizes, discharge.

Severe PE (≥160/110 mm Hg)

- Admit in hospital
- No need for strict bed rest
- Treat with oral labetelol (1st line drug) to keep DBP between 80–100 mm Hg and SBP lower than 150 mm Hg
- Measure BP more than 4 times/day
- Measure proteinuria
- Investigations: 3 times/week
    - KFT with electrolytes; CBC
    - LFT—only transaminases and bilirubin
- Deliver at 34 completed weeks after course of corticosteroids or earlier, if indicated.

Though edema is no longer included in the definition of pre eclampsia but rapid development of generalized edema should alert the clinician

Proteinuria is a poor predictor of either maternal or fetal complications in women with pre eclampsia.

Testing for Proteinuria
- Exclude UTI
- Clean catch urine sample
- Measure using automated reagent strip first
- Quantitation by laboratory methods if urine dipstick test is ≥ "1+"

Readings of Dipstick
- Trace → 0.1 gm/L
- 1+ → 0.3 gm/L
- 2+ → 1 gm/L
- 3+ → 3 gm/L
- 4+ → 10 gm/L

Advice on Discharge
- Regular diet (no salt restriction)
- Counsel woman and family about danger signals of PE and eclampsia
- Do not give anticonvulsants, sedatives and diuretics
- Maternal evaluation: Biweekly follow-up
- BP recording at every visit. Look for signs and symptoms of impending eclampsia
- Investigations biweekly
- Fetal evaluation: USG every 15 days; DFKC; NST weekly

Chapter 30

Chronic Hypertension

Tania G Singh

Other Features of Primary Hypertension:

- Mainly present in multiparous women of little older age group
- Family history often present
- Blood parameters usually remain unchanged
- Ophthalmic changes: may present as silver wiring of arterioles/ hypertensive retinopathy

Other Features of Secondary Hypertension:

- Can present at any age
- Parity is unrelated
- There is no family history
- Persists even after pregnancy
- Blood urea and creatinine often found elevated
- Urinary changes:
  - Low specific gravity
  - Presence of albumin and granular casts
- Ophthalmic changes:
  - Albuminuric retinopathy
  - Cotton wool patches
  - Flame-shaped hemorrhages

DEFINITION

Hypertension which is detected at less than 20 weeks period of gestation or was present preconceptionally. Can be:

Essential (Primary)

- Idiopathic
- Present in 90–95% of cases
- There is no accompanying proteinuria
- BP higher than 140/90 mm Hg preconceptionally or prior to 20 weeks without an underlying cause OR
- BP lower than 140/90 entering pregnancy on antihypertensives.

Secondary

Hypertension due to:
- Chronic kidney disease (e.g. glomerulonephritis, reflux nephropathy and adult polycystic kidney disease)
- Renal artery stenosis
- Pyelonephritis, tuberculosis or neoplasm
- Systemic disease with renal involvement (e.g. diabetes mellitus, systemic lupus erythematosus)
- Endocrine disorders (e.g. pheochromocytoma, Cushing's syndrome and primary hyperaldosteronism)
- Coarctation of the aorta.

Pre Eclampsia Superimposed on Chronic Hypertension

Diagnosed where a woman with pre-existing hypertension develops:
- Systemic features of pre eclampsia or proteinuria
- After 20 weeks gestation
- Occurs in ≈ 20% of women with chronic hypertension
- Risks for both mother and fetus are greater than for pre eclampsia or chronic hypertension alone
- Risk increases if:
  - Hypertensive for more than or equal to 4 years
  - History of pre eclampsia in previous pregnancy
  - Baseline diastolic BP more than 100 mm Hg.

Management of Chronic Hypertension

Maternal

- Preconceptional counseling
- Stop ACE inhibitors/ARBs (angiotensin receptor blockers) or chlor-thiazides (increased risk of congenital abnormalities) within 2 days of pregnancy detection
- Start labetelol (drug of choice) or nifedepine (start in 1st trimester)
- Methyldopa can be given 2nd trimester onwards
- Do not give:
  - Atenolol—associated with IUGR
  - Diuretics—not teratogenic, but may restrict the natural plasma volume expansion of pregnancy
- Maintain BP lower than 150/100 mm Hg
- Low sodium intake
- USG whole abdomen
- Spot urine protein: creatinine ratio where there is doubt about proteinuria on dipstick, i.e., +1 or +2 proteinuria
- Serum electrolytes
- 24-hour urine catecholamine, if there is severe hypertension
- Specialist (Obstetrician/Physician) opinion
- Ophthalmic examination
- Delivery at 37 completed weeks, if BP lower than 160/110 mm Hg or earlier if high
- Continue antenatal antihypertensives for 2 weeks after delivery
- If a woman has taken methyldopa to treat chronic hypertension during pregnancy, stop within 2 days of birth and restart the antihypertensive treatment taken before pregnancy
- Review long-term antihypertensive treatment 2 weeks after delivery
- Medical review at 6–8 weeks after delivery.

Fetal

- USG and Doppler at 28°30 weeks and between 32 and 34 weeks
- If results are normal, do not repeat further
- NST weekly from 30 weeks onwards or if ↓ DFKC.

Diagnosis of Chronic Hypertension can be Missed if:

- Patient approaches the doctor after mid pregnancy, when physiologic decrease in blood pressure may incorrectly label the patient as normotensive and
- When these physiologic effects will go, it will be labelled as gestational hypertension in 3rd trimester
- Such patients should be reassessed after 6 weeks of delivery to reclassify them

'White Coat Hypertension'

- Defined as hypertension in a clinical setting but normal blood pressure in nonclinical settings (e.g. home) using an appropriately validated device
- No medication given but BP monitoring done
- Office diastolic BP of ≥90 mm Hg but home BP of <135/85 mm Hg

Chapter 31

Intrauterine Growth Restriction

Tania G Singh

Gestational Age	Fundal Height
40 weeks	1-2 finger width below subcostal arch
36 weeks	At costal arch
32 weeks	Between umbilicus and xiphoid process
28 weeks	3 finger widths above umbilicus
24 weeks	At umbilicus
20 weeks	3 finger widths below umbilicus
16 weeks	3 finger widths above symphysis

CLINICAL EXAMINATION

- Prepregnancy weight less than 40 kg and BMI <19 kg/m^2 are more prone for IUGR
- Ideal weight gain depends upon prepregnancy BMI
- Check for any rise in BP (suggestive of hypertensive disorders)
- Fundal height (McDonald's Rule): It is a measure of the size of the uterus used to assess fetal growth and development during pregnancy. It is measured from the top of the mother's uterus to the top of the mother's pubic bone in centimetres
- In IUGR: fundal height is less than period of gestation (lag of ≥4 weeks) → but this is less sensitive
- Symphysis fundal height measurement: In IUGR, there is a lag of more than or equal to 3 cms (≈ ≥ 3 weeks)
    - If lag of 4 weeks → moderate IUGR
    - If lag of >6 weeks → severe IUGR.

Investigations

Less than 28 Weeks (Usually Symmetrical)

- Congenital abnormality → USG
- Chromosomal abnormality → Karyotyping.

More than 28 Weeks (Usually Asymmetrical)

- Rule out hypertensive disorders of pregnancy.

TREATMENT PROPER (2 BASIC STEPS)

I. Antepartum Fetal Surveillance (APFS)

Start at ≈ 32 weeks or 1–2 weeks before stillbirth in previous pregnancy. Methods:

Fetal Movement Count

- From 28 weeks onwards
- Loss of fetal movement is followed by disappearance of FHR within next 24 hours
- Most commonly used is Cardif 'count 10' formula:
    - Start counting from any particular time
    - Count ends when 10 movements are perceived
    - Report if,
        - Less than 10 movements during 12 hours on 2 successive days OR
        - No movement is perceived even after 12 hours in a single day

Common Investigations (To Both Symmetrical and Asymmetrical IUGR)

- TORCH
- Urine culture/ sensitivity
- Rule out malaria
- Investigate for present maternal status
    - Chronic hypertension
    - Chronic renal disease
    - Chronic DM
- Send APLA → if clinical profile of patient suggests
- History based → smoking, alcohol or other substance abuse

NST

Reactive NST
- Baseline FHR 110–160 bpm
- At least two accelerations of more than or equal to 15 beats lasting atleast 15 seconds
- If nonreactive in 20 minutes → extended to 40 minutes → if still nonreactive → BPP.

BPP (Manning Score)

Time consuming
- Does have a role in cases in which UA Doppler is abnormal
- Time required = 30 minutes (at least)
- Interpretation:
  - Score: 0 → if absent; 2 → if present; maximum → 10/10
  - Score: highter than or equal to 8/10 → no fetal asphyxia
  - Score: 6/10 → repeat test within 24 hours
  - Score: 0/10 to 4/10 → ↑ hypoxia
  - In 30 minutes:
    - Tone: 1 episode of active extension with return to flexion of limbs or trunk → 7th week (1st to come and last to go)
    - 3 discrete body/limb movements in 30 minutes → 8–9 weeks
    - 1 episode of breathing at least 30 seconds → 18–19 weeks
    - Amniotic fluid (1 pocket ≈ 2 cm in 2 perpendicular planes)
    - NST: Reactive (last to come and 1st to go, so if NST is REACTIVE, everything is there.

Modified BPP

- AFI and NST.

II. Determination of Optimum Time of Delivery

More than 28 weeks: Investigations + APFS + Steroids
Follow-up:
- UA/MCA Doppler weekly
- AFI weekly
- NST weekly (if gestation age >32 weeks)
- USG every 2 weeks for growth
- If RI/PI ↑ on USG:
  - UA and MCA Doppler biweekly
  - NST biweekly
  - AFI biweekly.

Modes of Termination

Termination by Induction, If

- ↑ resistance to flow
- Absent diastolic flow
- Severe oligohydramnios

Termination by Cesarean Section, If

- Reversal of flow
- Abnormal DV Doppler (i.e. absent 'a' wave and/or pulsations in umbilical vein).

NST Changes Consistent with Fetal Hypoxia
- Fixed baseline heart rate
- Poor baseline variability
- Loss of acceleration
- Spontaneous fetal heart decelerations

Indications for Termination
- Gestational age 37 weeks
- Absent diastolic flow in UA
- Reversal of flow in UA
- AFI <3 cm
- Absent 'a' wave on DV Doppler
- Nonreactive NST (>32 weeks)

Following has NO ROLE
- Bed rest
- β mimetics
- Ca^{2+} channel blockers
- TENS (Transcutaneous electrical nerve stimulation therapy)
- Estrogens (thought to increase blood flow)
- O_2 therapy
- Nutrient supply (carnitine – amino acid which releases energy from fat, solcoseryl – protein free calf blood extract, glucose and galactose—fruit, meat and milk sugars)
- Plasma volume expansion

Chapter 32

Intrauterine Fetal Death

Tania G Singh

RISK FACTORS

Maternal

- Maternal age more than 35 years
- Obesity
- Black race; low socioeconomic status
- Low education status
- Smoking/tobacco
- Nulliparity.

Fetal

- Congenital malformation
- Male sex.

Pregnancy Complications

- IUGR; Pre eclampsia; Abruptio
- Rh negative/Nonimmune hydrops
- Multiple pregnancy
- Post-term pregnancy; Infection
- Antepartum asphyxia
- Previous history of stillbirth
- Nuchal cord or knotted cord.

Medical Disorders

- Diabetes milletus; Hypertensive disorders
- Chronic nephritis; SLE
- Thrombophilias; Cholestasis of pregnancy
- Hyperpyrexia; Severe anemia
- Drugs (Quinine beyond therapeutic levels).

Infection

- Parvovirus B19; CMV
- *Listeria monocytogenes; E. coli*
- Group B streptococcus
- *Ureaplasma urealyticum.*

DIAGNOSIS (2 STEPS)

To Confirm IUD

- Symptoms: Fetal movements absent (which were present earlier)
- Signs: Retrogression of positive breast changes
- Per abdomen changes
- Ultrasound:
  - Fetal movements and fetal cardiac activities absent, which is observed for a period of 10 minutes
  - Look for oligohydramnios and collapsed cranial bones.
- Straight X-ray abdomen (rarely done).

To Find Cause of IUD

Antepartum

- Complete history (exclude all risk factors)
- Investigations (Lab.)
  - FBS/RBS; HbA$_1$C
  - TORCH; VDRL; APLA
  - Thyroid profile
  - Mini renals (urea/creatinine)
  - Kleiheuer Betke tests.
- Amniocentesis (if not done during pregnancy) → 10–25 mL of amniotic fluid taken
- Cord blood or cardiac blood for:
  - Cytogenetic studies
  - Bacterial culture
  - TORCH.

Postpartum

Newborn

- Photographs of unclothed infant
  - Views of whole body in frontal, dorsal and lateral views
  - Close up of face and any grossly abnormal part.
- X-ray
  - Single AP view of whole body (including hands and feet) with limbs extended
  - If dwarfism is present, additional AP and lateral views of infant limbs, head and spine.
- Autopsy
- MRI: If autopsy consent denied.

Placenta

- Gross and microscopic examination
- Culture for bacteria and viruses (with sterile sticks, cultures taken from under the amnion).

Management

- Spontaneous expulsion occurs in 80–90% (within 2 weeks)
- Refractory cases or cases where early termination is indicated:

X-ray Abdomen

- Appearance of gas shadow → Robert's sign (In chambers of heart and great vessels) as early as 12 hours
- Spalding sign → Liquefaction of brain matter + softening of ligamentous structure (supporting the vault) [can be seen on USG] → Irregular overlapping of cranial bones (7-10 days after death)
- Hyperflexion of spine (common) → due to loss of muscle tone (Ball sign)
- Hyperextension of neck (less common)
- Crowding of ribs shadow → loss of normal parallelism
- Accumulation of fluid in subaponeurotic space → elevation of thin, dark fat line around the head (Halo sign)

Grade of Maceration Time Since IUD

0	"Parboiled" reddened skin	<8 hours
I	Skin slippage and peeling	>8 hours
II	Extensive skin peeling; red serous effusions in chest and abdomen	2–7 days
III	Liver yellow-brown; turbid effusion	≥8 days

Indications for C. Section

- Major degree placenta previa
- ≥2 previous LSCS
- Transverse lie

- Psychological
- Infection (if membrane ruptured)
- ↓ Fibrinogen level
- Retained more than 2 weeks
- Hospitalization
- Proper counseling
- Investigations (Hb, blood group, PT /aPTT)
- Options for induction (prostaglandins/oxytocin).

Chapter 33

Diabetes in Pregnancy

Tania G Singh

At first one must be aware of the risk factors which lead to diabetes in pregnancy so that those patients can be checked for it timely.

Risk Factors

Low-risk

- Young (age <25 years)
- Non-Hispanic white
- Normal BMI ($\leq$25 kg/m^2)
- No history of previous glucose intolerance
- No history of adverse pregnancy outcomes associated with GDM
- No first degree relative with known diabetes.

Moderate risk

- Do not satisfy all criteria of women at low-risk, but they lack two or more risk factors for GDM.

High risk

Usually defined as having two or more risk factors:
- Age more than 35 years
- BMI more than 30 kg/m^2
- GDM in previous pregnancy
- Unexplained IUD in previous pregnancy
- Previous macrosomic baby (weight $\geq$4.5 kg)
- First degree relative with DM
- Previous bad obstetric history
- Large baby in present pregnancy
- Member of ethnic group with high-prevalence (South Asians, Black Caribbean, Middle Eastern countries)
- Polycystic ovary syndrome
- Polyhydramnios in present pregnancy
- Hypertension (more recently noted).

How To Screen

You should give the following general advice to all diabetic patients before testing for blood sugars by any of the methods described below:
- Unrestricted diet (carbohydrate $\geq$150 gm/day)
- Normal physical activity for 3 days prior to testing
- Ask her to fast for at least 8 hours

GDM is defined as carbohydrate intolerance of variable severity with onset or first recognition during the present pregnancy

Gestational Prediabetes
Absence of diabetes before pregnancy and the presence of blood glucose levels above normal but not high enough to meet the diagnostic criteria for GDM when tested in early pregnancy.
It should be considered as risk factor for diabetes and timely modifications like diet with reduced calorie intake, adequate physical exercise, adequate weight gain would help to prevent GDM

Do not start her immediately on diabetic diet before investigating. This will mask her diabetes.

- Take a fasting sample then give anhydrous glucose (5 level teaspoons, not heaped)
- Juice of half a lemon can be added to avoid nausea and vomiting, when taken on empty stomach
- During this, patient should remain seated and refrain from smoking throughout the test.

There are so many screening methods for diabetes. A few are described below with their normal values.

IADPSG (International Association of Diabetes and Pregnancy Study Group)

- Glucose—75 gm in 250–300 mL of water
- Criteria—when any one or more of the following is met or exceeded:
  - FBS → 92 mg/dL (5.1 mmol/L)
  - 1 hour → 180 mg/dL (10 mmol/L)
  - 2 hour → 153 mg/dL (8.5 mmol/L).

Carpenter and Coustan

It is a two step procedure.
- Step 1: GCT (glucose challenge test) → with 50 gm glucose (irrespective of the last meal) → after 1 hour → if higher than 140 mg/dL → OGTT
- Step 2 : OGTT → 4 samples are taken (any 2 values above cut off) with 100 gm glucose
  - Fasting → 95 mg/dL
  - 1 hour → 180 mg/dL
  - 2 hour → 155 mg/dL
  - 3 hour → 140 mg/dL.

WHO/NICE

- Glucose—75 gm
- Fasting higher than or equal to 126 mg/dL (≥7 mmol/L)
- 2 hour → higher than or equal to 140 mg/dL (≥7.8 mol/L).

DIPSI (Diabetes in Pregnancy Study Group India)

- Approved by Ministry of Health, Government of India
- Glucose—75 gm (irrespective of fasting or nonfasting state)
- 2 hour → higher than or equal to 140 mg/dL (7.8 mmol/L)
- Advantages:
  - Requires only 1 blood sample
  - Less costly as compared to IADPSG
  - No fasting
  - Both screening and diagnostic
  - Best for low resource settings.

Gestational Diabetes Milletus

- FBS higher than 92 mg/dL but less than 126 mg/dL

Once the patient is labeled as diabetic, advice her of the following risks associated.

Risks to Mother

- Pre eclampsia/gestational hypertension
- Increased weight gain in pregnancy

Impaired Fasting Glucose

FBS 100–125 mg/dL (5.6–6.9 mmol/L) OR

Impaired Glucose Tolerance

Give 75 gms glucose load
- 2 hr plasma glucose → 140–199 mg/dL (7.8–11.0 mmol/L) OR
- HbA$_{1c}$ → 5.7–6.4%

Pregestational Diabetes (Overt Diabetes)

Diabetes present before pregnancy (irrespective of the type)

Diagnosed if any of the following is found in pregnancy:
- FBS ≥126 mg/dL
- RBS ≥200 mg/dL
- HbA$_{1c}$ ≥6.5%

Advantages of Measuring FBS in 1st Trimester:
- No need for taking glucose
- Early detection of overt diabetes
- GDM and overt diabetes can be easily differentiated

- Increased risk of cesarean section
- Labor inductions are increased
- Obstructed labor
- Traumatic vaginal delivery
- PPH (traumatic)
- Interventional delivery
- Complications associated with coagulopathy (in cases of prolonged retention of dead fetus)
- Risk of developing postpartum prediabetes, Metabolic syndrome and Type 2 diabetes in future.

Risks to Fetus

- Fetal macrosomia/large for gestational age
- Fetal malformations (Type 1 DM)
- Stillbirth
- Preterm labor/Prematurity
- Intrapartum asphyxia
- Birth trauma
  - Shoulder dystocia
  - Bone fracture (clavicle)
  - Nerve palsy (brachial plexus injury).

Risks in Newborn

- Respiratory distress syndrome/Admission to NICU
- Hypoglycemia (because of high insulin levels in fetus)
- Hypocalcemia/Hypomagnesemia
- Hyperviscosity
- Polycythemia/Hyperbilirubinemia
- Hyperinsulinemia
- Cardiomyopathy.

Risk to Children Born to Diabetic Mothers

- Obesity/Metabolic syndrome
- Impaired glucose tolerance/Type 2 diabetes in adulthood.

TREATMENT

In Pregnancy

Treat even a milder form of GDM

Diet and Nutrition Therapy

Nutritional Therapy—for 2 Weeks

- Diet plan with visit to dietician every 4 weekly
- Blood glucose is reassessed for 2-3 days with checking of FBS, premeals and post meal monitoring (1-2 hrs)
- If it fails, i.e. FBS—90 mg/dL and/or postmeal—120 mg/dL → start insulin or oral hypoglycemic agents
- If blood sugars are in range, wait for another 2 weeks and reassess
- Recommended calorie intake:
  - Underweight: 35–40 kcal/kg
  - Normal weight: 30–35 kcal/kg
  - Overweight: 25–30 kcal/kg

As there are so many classifications, and no one criteria, therefore, Fasting Blood Sugar should be done for all women presenting in 1st trimester.

- If FBS is ≥126 mg/dL → overt diabetes
- If it is >92 but <126 mg/dL → GDM
- If <92 mg/dL → no diabetes

For those at high-risk, screen using OGTT at first prenatal visit.
Those presenting for the first time in 2nd trimester, screen with OGTT at 24–28 weeks.
Role of HbA$_{1C}$ – only in predicting risk of fetal malformations when performed periconceptionally

Modest calorie restriction, 1600–1800 calories/day or a 33% reduction in intake, does not lead to ketosis but controls weight gain and glucose levels in obese women and has been more successful

<table>
<tr><td>

Recommended Weight Gain in Pregnancy
- Normal BMI (19.8–26.0 kg/m^2) → 11.4–15.9 kg
- Overweight (BMI 26.1–29.0 kg/m^2) → 6.8–11.4 kg
- Obese women (BMI >29 kg/m^2) → up to 7 kg

</td><td>

Medical Nutrition Therapy (MNT)

Defined as carbohydrate-controlled meal plan that promotes adequate nutrition with appropriate weight gain, normoglycemia and the absence of ketosis. It primarily targets postprandial glucose levels.

Recommended calorie intake according to trimester as follows:
- 1st trimester → no increase in calories
- 2nd trimester → an additional 340 kcal/day
- 3rd trimester → an additional 452 kcal/day.

</td></tr>
</table>

Carbohydrate

- One of the most important component especially playing role in diabetic patients
- Requirements:
  - In nonpregnant state—130 gm/day
  - Pregnancy—175 gm/day (this additional is for fetal brain development and functioning)
- In GDM, the carbohydrate intake has to be manipulated by:
  - Controlling the total amount of carbohydrate
  - Its distribution over several meals and snacks
  - Type of carbohydrate.

Recommended Calorie Intake According to Body Weight
- Underweight → 35–40 kcal/kg
- Normal BMI → 30–35 kcal/kg
- Overweight → 25–30 kcal/kg
- 60:20:20 → carbohydrate: protein: fat

Diet in Diabetes

- High-fiber foods: Whole grains, oats, gram flour, millets
- Must contain milk without cream (minimum 2 servings) → right combination of carbohydrates and proteins
- Fruits high in fiber: apple, orange, pear, guava
- Fruits avoided or eaten in moderation: mangoes, bananas, grapes
- High-fibre green vegetables: Peas, beans, broccoli, spinach, green leafy vegetables
- Pulses; Good fats (Omega 3, MUFA, etc.).

Insulin Therapy

Source of Exogenous Insulin

- Three types exist: Bovine, Porcine and Human insulin
- Pork insulin is more homologous to human insulin
- Only difference between them is that the 30th amino acid in the β chain in pork insulin is alanine whereas it is threonine in human insulin
- Human insulin:
  - Made by replacement of 30-alanine in β chain of porcine insulin by threonine
  - Less expensive, less immunogenic
  - Production by recombinant DNA technology in *E. coli* and in yeast or by enzymatic modification of porcine insulin
  - More water soluble and hydrophobic than porcine or bovine insulin
  - More rapid subcutaneous absorption
  - Has an earlier and more defined peak
  - Has slightly shorter duration of action.

Role of Glycemic Index

Even if total carbohydrates are controlled, low glycemic index (<55) foods produce a lower postmeal glucose elevation, whereas foods with a high glycemic index (>70) show higher postprandial values

Administration

- Subcutaneous route
- Intravenous (only regular insulin)

Disadvantages/Adverse Reactions

- Insulin allergy (IgE antibodies): Itching, redness, swelling, anaphylaxis, shock
- Pain at the injection site
- Need for multiple injections
- Insulin resistance (IgG antibodies)
- Need for refrigeration
- Potential for hypoglycemia: Nausea, hunger, tachycardia, sweating
- Skillful handling of syringes (problem in low resource countries)
- High-cost
- Poor patient compliance
- Lipodystrophy at injection site: Atrophy.

Available Types

Short Acting Insulin (Regular or Soluble)

- Onset of action: 30 minutes to 1 hour after injection
- Therefore, should be injected 30 minutes before planned meal
- Peak action → in 2–4 hours
- Duration of action → 6–8 hours
- Vial has a yellow color strip for identification
- Brand names: Actrapid, Huminsulin, Insugen R.

Intermediate Acting

Lente insulin (insulin zinc suspension)
- Mixture of 30% semilente with 70% ultralente insulin → provide a combination of relatively rapid absorption with sustained long action
- Onset of action: 1–2 hours
- Peak action: 8–10 hours
- Duration of action: 20–24 hours.

Isophane insulin (neutral protamine hagedorn, NPH)
- Absorption and onset of action is delayed by combining appropriate amounts of insulin and protamine
- 6 molecules of insulin per molecule of protamine
- Onset of action: 1–2 hours after injection
- Peak action: 8–10 hours
- Duration of action: 20–24 hours
- Vial has a green color strip for identification

Ultrashort-acting (modified insulin with minor changes)
- Onset of action: within few minutes after injection (very fast)
- Permit more physiologic prandial insulin replacement
- Injected just before meal or sometimes immediately after the meal
- Peak in 30 minutes
- Duration of action: 2 hours
- The only type that should be administered intravenously
- Brand names: Lispro and Aspart.

Ultralong-acting
- Not approved to use in pregnancy
- Concern: they bind with IGF-1 receptor and possible teratogenicity
- Brand names: Glargine and Detemir.
a. Extended insulin zinc suspension (Crystalline)
   - Slower onset: 4–6 hours

Exercise in Diabetes
- Physical activity ≈ 30 min/day is recommended
- Brisk walk or arm exercises while sitting on a chair for at least 10 minutes after each meal

Degradation of Insulin:
- Endogenous Insulin: Liver (60%) and kidney (35–40%)
- Exogenous Insulin: Liver (35–40%) and kidney (60%)

Concentration of Insulin in Pregnancy: Not always same in different trimesters
- ↑ in very early pregnancy
- ↓ in second half of 1st trimester
- ↑ in 2nd and 3rd trimester
- After 32 weeks stays constant or even decline, which may manifest as hypoglycemia

- Prolonged peak of action: 14–18 hours
- Duration: 24–36 hours.

b. Protamine zinc insulin (Ultralente)
- Onset (4–6 hours) and a prolonged peak (14–20 hours)
- Duration: 24–36 hours
- Recommended dose to be taken in 2 or more divided doses.

c. Glargine
- Soluble, peakless, ultralong-acting insulin analog
- Designed to provide reproducible, convenient, background insulin replacement
- Has a slow onset of action (1–1.5 hours)
- Achieves a maximum effect after 4–5 hours and maintained for 11–24 hours or longer
- Given once a day.

REGIMENS FOR ADMINISTRATION OF INSULIN

Regimen I (Split Mix Regimen)

- Total dose → 2/3rd in morning and 1/3rd in evening (with ≈ 12 hours gap).
- Check before lunch—if out of target range, give 4–8 units of regular insulin
- Out of the total dose to be given in morning (before breakfast)
  - 2/3rd—isophane (long acting)
  - 1/3rd—actrapid (regular)
- Out of 1/3rd in evening (before dinner)
  - 1/2—isophane
  - 1/2—actrapid

Try to start with 0.2–0.4 U/kg body weight, i.e. 12–24 units

- 24 units →16 units in morning and 8 units in evening
- 16 units →10 units long acting and 6 units regular insulin
- 8 units → 5 units long acting and 3 units regular insulin.

Regimen II (Multiple Subcutaneous Injections)

- Before meals—short-acting
- Bedtime—long-acting or intermediate acting
- Try to start with 0.2–0.4 units/kg body weight
- Start Inj. Actrapid 4 units before meals
- Bedtime—6–10 units Inj. Insulatard
- Check FBS, pre and post each meal sugars—Observe for 2–3 days
- Dose can be increased by 2 units at a time.

Oral Hypoglycemic Agents (OHAs)

There are many but of use in pregnancy is second generation:
Biguanide/Insulin sensitizer Metformin

Metformin

- Category B drug
- It does not stimulate endogenous insulin secretion, therefore, hypoglycemia does not occur with it
- Hypoglycemia may occur when metformin is taken with
  - Insulin
  - A sulfonylurea
  - Excessive amount of alcohol.

- Beneficial effects:
  - Lowers triglyceride and LDL cholesterol
  - Increases HDL cholesterol
  - Weight loss or no weight gain
  - Useful in PCOS patients.
- Side effects:
  - GI upset (diarrhea, bloating)—start with low dose, increase gradually and take with meals
  - Metallic taste
  - Effect on vitamin B_{12} levels
  - Decrease in appetite
  - Lactic acidosis (rare)—excreted by kidneys, therefore, serum creatinine is to be monitored periodically
  - Serum creatinine more than 1.4 mg% → stop medication.
- Contraindicated in: Significant hepatic disease, cardiac insufficiency, alcohol abuse, hypoxic conditions, history of lactic acidosis
- Temporarily discontinued 1–2 days before any dye studies
- t ½ :1.5–3 hours; duration of action: 6–8 hours
- Cleared by kidneys and is not bound to plasma proteins
- Daily dose: 0.5–2.0 gm
- Not metabolized at all. GFR increases in pregnancy, therefore, dose adjustment is required as it's excretion is mainly through renal tubules
- Crosses placenta
- Studies have proved it's role in PCOS patients who got pregnant while on metformin. Rates of early pregnancy loss, gestational diabetes, neonatal morbidity and mortality was significantly lower in metformin group
- Concentration in breast milk is low making it safe while breastfeeding.

Management Proper

Prepregnancy Counseling (In Cases of Pre-existing Diabetes)

- Pregnancy need to be started with a good glycemic control
- Explain the patient the risks (maternal and fetal) and fetal malformations with Type 1 diabetes
- In cases of PCOS well-controlled on metformin, the drug need not be stopped at conception
- Weight reduction in cases of obese patients
- Folic acid 4 mg/day at least 3 months prior to conception
- Oral hypoglycemics to be switched over to insulin (studies on complete safety of glyburide still awaited)
- To lay stress on diet and exercise
- Systemic examinations to be done (in case of Type 1 diabetes)
  - Fundus examination, renal function tests, hypertension
  - Any infections to be treated well before (UTI, dental caries)
- Immunity to rubella should be checked
- Patients with IGT, IFG, or an HBA_{1C} of 5.7–6.4% should undergo following interventions before pregnancy:
  - Weight loss ≈ 7% of body weight
  - Increasing physical activity to at least 150 minutes/week of moderate activity, such as walking
  - Metformin therapy for prevention of Type 2 diabetes may be considered in those with:
    - BMI more than 35 kg/m^2 and in women with prior GDM.

Home Glucose Monitoring
- Check by glucometer
- Check FBS, pre- and postmeal (1-hour) sugars
- Check late night sugars between 2 am–4 am (2–3 times/week)
- Charting of each day's value

<table>
<tr><td valign="top">

FBS (in all antepartum women irrespective of risk category)

⤷ To exclude any hidden cases of pregestational diabetes

⤷ To rule out cases of gestational prediabetes so that proper management, to avoid their progression to GDM, can be done timely

</td><td valign="top">

Antenatal Management

First Trimester (Prediabetics)

- All routine investigations (CBC, ABO Rh, HIV, HbsAg, Anti-HCV, Urine routine)
- HbA$_{1C}$ and OGTT
- Kidney function tests with electrolytes
- 24-hour urine albumin and creatinine
- Fundus examination
- Metformin to be continued
- ACE inhibitors to be discontinued and switch on to safer drugs
- Folic acid 4 mg/day
- Regular BP monitoring (in case of hypertensive patients)
- Oral hypoglycemics to be switched over to insulin
- Diet/exercise
- USG for nuchal translucency and congenital anamolies
- Dental checkup (optional, if required)
- BP, weight and urine examination to be done at each visit
- ANCs:
    - 1st and 2nd trimesters → every 15 days
    - 3rd trimester → weekly.

</td></tr>
</table>

Second Trimester

- Triple screen at 16–18 weeks
- Level II scan at 18–22 weeks
- Fetal echocardiography at 20–24 weeks (especially in cases of overt diabetes)
- USG for growth and liquor at ≈ 26–28 weeks
- Injection tetanus toxoid
- Iron and calcium supplements
- Fundus examination in Type 1 diabetes
- Signs and symptoms of hypoglycemia to be explained
- Hypocare.

<table>
<tr><td valign="top">

Fetal macrosomia or polyhydramnios is not an indication to start insulin in patients of GDM, being managed on diet alone

</td></tr>
</table>

Third Trimester

- Serial USG to exclude
    - Large for date fetus/Excessive liquor
    - IUGR (in cases of diabetic vasculopathy).
- In patient with uncontrolled diabetes, risk of sudden IUD should be kept in mind and well-explained to patient before
- Fetal monitoring (in all cases):
    - Daily fetal kick count; NST twice weekly from 32 weeks onwards
    - BPP weekly; Doppler in cases of IUGR.

Chapter 34

Intrahepatic Cholestasis of Pregnancy

Tania G Singh

INTRAHEPATIC CHOLESTASIS

It is defined as a multifactorial condition characterized by:

- Pruritis without rash
- Abnormal liver function in the absence of other liver disease
- Progression with pregnancy
- Resolves following delivery (within 48 hours).

Diagnosis is made only after excluding other causes.

Clinical Features

Effects on Mother

- PRURITIS (an unpleasant sensation that evokes the desire to scratch)—most common symptom
- After 30 weeks, but may occur as early as 8 weeks
- Palms of hands and soles of feet—most common sites, but can be generalized in few cases.

Usually presents at night, sometimes causing insomnia

- O/E: excoriation marks on skin (dermatographia artefacta)
- Other skin conditions MUST be excluded like eczema or atopic eruption of pregnancy
- Jaundice—rare
- Anorexia, malaise and abdominal pain may occur
- Rarely—pale stools, dark urine and steatorrhea is seen
- Itch may present either before or after abnormal liver function is detected and usually resolves within 2–8 weeks of delivery.

Effects on Fetus

- Passage of meconium in ≈16–58% cases, mostly with ↑↑ maternal serum bile acids
- CTG abnormalities (Both ante- and intrapartum)
- Preterm labor, mainly when fasting serum bile acids higher than 40 micromol/lit
- Sudden IUD, which can be reduced by:
  - Increased fetal monitoring
  - Frequent biochemical testing
  - Pharmacotherapy with ursodeoxycholic acid (UDCA)
  - Delivery at 37–38 weeks gestation

Incidence Increases
- After IVF
- In twin pregnancies
- Age ≥35 years
- Risk factor—Hepatitis C seropositivity leading to early onset of the condition

CTG Abnormalities (Both Ante- and Intrapartum)
- Reduced FHR variability
- Tachycardia
- Bradycardia (<100 bpm)

Glutathione S-transferase alpha (GSTA) is considered to be more sensitive and specific marker of hepatic integrity than standard LFT

Investigations

Bile Acids

- Serum bile acid levels—most suitable biochemical marker for both the diagnosis and monitoring of ICP
- CA level or the CA: CDCA—most sensitive indicator for early diagnosis
- $\uparrow$ DCA—impairment of enterohepatic circulation
- Maternal cholestasis →$\uparrow$ bile acids in the fetal circulation
- Though random bile acid levels are used in routine practice, it's significant rise after a meal and fall after fasting should be kept in mind.

Liver Function Tests

- ALT—most sensitive marker ($\uparrow$ by 2–10-folds)
  - $\uparrow$ AST
  - Bilirubin—usually normal. If raised, it tends to be a conjugated hyperbilirubinemia
  - GGT→ normal or raised
  - Alkaline phosphatase may $\uparrow$
  - LFTs may increase in the first 10 days of puerperium, therefore, should be deferred for at least 10 days postnatally.

Urine Routine/Microscopy

- $\uparrow$excretion of total bile acids
- 10–100-folds $\uparrow$ in CA and CDCA
- $\downarrow$ excretion of DCA and LCA.

Ultrasonography

- Features of cholelithiasis
- In ICP, the intrahepatic bile ducts appear normal
- Fasting and ejection volumes of gallbladder are greater, predisposing these women to formation of gallstones.

Management of ICP

- Fetal surveillance (CTG, fetal movement count) do not actually prevent IUD
- Elective delivery: Good outcome with induction of labor at 37–38 weeks.

Drugs

Ursodeoxycholic Acid

- Naturally occurring hydrophilic bile acid
- Constitutes less than 3% of the physiological bile acid pool in humans
- UDCA lowers serum levels of ethinyl-estradiol 17 β-glucuronide, a major cholestatic metabolite of estrogen
- UDCA 300 mg BD show significant reduction in pruritis and LFTs, including bile acids, compared to baseline
- Results in normalization of CA: CDCA and glycine: taurine ratios and a reduction in urinary excretion of sulfated progesterone metabolites
- Does not harm the fetus
- Levels of bile acids in meconium is considerably elevated in ICP and this is not influenced by treatment with UDCA.

Asymptomatic Hypercholanemia of Pregnancy (AHP)

- Raised serum bile acids in the absence of symptoms and other biochemical markers of ICP
- It has: $\uparrow$ CA; unchanged CDCA
- Affects ≈ 10% of pregnancies
- 2-3% of patients with AHP during 2nd trimester subsequently develop ICP

Complications

- Meconium passage
- CTG abnormalities
- Spontaneous preterm labor
- RDS
- Intrauterine death

There is an increased risk of RDS if iatrogenic delivery is anticipated at 37 weeks with either induction of labor or elective C. section

Prognosis

- ICP recurs in the majority of cases, with variations in intensity in subsequent pregnancies
- Recurrence is less likely following multiple pregnancy
- Women with the history of ICP may also develop symptoms, if taking COCs or in 2nd half of menstrual cycle
    - There is an increased risk of gallstones, nonalcoholic cirrhosis and pancreatitis, Hepatitis C and autoimmune hepatitis in future.

Chapter 35

Antiphospholipid Antibody Syndrome (APAS)

Tania G Singh

- Antiphospholipid Antibody (APLA) is a family of antibodies that bind to negatively charged phospholipids, phospholipid binding proteins or combination of the two
- Antibodies include:
  - LA- IgG and IgM
  - aCL- IgG, IgM, IgA
  - Anti-β_2 glycoprotein 1—IgG/IgM titers.

Lupus Anticoagulant (LA)

- Antibody directed against prothrombin or annexin V
- Causes prolonged APTT (abnormally)
- Requires prothrombin to exert their action.

Anticardiolipin Antibodies (aCL)

- Not all aCL are pathogenic—IgM aCL may not be pathogenic
  - Can be detected after syphilis, adenovirus, chickenpox, mumps, Q fever, TB, Parvovirus, HIV, CMV
  - Drugs: Procainamide, Chlorpromazine, Sodium valproate
- aCL require β GP1 to exert their action.

Anti-β_2 Glycoprotein1

- β_2 GP1$\rightarrow$ a phospholipid binding protein which inhibits prothrombinase activity
- New addition to diagnostic criteria
- Considered more specific.

Complications of APAS

Obstetric

- Thrombotic complications—70% in venous system (mainly lower limb deep vein thrombosis and/or pulmonary embolism)
- Gestational hypertension/pre eclampsia
- IUGR/Preterm
- RPL
- IUD
- Chorea gravidarum
- Neonatal thrombosis.

APAS and Pregnancy

- LA has a stronger association with pregnancy loss than the other antiphospholipid antibodies
- Association of anti-β_2GP1 and pregnancy loss is uncertain
- Both IgG and IgM aCL are associated with recurrent fetal loss
- Testing for IgA aCL antibodies is not recommended.

MANAGEMENT

Low Dose Aspirin (75-80 mg)

- Mechanism of action: selectively inhibit thrombaxane A_2 without affecting prostacyclin production
- Started as soon as UPT comes positive
- Success rate (with aspirin alone): 40%
- Stopped at 34 weeks: why?
  - Closure of ductus arteriosus when used near term
  - Oligohydramnios
  - Neonates: hemolysis, increased blood transfusion, metabolic acidosis.
- Side effects:
  - Increased bleeding during surgery
  - Fetal gastroschisis.

Heparin (1st Line Therapy)

- Unfractionated heparin 5,000 IU s/c BD
- Formation of irreversible complexes between antithrombin III and coagulation factors complex
- Started when cardiac activity is seen on USG
- aPTT is done weekly and dose adjusted until anticoagulation is achieved (it inactivates factors IIa and Xa and affects aPTT, a measure of thrombin activity)
- Platelet count—1 week after starting and monthly thereafter
- Regimens in 1st trimester:
  - Prophylactic: 7,500–10,000 IU every 12 hourly
  - Anticoagulation: every 8–12 hours.
- Regimen in 2nd and 3rd trimester: 10,000 IU every 12 hourly maintaining levels
- Monitoring:
  - Maintain aPTT values between 1.5–2 times control
  - aPTT not used in case of LA positive patients
  - Success rate (aspirin + UFH)—70%.

Low Molecular Weight Heparin

Enoxaparin 20–40 mg/day s/c.

Advantages

- Once daily administration
- Less laboratory monitoring—response much more predictable
- Increased bioavailability because binds less to plasma proteins
- Lesser degree of osteopenia and bleeding
- Decreased risk of heparin-induced thrombocytopenia because of lower affinity to platelets and vWF

The best predictor of pregnancy outcome in women with APAS is past obstetric history

HIT Type I (Nonimmune)
- Mild and reversible
- Occurs within 1st few days of treatment
- Common after high dose UFH
- Patients do not exhibit symptoms, recover over following 3–4 days

HIT Type II (Immune)
- Rapid drop of platelet count
- Occurs between 6–10 days of treatment
- Formation of heparin dependent antibodies can result in platelet activation

Complications with Heparin
Osteopenia
- Reversible on stopping therapy
- In 1–2% of cases
- Advice: calcium, vitamin B, weight bearing exercises, graduated elastic compression stockings
Symptomatic vertebral fracture in 2.2–3% patients
Heparin-induced thrombocytopenia (HIT)
- In 0.5% of cases
- Manifests between 3–21 days
- If severe, can cause limb ischemia, cerebrovascular accidents and myocardial infarction
- Uncommon with prophylactic dose

Regimens

Enoxaparin

- Prophylactic: 40 mg OD (20 mg if body wt <50 kg)
- Anticoagulant: 1mg/kg BD
- Intermediate dose: 40 mg OD until 16 weeks

Dalteparin

- Prophylactic: 5000 IU OD
- Anticoagulant: 20 U/kg BD
- Intermediate dose: 5,000 IU OD until 16 weeks
- 12 hourly monitoring with Anti factor Xa

- Molecular weight: 2,000–8,000 daltons
- Single chain: 13–22 saccharide units
- Ratio of anti Xa: IIa varies between 2:1 and 4:1
- Minimum alteration in microvascular bleeding
- Bioavailability 70% after s/c administration
- Longer $t_{1/2}$ can be given as OD dose.
- It inhibits factor Xa and augments tissue factor pathway inhibitor
- Has minimal effect on thrombin (factor IIa)
- Therefore, monitoring requires anti-Xa assay and not aPTT
- Metabolized in liver by heparinize
- Fragments excreted in urine
- $t_{1/2}$ is increased in cirrhotic and renal failure cases.

Unfractionated Heparin

- Molecular weight: 5000-35000 daltons
- Single chain: 40–50 saccharide units
- Ratio of anti Xa:IIa—1:1
- Augments microvascular bleeding
- Bioavailability 30% after s/c injection
- Short $t_{1/2}$ doses every 8–12 hours.

Scheme of Management in Case of APLA Positive

With Previous History of Thrombosis

- Anticoagulation (in therapeutic doses) throughout pregnancy and 6 weeks postpartum.

With Previous Pregnancy Mishap

- Aspirin + Heparin (standard treatment)
- aPTT and factor Xa levels weekly (till adjustment of dose)
- Platelet count 1–2 weeks after initiating therapy
- Routine monitoring with aPTT or serum Xa levels is not required
- Antenatal visits:
  - Up to 20 weeks—every 2–4 weeks
  - Thereafter 1–2 weeks
  - Serial USG 3–4 weeks after 20 weeks (for IUGR and oligohydramnios)
  - 2nd trimester: uterine artery velocity waveform on USG (for predicting adverse fetal and neonatal outcomes).
- Close maternal and fetal surveillance due to increased risk of pre eclampsia, IUGR, abruption
- At 32 weeks—fetal kick count, weekly NST and BPP
- Induction at 38–39 weeks (warfarin stopped; start heparin 7–10 days earlier)
- Heparin discontinued anytime with:
  - Uterine contractions
  - Elective induction is planned.
- No specific neonatal complications per se because of APAS (only secondary to IUGR or IUD)
- Postpartum period:
  - Heparin × 6 weeks
  - Warfarin after 2–3 days and heparin discontinued once adequate INR is achieved
- OCPs contraindicated (risk of thrombosis).

Warfarin

- Patient with history of recurrent thrombosis or cerebral thrombotic events
- Can be given between 13–36 weeks
- MOA: interfering with synthesis of vitamin K dependent clotting factors in liver
- Anticoagulant effect develops within 1–3 days
- Secreted in milk. However, quantity of active form is insufficient to affect the suckling infant
- $t_{1/2}$ is 36–48 hours, thus single dose 3–5 mg OD
- Start of therapy:Warfarin + Heparin→ INR done after 2 days of initiating the therapy→ repeat daily → INR more than 2 (2 continuous days) → stop Heparin
- INR values maintained between 1.5 and 2.5
- Started on postnatal day 2.

Glucocorticoids

- Generally used in secondary APAS
- Prednisone 40 mg/day
- Successful pregnancy rate 60–70%.

Intravenous Immunoglobulins

- Used when 1st line of management fails
- Cases of HIT
- Doses:
    - 0.4 gm/kg IV × 5 days monthly OR 1 gm/kg IV monthly
    - 0.3 gm/kg every 4 weekly till 32 weeks.
- Associated with anaphylactic reaction
- Inhibits APA themselves and decrease their further production
- Helps mainly in refractory cases, i.e. pregnancy failure despite heparin use
- Disadvantage: Cost
- Side effect: Anaphylaxis (particularly in patients with IgA deficiency)
- No added benefit, if added to heparin treatment
- Decrease in number of IUGR babies.

Side Effects of Glucocorticoids

- Osteopenia/ Osteoporosis/ Pathological fractures
- Delayed wound healing
- Overt/Gestational DM
- Preterm delivery/ PROM
- Cushinoid features
- Vertebral body collapse
- Significant infection

Chapter 36

Post Term Pregnancy

Tania G Singh

Fetal and Neonatal Risks in Post Term Pregnancy

Fetal Risks

- Perinatal mortality (defined as stillbirths + early neonatal deaths)
- Meconium aspiration syndrome (tachypnea, cyanosis and reduced pulmonary compliance in newborns → chemical pneumonitis
- Placental insufficiency—calcium deposition on walls of blood vessels and protein deposition on surface of placenta
- Fetal distress
- Low umbilical artery pH levels at delivery
- Neonatal acidemia
- Low Apgar scores
- Macrosomia and subsequent prolonged labor, CPD, shoulder dystocia, birth injury (orthopedic or neurological)
- Dysmaturity (postmaturity) syndrome in about 20% of infants with characteristics of chronic IUGR from uteroplacental insufficiency. These pregnancies are at increased risk of:
  - Oligohydramnios
  - Umbilical cord compression
  - Nonreassuring CTG (both ante- and intrapartum)
  - Meconium
  - Short-term neonatal complications—hypoglycemia, seizures, respiratory insufficiency.
- Neonatal encephalopathy
- Intermittent Positive Pressure Ventilation (IPPV with intubation)
- Cerebral palsy, if delivered at more than or equal to 42 weeks
- Increased risk of death within first year of life.

Maternal Risks

- Increase in labor dystocia (9–12%)
- Increase in severe perineal injury (3rd and 4th degree perineal tears) related to macrosomia
- Operative vaginal delivery
- Increase in number of labor inductions with unfavorable cervices
- Increase in rate of cesarean section by 2-folds → increased risks of endometritis, hemorrhage, thromboembolic disease
- Intrauterine infections
- Postpartum hemorrhage
- Anxiety and frustration of carrying a pregnancy more for 1–2 weeks beyond due date.

Management of Post-term Pregnancy

Place of Induction of Labor (IOL)

- IOL is typically recommended when the risks to the fetus by continuing pregnancy are greater than those faced by the neonate after birth (selective IOL)
- Medical expert consensus favors IOL around 38^{+0} to 39^{+0} weeks of gestation for women with significant perinatal complications of pregnancy
- At term, low-risk women should be counseled about the risks and benefits of an IOL at 41^{+0} to 41^{+3} weeks of gestation compared with expectant management
- When determining timing of delivery, consider:
  - Identifying perinatal complications of pregnancy, e.g. pre eclampsia, gestational diabetes, intrauterine growth restriction
  - Results of antepartum fetal surveillance
  - Favorability of the cervix
  - Gestational age
  - Maternal preference and risks if the woman chooses expectant management.

Management Proper

During Pregnancy

- Establish appropriate gestational age
- Ensure fetal maturity
- Rule out other obstetric complications → if present → terminate pregnancy
- Discussion with patient explaining risks and benefits of induction and expectant management
- Offer induction at 40 completed weeks in all healthy uncomplicated pregnancies
- If willing for induction → induce
- If patient has opted for expectant management, monitor with:
  - Daily fetal kick count by the mother
  - Biweekly modified BPP (NST and AFI assessment)
  - BPP weekly (though Modified BPP is as sensitive as complete BPP)
  - Doppler → role in post-term pregnancy is not supported by evidence.
- Terminate at 42 weeks.

Intrapartum

- Left lateral position
- Watch for complications:
  Meconium
  - ↑ uteroplacental insufficiency (also contributed by ↓ liquor) → hypoxia in labor → activation of vagal stimulation
  - Early ARM in active phase may help.
  Macrosomia
  - Maternal and fetal birth trauma → one should be prepared to manage shoulder dystocia
  - Arrest of 1st and 2nd stage.
  Nonreassuring CTG
  - Continuous CTG monitoring
  - Should not lead to acidosis
  - In cases of equivocal tracings › fetal scalp stimulation and/or fetal scalp blood sampling may provide reassurance
  - Neonatologist → at the time of delivery.

Chapter 37

Polyhydramnios

Tania G Singh

Excessive accumulation of amniotic fluid, more than that expected for that gestational age. It is generally defined as:

- Amniotic fluid index (AFI) >20–25 cm
- Largest fluid pocket depth (maximal vertical pocket (MVP) >8 cm
- Overall amniotic fluid volume >1,500–2,000 cc^3
- Two diameter pocket (TDP) >50 cm^2

Classification

- Acute: within days, occurring usually in 2nd trimester
- Chronic: gradual, asymptomatic and occurs in 3rd trimester

Acute Polyhydramnios
Management:

- Spontaneous abortion occurs (most common)
- Relieve distress—decompression done
- Pregnancy terminated by low ROM → allow slow escape of fluid (head should be well-stabilized)
- If very precious pregnancy (though every pregnancy is precious) → repeated abdominal amniocentesis after ruling out fetal congenital abnormalities

Causes

Maternal (25–30%)

- Diabetes: commonly gestational diabetes
- Hypertension/pre eclampsia
- Maternal congestive heart failure.

Fetal (10–20%); Idiopathic (60–65%)

Clinical

Chief Complaints

- Unmanageable girth
- Shortness of breath
- Digestive discomfort
- Edema of lower extremities
- Increasing troublesome varicose veins
- Hyperemesis (in late pregnancy).

Signs

- Dyspnea even in lying position
- Evidence of pre eclampsia (hypertension, proteinuria/edema).

GPE

Per abdomen

Inspection

- Abdomen markedly enlarged, globular, fullness at flanks (like in ascites)
- Skin: tense, shiny, large striae.

Palpation

- Height of uterus more than period of gestation
- Girth of abdomen (round umbilicus) more than normal
- Fetus freely balloted
- Fluid thrill present
- Fetal parts may not be easily palpable
- External ballottment → more easily elicited
- Malpresentation common
- Lie: Unstable (may)
- If vertex presentation: Head likely to be high.

Auscultation

- FHS not well heard.

Investigations

USG

- For diagnosis
- Any associated fetal malformations should be looked for.

USG Criteria

The AFV can be assessed by ultrasound by using three main indirect parameters:
- Single deepest (maximum vertical) pocket method
- Amniotic fluid index
- Two diameter pocket method.

Largest Vertical Pocket (Deepest Pocket)

- Considered the best method of assessing amniotic fluid volume
- Performed by assessing a maximal depth of amniotic fluid which is free of umbilical cord
- The usually accepted values are:
    - less than 2 cm → indicative of oligohydramnios
    - 2–8 cm → normal but should be taken in the context of subjective volume
    - more than 8 cm → indicative of polyhydramnios
        - 8–11 cm → mild
        - 12–15 cm → moderate
        - more than 16 cm → severe.

Amniotic Fluid Index

- Sum of deepest pocket in 4 cord and extremity free quadrants in gravid uterus (using external maternal landmarks of umbilicus and linea nigra)
- Polyhydramnios, if AFI more than 24 cm
- Best definition: AFI more than 95th percentile (for Indian women at term ≈ 18.2 cm)
- More than 5 cm and less than 18–20 cm → considered normal (by most).

Management Options

Usually, minimal or no intervention required for idiopathic mild uncomplicated cases.
Options include:
- Improved maternal diabetes control
- Cesarean section, if there is profound macrosomia
- Therapeutic amniocentesis/amnioreduction
- Indomethacin antenatally for a short period.

Chapter 38

Oligohydramnios

Tania G Singh

Oligohydramnios

- Amniotic fluid volume <300–500 mL after midtrimester (≈ 24 weeks) because before that normal AFV is <500 mL
- AFI <5 cm
- Single vertical pocket <2 cm
- Two diameter pocket method <1 × 1 cm or <15 cm^2

FETAL CAUSES

Renal Tract Abnormalities

Bilateral Renal Agenesis

- Amniotic fluid volume will be normal until 20 weeks (due to other sources)
- Oligohydramnios mainly occur after 20 weeks when fetal urine becomes the prime source of amniotic fluid
- Number of dysmorphic characteristics develop over remaining weeks, as:
    - Potter's Facies
    - Marked pulmonary hypoplasia
    - Limb deformities
    - Generalized growth retardation.

Urinary Tract Obstruction

- Urethral obstruction and PUJ obstruction → bladder overdistention (MEGA CYSTITIS) with back pressure upon the kidneys
- There is progressive renal damage and bladder rupture
- Subsequently, renal failure and urinary ascites develop.

Genetic Abnormalities

Smith Lemli-Opitz syndrome; Meckel-Gruber syndrome.

GI Conditions

Aneuploidies, Chromosome Abnormalities, Genetic and Structural Defects and Metabolic Disorders

IUGR and Placental Insufficiency

Fetal Presentation (Breech)

Isolated (≈ 50%)

MATERNAL CAUSES

- Postdated pregnancy
- PROM (25% of cases) → but not all cases of PROM will have less liquor
- Hypertension

- Indomethacin (especially when used for prolonged periods) → ↓ in fetal urine production
- Autoimmune disorders
- Maternal hydration.

Clinical Features

- Uterus appears small for dates (with moderate to severe oligohydramnios)
- If IUGR is also present:
  - Fetal parts are easily palpated
  - Uterus feels as if clamped over fetal parts
  - Little ballotment.

USG

- Oligohydramnios diagnosis may be difficult, give amnioinfusion with normal saline and do detailed examination. Look for:
  - Fetal anatomy (mainly renal tract)
  - Fetal growth, parameters (for IUGR).
- Doppler: Umbilical artery (must be performed) → If ↑ S/D ratio → fetus at risk. If normal → ↓ iatrogenic morbidity.

Management

- Remote from term → prolong pregnancy, if possible with close fetal monitoring
- Near term → If there is associated IUGR (and/or hypertension) OR Abnormal UA Doppler in otherwise uncomplicated pregnancy, follow protocol for IUGR and termination planned accordingly
- If there is isolated oligohydramnios and normal FHR (but no maternal indication), induce electively
- While terminating pregnancy, monitor with continuous intrapartum FHR monitoring +/– amnioinfusion.

Role of Maternal Hydration

- Oral or IV → increases AFI up to 30% (But temporary)
- Oral → 2–4 litres of water/day
- IV → 2 litres of hypotonic (diluted) Ringer's lactate, but not isotonic (undiluted)
- Amino acid infusion (e.g. alamine SN) IV thrice/week. May be repeated after 3–4 weeks, if necessary
- Amnioinfusion: 250–500 mL RL
  - Transabdominally → antepartum
  - Transcervical → intrapartum
  - Uses: increases accuracy of USG diagnosis.

Complications

- Fetal distress; fetal death
- Pulmonary hypoplasia; Prematurity
- Pressure effects; Talipes
- Dislocated hips; Ankylosis of joints
- Intrauterine constriction of limb or amputation

Chapter 39

Cardiac Disease in Pregnancy

Tania G Singh

Symptoms in Pregnancy that Mimic Cardiac Disease

Pathological Symptoms
- Dyspnea on rest
- Paroxysmal nocturnal dyspnea
- Chest pain
- Cough/expectoration
- Syncopal attacks
- Hemoptysis

- Fatigue
- Decreased exercise capacity
- Palpitations
- Orthopnea
- Light-headedness
- Hyperventilation
- Breathlessness
- Ankle edema.

Signs in Pregnancy that Mimic Cardiac Disease

Pathological Signs
- Cyanosis
- S3/S4
- Diastolic murmur
- Pansystolic murmur
- Continuous murmur
- Atrial flutter or fibrillation
- Harsh basal murmur (with thrill)
- Cardiac enlargement

- JVP—Mildly distended
- Enlargement of heart with increase in LV volume
- Ejection fraction—not changed
- Apex beat displaced upwards into 4th intercostal space and may reach midclavicular line.

Approach to the Pregnant Patient

- Careful frequent history and physical examination at least once per trimester
- Functional class to be decided during 1st 4 months
- Diet/folic acid/vitamin B complex/calcium
- Investigations and referral:
    - All routine investigations
    - ECG—in diagnosis of arrhythmias (and not for structural abnormalities)
    - 2D echo—investigation of choice
    - CXR—not much useful
    - Refer to cardiologist at the first visit.
- Bed rest (class II and III) →12 hours at night and 2 hours during day
- Early part of pregnancy
    - Class I and II → seen monthly
    - Severe cases → weekly.
- More frequent monitoring if:
    - New symptoms develop
    - Changes in functional class.
- In case of valvular lesions
    - Mild valvular disease → monthly till 28–30 weeks, thereafter every 2 weeks or weekly

- – Moderate to severe valvular disease → every 2 weeks until 28–30 weeks, thereafter weekly
- – Hemodynamic changes intensify after the 26th–28th week, which is the most critical period along with the delivery.
- Following illnesses avoided and promptly attended to:
  - – Anemia—Hemoglobin at least once in each trimester
  - – UTI—urine culture in all cases (to exclude asymptomatic bacteriuria)
  - – Pre eclampsia—very serious.
- Any febrile illness, even in mild cold, patient should take rest
- Any dental procedures—prophylactic antibiotics as follows:
  High-risk patients:
  - – Ampicillin 2 gm IM or IV +
  - – Gentamycin 1.5 mg/kg (not >120 mg) within 30 minutes of starting procedure
  - – After 6 hours—ampicillin 1 gm IM or IV or amoxicillin 1 mg per os.
  High-risk (allergic to Penicillin):
  - – Vancomycin 1 mg over 1–2 hour + Gentamycin 1.5 mg/kg: complete infusion within 30 minutes of starting procedure.
  Moderate risk:
  - – Amoxicillin 2 gm per os (1 hour before procedure) OR
  - – Ampicillin 2 gm IM/IV (within 30 minutes of starting procedure).
  Moderate risk (allergic to Penicillin):
  - – Vancomycin 1 gm IV over 1–2 hour: complete infusion within 30 min of starting procedure.
- Weight gain not to exceed 0.6 kg in any one week
- Watch for earliest signs of failure—particular attention to lung bases
- Hydramnios may complicate the picture, therefore bed rest, diuretics, abdominal paracentesis, if required
- Reassessment by cardiologist at 28–32 weeks. Why?
  - – In later half of pregnancy, enlarging uterus causes displacement and rotation of heart and to some extent, splints diaphragm
  - – Inspite of splinting of diaphragm, vital capacity is not reduced but some compensation is provided by increase in diameter of thoracic cage
  - – Therefore, if checked between 28–32 weeks, one can make a reasonable estimate of how heart will behave during labor.
- Hospitalization:
  - – Class I and II with no other complications → admitted during last fortnight (dangers of transportation avoided)
  - – Severe cases (NYHA class III or in failure) → throughout pregnancy.
- Diuretics: if intravenous volume expansion is not normal
- Prophylactic digitalization :
  - – Improves contractility of heart
  - – Relieves fatigue ability/ orthopnea/ weakness
  - – Avoid ventricular tachycardia and rapid atrial rhythm.
- Anticoagulation in case of:
  - – CHD
  - – Artificial mechanical valve prosthesis
  - – Chronic or recurrent arrhythmias.
- Fetal echocardiography at 20–24 weeks
- ACE inhibitors are contraindicated
- Inj. Penidure LA12 (Benzathine Penicillin) at interval of 3–4 weeks throughout pregnancy to prevent risk of rheumatic fever

---

"NYHA Classification"

Grade I: No limitations of physical exercise; ordinary activity does not cause undue fatigue, palpitations, dyspnea or angina

Grade II: Slight limitations of physical exercise; ordinary activity results in fatigue, palpitations, dyspnea or angina

Grade III: Marked limitations of physical activity, less than ordinary activity causes symptoms

Grade IV: Inability to carry out physical activity without symptoms

3Es: Elevation of JVP + Enlarged liver + Edema of ankles are signs and symptoms of systemic or pulmonary venous congestion and are labeled as CHF

Pulse rate is best measured using a stethoscope and auscultating the heart because when the pulse becomes fast, irregular or faint, the radial pulse is often difficult to measure accurately

- Diagnosis should be made as per the present NYHA class (in case deterioration has occurred)
- A rising pulse rate can be one of the first signs of cardiac decompensation
- BP should be measured using a manual sphygmomanometer in a sitting, not talking position with appropriately sized cuff placed on the correct arm (for example, the right arm is usually used in women with coarctation of the aorta, 80% of whom will also have a bicuspid aortic valve) at the level of the left atrium
- Auscultation:
    - Murmur may increase by one grade as pregnancy advances because of increase in cardiac output
    - Sudden increase in loudness → suggests development of vegetations from endocarditis
    - Appearance of a new murmur is nearly always significant and requires urgent diagnosis and intervention
    - Lung bases posteriorly should be auscultated at each visit to check for crackles, which can indicate developing pulmonary edema (incipient heart failure).
- Apart from routine investigations in a cardiac case, others include:
    - Complains of chest pain → check troponin I levels and repeat after 24 hours
    - Suspicion of CAD → Treadmill test, first noninvasive test of choice
    - Suspicion of pulmonary embolism → measure of d-dimer levels → if ↑, anticoagulation
    - Doppler examination of leg vessels → to identify any DVT.

C h a p t e r 40

Macrosomia

Tania G Singh

UNDERSTANDING MACROSOMIA

- Generalized fetal enlargement
- Rare before 37 weeks of gestation and is more common in postdated pregnancy (≥42 weeks).

Causes

- Size of parents (especially mother → obesity)
- Poorly controlled diabetes milletus/GDM
- Postmaturity (>42 weeks)
- Multiparity
- Male fetus
- Erythroblastosis fetalis and other causes of hydrops
- Prior macrosomic infant.

Refers to fetal growth where EFW has surpassed a specific weight (4000 gms) regardless of gestational age, whereas large for gestational age is where the EFW >90th percentile for gestational age

Fetal Hazards

- Surprise dystocia due to CPD
- Shoulder dystocia
- Brachial plexus injury
- Asphyxia
- Birth trauma
- Meconium aspiration
- Clavicle fracture
- Humerus fracture
- HI encephalopathy
- Death.

USG

- Early clue to macrosomia may be provided by decreased FL/AC ratio (N → 22% ± 2). This ratio is quiet accurate provided abnormally small femur is ruled out
- Increased subcutaneous fat (may) → as a sonolucency separating scalp from skull by ≥4 mm (Diabetic Halo)

Maternal Hazards

- Injury to maternal soft tissues (vagina, perineum)
- PPH
- Puerperal sepsis
- Increased number of cesarean section.

Treatment

- Prophylactic (preterm) induction of labor to decrease risk of shoulder dystocia
- Elective cesarean section in diabetic mother with big baby.

Section III:

Attending Obstetric Emergencies

Chapter 41

Management of Incomplete Abortion

Tania G Singh

Assessment (Incomplete Abortion or Ectopic?)

Incomplete Abortion

- Reproductive age woman
- Presence of vaginal bleeding and/or abdominal pain
- One or more missed menstrual periods.

Ectopic Pregnancy

- Uterus is small
- Cervix is closed and/or there is an adnexal mass.

Management

If There is no Suspicion of Infection and Uterine Size is Less than 14 Weeks

- Uterine evacuation with vacuum aspiration OR
- Misoprostol 600 micrograms orally or 400 micrograms sublingually.

If There is no Suspicion of Infection and Uterine Size is 14 Weeks or Larger

- Evacuation using vacuum aspiration and blunt forceps if necessary OR
- Misoprostol:
  - 14–28 weeks: 200 micrograms administered vaginally, sublingually or buccally at least 6-hourly
  - If possible, mifepristone 200 mg orally should be administered 12–48 hours before misoprostol
  - After 28 weeks: 25 micrograms vaginally 6-hourly or 25 micrograms orally 2-hourly.

> Antibiotic prophylaxis should be given before surgical evacuation—200 mg doxycycline within 2 hours before the procedure or a single dose of 500 mg azithromycin within 2 hours before the procedure

Instructions before Discharging

- In case of persistent and/or heavy bleeding or pain abdomen, report immediately
- Wait for at least one normal menstrual period or longer in case of severe anemia, if further conception is required
- Adequate contraception advice to be given and all methods should be discussed with the patient
- IUD insertion or female sterilization should be delayed until the woman's health is restored and any infection is resolved
- Interim contraception should be provided using the most effective acceptable method until an IUD can be inserted or sterilization performed
- If available, anti-D IgG should be given intramuscularly to all nonsensitized RhD-negative women within 72 hours following abortion.

Chapter 42

Ruptured Ectopic Pregnancy

Tania G Singh

- Surgical route is the option in case of ruptured ectopic pregnancy
- There are two options—Laparotomy and laparoscopic surgery.

Laparotomy

- If patient is unstable → Laparotomy (preferred and is an absolute indication)
- Also indicated when location is other than tubal pregnancy (ovarian, cervical, interstitial pregnancy).

Laparoscopic Approach

- Usually employed in hemodynamically (with obvious abdominal hemorrhage that requires definitive treatment) stable patient
- In unruptured ectopic (cases where medical management is either not possible or not opted)
- Advantages:
  - Faster recovery
  - Shorter hospitalization
  - Reduced overall costs
  - Less pain, bleeding and adhesion formation
  - Lower analgesic requirements.

Laparoscopy Versus Open Approach

- No difference in overall tubal patency rates
- No difference in subsequent intrauterine pregnancy rates
- But there is a trend towards lower repeat ectopic pregnancy rates with laparoscopy.

Salphingectomy

- Segmental or entire removal of fallopian tube
- Indications:
  - Recurrent ectopic pregnancy in the same tube
  - Severely damaged tube
  - Uncontrolled bleeding (before or after salphingostomy) both for ruptured or unruptured ectopics
  - Heterotopic pregnancy
  - Lack of desire to bear more children.
- Partial salphingectomy can be performed when ectopic pregnancy is small and fimbriae appear healthy.

Surgery can be offered as the 1st line of management in the following cases:

- Ectopic pregnancy with significant pain
- Ectopic pregnancy with adnexal mass of ≥35 mm
- Ectopic pregnancy with cardiac activity
- Ectopic pregnancy with serum hCG ≥5,000 mIU/mL
- When patient is hemodynamically unstable
- When patient is not compliant
- When patient is breastfeeding
- Heterotopic pregnancy in hemodynamically stable patient
- Tubal rupture in hemodynamically stable patient
- Imminent risk of rupture
- No desire for or an inability to comply with medical management
- Contraindication to methotrexate
- Failure of medical management such as tubal pregnancy >5 cm or fetal cardiac activity seen on TVS

Salphingostomy

- Method of choice in women of reproductive age who wish to preserve their fertility
- For removing pregnancy less than 2 cm in length and located in distal 1/3rd of fallopian tube
- Typically performed by making a linear incision ($\approx$ 10–15 mm) on the antimesenteric border of the fallopian tube at the point of maximal distention (i.e. over the ectopic)
- Removing the products of conception by hydrodissection is recommended, avoiding:
  - Excessive handling of the tube
  - Excessive cautery to prevent further damage to the fallopian tube.
- Incision left unsutured to heal by 2° intention
- Rate of intrauterine pregnancy is improved in patients having linear salpingostomy but recurrent ectopic rate is also higher
- Readily performed through laparoscope
- Drawback: Risk of persistent trophoblast (incomplete removal of trophoblastic tissue, resulting in rising or plateauing serum β hCG postoperatively) and repeat ectopic pregnancy.

Salphingotomy

- Same procedure as salphingostomy except that incision is closed with 7-0 vicryl or similar suture.

Preliminaries before and after the Surgery

- Quick thorough history
- Physical examination
- Vitals
- Secure IV line and start IV fluids till blood and blood products are made available
- Foley catheter insertion
- Minimum required investigations before the surgery: CBC, ABO Rh, HIV, HbsAg, TVS
- Arrange at least 2 units of blood initially
- Anti-D within 72 hours of surgery, if Rhesus negative
- In cases of salphingectomy, perform UPT after 3 weeks
- In cases of salphingotomy, perform serum hCG after 1 week and then weekly until the results are negative
- Contraception advised
- Risk of recurrence and future pregnancy rates discussed before discharge.

Surgery can be:
Conservative
- Salphingostomy
- Salphingotomy
- Fimbrial expression of ectopic pregnancy

Radical: Salphingectomy

Key Points
- In the presence of a healthy contralateral tube, there is no clear evidence that salphingostomy should be used in preference to salphingectomy
- Laparoscopic salphingostomy should be considered as primary treatment when managing tubal pregnancy in the presence of contralateral tubal disease and the desire for future fertility

Chapter 43

Abruptio Placenta

Tania G Singh

Abruptio Placenta
Partial or complete separation of a normally implanted placenta from it's attachment on the uterine wall, after the 20th week of pregnancy but before delivery

RISK FACTORS

- Prior abruption
- Maternal hypertensive disorders
- IUGR (fetal growth restriction)
- Rapid uterine decompression as in case of
  - Polyhydramnios and twin gestation.
- Nonvertex presentations
- Increasing parity
- Trauma (Blunt or penetrating)
- Bleeding in the 1st trimester
- Preterm premature rupture of membranes
- Low body mass index (BMI)
- Inherited or acquired thrombophilia
- Uterine and placental factors
  - Placental implantation over a uterine malformation (e.g. septum or fibroid)
  - Placental abnormalities (e.g. circumvallate placenta).
- Pregnancy following assisted reproductive technique
- Intrauterine infection
- Smoking
- Cocaine abuse during pregnancy.

Predominant Locations for Placental Abruption
Retroplacental abruption: Blood collection behind the placenta (between placenta and myometrium)
Subchorionic abruption: Between placenta and membranes
Preplacental abruption:
- Between placenta and amniotic fluid
- Anterior to the placenta within amnion and chorion

CLASSIFICATION
Ernest Page's Classification

There are 4 grades:

Grade 0

- No symptoms
- Retrospective diagnosis by finding an organized blood clot or a depressed area on the delivered placenta.

Grade I

- Mild abruption
- Variable bleeding per vaginum
- Slightly tender/irritable uterus
- Normal maternal BP and heart rates
- No coagulopathy.

- No fetal distress
- Constitutes ≈ 40–48%.

Grade II

- Partial abruption
- Mild to moderate vaginal bleeding
- Moderate-to-severe uterine tenderness with possible tetanic contractions
- Maternal tachycardia with orthostatic changes in BP and heart rate
- Fetal distress
- Hypofibrinogenemia may be present
- Account for ≈ 45% of all placental abruptions.

Grade III

- Large to complete abruption
- Moderate to heavy vaginal bleeding
- Very painful tetanic uterus
- Maternal
  - Shock; coagulopathy
  - Anuria; fetal death—is a rule.
- Constitutes 15%.

CLINICAL FEATURES

- Although vaginal bleeding is the hallmark of placental abruption, in 10–20% cases, it may be occult or concealed
- Pain—prominent feature, which may be due to:
  - Extravasation of blood into the myometrium
  - Overdistension of the uterus due to retroplacental bleeding
  - Frequent contractions associated with the release of prostaglandins.
- Uterine contractions may start causing additional, intermittent pain
- Contractions characteristically have a:
  - High frequency but
  - Low amplitude (5 per 10 minutes → "sawtooth" pattern)
  - An elevated baseline tone.
- Uterus → extremely hard and tender, it does not relax
- Fetal parts are difficult to palpate especially when blood is accumulating inside
- If the membranes are ruptured, blood-stained liquor may be seen
- FHR inaudible, if death has occurred
- Fetal head may have entered the pelvic brim
- Pre eclampsia may be associated in 1/3rd of cases
- Faintness and collapse, in severe cases.

MANAGEMENT

Active Management

- Resuscitation
  - IV access (large wide bore cannulas)
  - Crystalloids followed by transfusion of blood and blood products.
- O_2 by mask
- Investigations
  - Hemoglobin; hematocrit; platelet count; fibrinogen

Important Observations in Grade III Abruption

- About 40% of patients will demonstrate signs of DIC
- Within 8 hours of initial symptoms in such women, hypofibrinogenemia will be present
- It will not recover without blood products
- Hypofibrinogenemia recovery is 10 mg/dL/hr after delivery of fetus and placenta

Sher's Classification

Stage I: Mild form with
- Unexplained vaginal bleeding
- Retrospective diagnosis of a small hematoma postpartum

Stage II: Intermediate form with
- A hypertonic uterus
- A live fetus

Stage III: Severe form with
- Intrauterine death of the fetus
- IIIa → Without coagulopathy
- IIIb → With coagulopathy

- LFT; RFT with electrolytes
- Blood group and typing; coagulation profile
- Continuous FHR monitoring
- Expedite delivery once mother stabilizes
- Prevention of complications.

Expectant Management

If abruption is mild and self-limiting or diagnosis of abruption is not conclusive.

Management Proper

- Stabilization of mother is most important
- Maternal hemodynamic and clotting parameters must be followed closely.

Scenario I

- Grade I abruption; preterm; mother and fetus → stable
- Hospitalization
- Tocolysis
- Steroids.

Scenario II

- Fetus is already dead (term or preterm) → aim for vaginal delivery
- Induction or augmentation of labor is not contraindicated but with close surveillance.

Scenario III

- Fetus is alive; not in labor
- Gestation not so early as to make fetal survival extremely unlikely
- Deliver by cesarean section.

Scenario IV

- Fetus is alive and patient in established labor
- Augmentation (ARM + oxytocin)
- Expedite delivery with strict monitoring and continuous
- Continuous FHR monitoring is recommended because 60% of fetuses may exhibit nonreassuring heart rate.

Massive and/or Repeated Hemorrhage in Placenta Previa

Tania G Singh

- Hospitalize the patient
- Written and informed consent
- General condition and vitals of the patient and assessment of degree of shock
- Estimation of amount of bleeding (number of pads used/soiled clothes)
- Wide bore cannula
- Immediately start IV fluids
- Draw blood for investigations
- Catheterize the patient
- Foot-end elevation
- Per abdominal examination (uterine activity, tenderness, FHS)
- Give corticosteroids, if gestation is less than 34 completed weeks
- Blood and blood products arranged and transfused according to laboratory reports
- Bleeding stops:
  - Expectant management (Macafee regime)
  - Per speculum examination to rule out any local cause.
- Bleeding continues:
  - Immediate intervention
  - Fluids on flow
  - Blood made available
  - Shift the patient to OT.
- USG assessment of:
  - Fetal well-being
  - Placental localization and distance from internal os
  - Fetal abnormality (contraindication to expectant Rx)
- In operation theatre (Double set-up examination)
  - Anesthetist with arrangements for general anesthesia ready
  - Lithotomy position—according to surgeon's preference
  - Per speculum examination—to rule out any local lesions
  - Per vaginal examination:
    - Index and middle fingers are introduced uptil fornices
    - Push fetal head into brim from above.
- If head is felt through all fornices:
  - No placenta previa or minor degree previa
  - Insert fingers gently into cervix
  - Explore (any soft and friable tissue may be a simple blood clot)
  - Sweep the finger 360° around internal os,
    - If slight bleed is present—rupture the membranes and try to bring the head down

> **If patient is Rh negative,** Kleiheuer-Betke test is done to know the amount of fetomaternal bleed and anti-D immunoglobulin is given accordingly

Low Transverse Skin Incision

Allows access to the lower half of the uterus.

Can be given in cases where the upper margin of the anterior aspect of placenta does not rise into the upper segment of the uterus

Midline Skin Incision

When placenta is anterior and is extending towards the level of the umbilicus.

Uterine incision— high upper segment longitudinal uterine incision or high transverse incision or a fundal incision

Consequences of Leaving the Placenta in Situ

Can have a normal subsequent pregnancy.

Elective evacuation of retained products of conception.

Increased chances of infection → can even lead to sepsis.

Heavy bleeding requiring hysterectomy

- If bleeding has stopped: Shift out of OT
- If heavy bleeding present—keep the fingers in the cervix (act as a plug), pack vagina with roller gauze, change gloves and proceed with cesarean section.

- If any overriding mass/thickness is felt:
  - Placenta previa present
  - Proceed with C. section.

Delivery by Cesarean Section

- Choice of skin and uterine incisions solely depends upon the location of placenta, hence the need for USG before surgery
- The baby may also be delivered by passing a hand round the margins of the placenta, or by incising the placenta
- Breech extraction can also be performed by grasping one of the baby's feet and pulling, which would be better than to struggle for quiet a high-head
- If the placenta is cut, immediate clamping of the cord is recommended
- Troublesome separation of placenta
  - Do not continue attempting separation of placenta, if it is not separating with the usual methods (which will eventually land up in hysterectomy)
  - Two options, that can be attempted are:
    - Leaving the placenta in place and closing
    - Leaving the placenta in place, closing the uterus and performing hysterectomy.
- If the placenta separates partially (partial accreta)
  - Remove the separated part
  - Leave the nonseparated part in situ
  - But massive hemorrhage may ensue—all measures to combat the problem should be ready, saving the patient from DIC.
- Management of retained placenta:
  - Risks of increased bleeding and infection should be explained
  - Appropriate antibiotics started from the immediate postpartum period
  - Neither methotrexate nor arterial embolization helps in avoiding the above complications, therefore, not recommended routinely
  - Patient should be followed up by serial USG and measurement of β-hCG on weekly basis, to see for placental resolution.

Chapter 45

Impending Eclampsia

Tania G Singh

Symptoms/Signs of Impending Eclampsia

- Severe hypertension with proteinuria
- Persistent neurological symptoms—Headache (occipital or frontal), restlessness, agitation, phosphene signals, tinnitus, and brisk, diffuse, polykinetic tendon reflexes
- Visual disturbance—blurred vision, photophobia
- Fundoscopy—marked retinal edema, severe hemorrhages, exudates and papilloedema
- Epigastric and/or RUQ pain
- Nausea/vomiting
- Oliguria
- Renal impairment—Serum creatinine higher than 106 μmol/L
- Laboratory evidence of DIC/HELLP syndrome
- Sudden swelling of face, hands or feet
- Signs of clonus (≥3 beats)
- Platelets less than 1 lakh/mm^3
- Liver enzymes more than 70 IU/lit
- Pulmonary edema
- "Pre eclamptic angina"—severe epigastric pain and/or vomiting with abnormal liver enzymes.

Management

- Main aim—to prevent seizures
- No role of ambulatory management
- Expectant management at tertiary care centre
- If symptoms developed at home—keep in bed; sedate and transfer
- On admission to hospital:
    - Quiet darkened room
    - Sedated, if required
    - IV access.
- Antihypertensives
- Prophylactic MgSO$_4$ (after catheterization)
    - Pritchard regime (× 24 hours) or stat dose according to progress
    - Look for signs of magnesium toxicity
- Investigations
- Maintain O$_2$ saturation
- Fluids—use judiciously.

But eclampsia may not develop even in the presence of following signs:

- Severe headaches (especially occipital)
- Brisk reflexes >3+
    - 3+ is hyperactive without clonus
    - 4+ is hyperactive with unsustained clonus
    - 5+ is hyperactive with sustained clonus
- Visual disturbances

Antihypertensive in Hospital

- At '0'hrs: Inj. Labetelol 20 mg IV (over 2 min)
- At '20' min.: If BP> 150/100 mm Hg, double the dose every 20 min (20 mg, 40 mg, 80 mg, 80 mg) till a maximum dose of 220 mg/hour

Signs of Magnesium Toxicity

- Respiratory rate <16/minutes
- Urine output <30 mL/hr or <100 mL in 4 hours
- Absent patellar reflexes

Fundus Changes in Hypertensive Disorders

Grade I
- Mild arteriolar constriction
- Broadening of light reflex

Grade II
- Attenuation of vessels
- Deflection at A-V crossings (Salu's sign)

Grade III
- Salu's sign
- Banking of veins (Bonnet)
- Tappering of veins (Gunns)
- Copper wire vessels
- Cotton wool spots
- Hard exudates

Grade IV
- Silver wire papilloedema

Excessive fluid administration can result in pulmonary edema, ascites and cardiopulmonary overload, whereas too little fluid exacerbates an already constricted intravascular volume and leads to further end-organ ischemia.

Urine output should be >30 mL per hour and intravenous fluids limited to 100 mL/ hour (≈ 1 mL/kg/hour, using present weight) unless there are other ongoing losses (input/output charting)

Maternal

- CBC with platelets
- Urine protein (midstream urine sample)
- 24 hour urinary protein
- KFT with electrolytes
- LFT (AST, ALT, LDH and bilirubin)
- If platelet count is less than 1 lakh/mm^3 → coagulation profile and peripheral smear
- Fundoscopy.

Fetal

- NST, if gestational age more than 32 weeks
- USG (gestational age, AFI, abruption, IUGR)
- Doppler, if IUGR
- Depending upon gestational age
  Less than 28 weeks (EFW<1 kg) or more than 34 weeks
  - Antihypertensives
  - Prophylactic MgSO$_4$
  - Termination (induction with prostaglandins).
  28–34 weeks
  - Antihypertensives; steroids
  - Prophylactic MgSO$_4$
  - Investigations
  - After 48–72 hours: manage as below, depending upon BP readings.
- BP Controlled → Expectant Management
  Maternal:
  - Bed rest; 4 hourly BP Daily
  - I/O charting
  - Daily LFT, KFT, platelet count
  - Daily urine albumin.
  Fetal:
  - DFKC; Daily NST; Biweekly Doppler and AFI
  - USG for fetal growth every 2 weeks.
- Stable → terminate at 34 weeks
- BP uncontrolled → termination.

Factors Mandating Immediate Delivery

Maternal

- Uncontrolled Hypertension
- Progressive deterioration of hepatic and/or renal function
- HELLP syndrome
- Eclampsia/Persistent neurologic signs
- Labor
- Gestational age more than or equal to 37 weeks
- Acute pulmonary edema.

Fetal

- Nonreassuring NST
- Severe IUGR with abnormal Doppler
- Placental Abruption
- AFI lower than 5 cms.

Chapter 46

Eclampsia

Tania G Singh

Risk Factors

- Primary prevention of eclampsia → Prevent women from developing pre eclampsia
- Family history
- Little or no antenatal care
- Age less than 20 years
- Having had more than or equal to 4 previous pregnancies
- More than or equal to 2 signs and symptoms of imminent eclampsia (such as headache, epigastric pain, hyperreflexia, visual disturbances and severe hypertension).

Time of Occurrence

- Antepartum—50% (mostly in T3)
- Intrapartum—10-20%
- Postpartum—30% (Fits occurring beyond 7 days of delivery rules out eclampsia).

Status Eclampticus

- When the fits occur in quick succession
- Give Inj. Thiopentone sodium 0.5 mg in 20 mL of 5% D IV slowly.

Clinical Features

Eclamptic Fit (Grandmal Seizures).

Stage I: Premonitory Stage (10–20 seconds)

- Eyes roll or stare
- Muscles of face and hand may twitch
- Loss of consciousness.

Stage II: Tonic Stage (10–20 seconds)

- Muscle—stiff or rigid
- Spasm of diaphragm, breathing stops and cyanosis occurs (1-2 minute)
- Back arched
- Teeth clenched
- Eyes bulge.

Definition

Occurrence of convulsions or coma unrelated to other cerebral conditions with signs and symptoms of pre eclampsia during pregnancy or postpartum

Convulsions Occur due to:

- Cerebral vasospasm
- Cerebral hemorrhage
- Cerebral ischemia
- Cerebral edema
- Hypertensive encephalopathy

Intercurrent (Antenatal) Fits

When patient becomes conscious after recovery from convulsions and pregnancy continues beyond 48 hours

Atypical Eclampsia

Occurring before 20 weeks gestation or >48 hours postpartum Before 20 weeks:

- Molar pregnancy or hydropic degeneration of placenta
- Multiple gestation
- Antiphospholipid antibody syndrome

Stage III: Clonic Stage (1–2 minute)

- Violent contraction and relaxation of muscles
- Increased salivation and frothing
- Deep, noisy breathing
- Face looks congested and swollen
- Tongue may be bitten.

Stage IV: Coma Stage (several minutes to hours)

- Deep unconsciousness
- Breathing—noisy and rapid
- Cyanosis fades but face remains congested and swollen
- Further fits may occur before woman regains consciousness.

Other Features

- Absence of other neurologic conditions
- Almost always associated with hypertension and proteinuria
- Convulsions can occur even with diastolic BP of 90–100 mm Hg
- Proteinuria → can be as high as 15–20 g/day to even very low amounts
- Most cases, occurring before or shortly (<24 hours) after onset of labor → rapid progression to delivery
- Late postpartum eclampsia: more than 48 hours but within 4 weeks postpartum
- Fits can be 1 or occurring at regular intervals → status epilepticus
- Fetus at the time of fit: Profound hypoxia and lactic acidemia after convulsions adversely affects the fetus → fetal bradycardia even up to 3–5 minutes can lead to intrauterine fetal death.

MANAGEMENT OF ECLAMPSIA

Management of Convulsion

Referral

- If symptoms developed at home, patient is kept in bed
- Sedate the patient
- Transferred to tertiary care centre
- A doctor or midwife or paramedical worker should accompany the patient and her relatives
- Inform place of referral by telephone (so that proper arrangements can be made and treatment is not delayed)
- Semiprone position with mouth gag in situ
- Give loading dose of $MgSO_4$ at PHC, if possible
- Nifedepine 10 mg orally, if BP more than or equal to 160/110 mm Hg
- Maintain IV line with Ringers lactate at a very slow rate.

On Admission to Hospital

- Work with speed → it takes only 4 minutes for permanent brain damage, if the brain is deprived of oxygen
- If the woman is anemic, she will withstand lack of oxygen less well
- Keep the patient in quiet, darkened room
- Any stimulus (noise, bright light, handling the woman) may precipitate a fit, so external stimuli are reduced to a minimum

---

Intrauterine fetal death at the time of fit may be due to:
- Intrauterine anoxia
- Cerebral hemorrhage
- Prematurity

Fluid Management

Extremely important in case of pre eclampsia and eclampsia. In these patients, though there is hypovolemia, the tissues are overloaded and any excess fluid will aggravate tissue overload → pulmonary edema and ARDS

Ringer lactate – fluid of choice

Total fluids → urine output (In previous 24 hours) + 1000 mL (Insensible loss through lungs and skin)

Normally ≤2 litres/24 hours, that is ≈ 75–100 mL/hr

- Sedated, if required but not to be left alone
- To be kept NPO
- Do not try to stop the convulsion
- Duration of convulsion to be noted
- Minimize risk of aspiration
- Lateral decubitus position
- Vomitus/oral secretion sucked out (suction apparatus in easy approach)
- Oxygenation 8–10 L/min after auscultating lung bases for rales
- Prevent tongue bite (insert a padded tongue blade between teeth)
- Prevent maternal injury from fall off the bed. Bed side rails should be padded and elevated
- Establish 2 IV lines
  - Draw blood for investigations from one
  - Administer $MgSO_4$ from other.
- Fluids very slowly at the rate of 75–100 mL/hour
- Catheterize the patient with Foley's catheter attached to a urometer/ urobag and hourly input/output charting should be maintained
- If BP ≥ 50/100 mm Hg, give IV labetalol or Nifedepine
- Reassure relatives and explain the prognosis
- Monitoring:
  - Pulse rate, BP using pulse oximeter
  - Sudden drop in BP may indicate either abruption or an IUD
  - Respiratory rate and FHS monitored hourly
  - RR should not be less than 12/minutes which may indicate cerebral hemorrhage
  - Temperature checked every 4 hourly
  - Turn the woman every 2 hourly to avoid hypostatic pneumonia
  - Intermittent chest auscultation
  - Level of consciousness should be noted
  - Urine output hourly (should be minimum 30 mL/hour or 100 mL in 4 hours)
  - Any signs of twitching or restlessness are to be looked for
  - Sudden cyanosis may indicate cardiac failure.
- Stabilize the patient before delivery
- Arterial blood gas analysis (ABG), if saturation lower than 92%
- P/V → assess cervical status
- Never be in a haste to deliver.

Investigations

Maternal

- Hematocrit; urine (albumin/microscopy); 24 hour urine protein
- Renal function tests with electrolytes
- Liver function tests
- Platelet count, if count less than 1 lakh/mm^3, send
  - Coagulation profile/serum fibrinogen
  - Peripheral smear.
- Blood film to rule out malaria (as a part of initial investigation in all patients presenting with a convulsion)
- Fundoscopy
- NST, if less than 32 weeks (optional).

Labetelol Dose

- '0' hours: Inj. Labetelol 20 mg IV (over 2 minutes)
- If BP >150/100 mm Hg, double the dose every 20 minutes
- After '20 minutes' of first dose: Inj. Labetelol 40 mg IV
- At '40 minutes': Inj. Labetelol 80 mg IV
- '60 minutes': Inj. Labetelol 80 mg IV
- Total → 220 mg/hour

Nifedepine Dose

- '0 hours': Nifedepine 10 mg orally stat
- After '30 minutes': If BP >150/100, opt 10 mg every 30 minutes (check BP every 15 minutes)
- Once BP is controlled (≤150/100 mm Hg), maintain with nifedepine 10 mg every 6 hourly till maximum of 120 mg/day

<table>
<tr><td valign="top" width="30%">

Magnesium Infusion (Continuous IV Regimen)

- 4 g loading dose IV over 15–20 minutes [can be repeated at a half dose (2 g) if convulsion recurs] followed by infusion of 1g/hour maintained for 24 hours

Zuspan Regimen

- Loading dose: Inj. $MgSO_4$ 4 gm IV over 15–20 minutes
- Maintenance dose: IV Infusion 1gm/hour
- Total duration of therapy = 24 hours

Sibai Regimen

- 6 gm $MgSO_4$ over 20 minutes followed by 2 gm $MgSO_4$ IV infusion
- Overall maternal mortality: 0.4%

</td><td valign="top">

Fetal

- USG for
  - Gestational age; fetal heart rate; AFI; Lie and presentation in case immediate delivery is anticipated
  - Placental localization
  - To rule out IUGR and abruption.
- Doppler, if IUGR
- Cerebral imaging in women with
  - Neurological deficits
  - Prolonged coma
  - Convulsions less than 20 weeks or more than 48 hours after delivery
  - Eclampsia refractory to $MgSO_4$ regimen.

Control of convulsions → $MgSO_4$ therapy.

Different Regimens Using MgSO$_4$

Pritchard's Regimen

Loading dose: IV (with 1 mL, 2% lidocaine solution)

- 8 mL $MgSO_4$ (4 gm) + 12 mL DW → Inj. 20 mL sol (slow over 20 minutes) IM
- 10 gm drug → 20 mL
- 5 gm + 5 gm in each buttock.

Maintenance dose:

- 5 gm deep IM in alternate buttock x 4 hourly
- Total → 39 gm.

</td></tr>
</table>

<table>
<tr><td valign="top" width="30%">

Signs	Magnesium Levels (mg/dL)
Loss of patellar reflex	10–12
Respiratory arrest	14.6
Paralysis	15.0
Cardiac arrest	30

</td><td valign="top">

Precautions while Giving Magnesium Sulphate

- Do not give nifedepine sublingually
- Do not give nifedepine with $MgSO_4$ → marked hypotension because of synergistic effect of Mg^{2+} ions on Ca^{2+} channel function
- Side effects: Palpitations, flushing, headache, ankle edema, nausea, hypotension
- Look for signs of magnesium toxicity
- Routine monitoring of magnesium levels is not necessary as it is costly and unnecessary (but may be done in women with impaired renal function →↑ magnesium toxicity)
- Withhold drug, if the following is observed:
  - Loss of patellar reflex
  - Urine output <100 mL in previous 4 hours
  - Respiratory rate <16/min.
- Antidote:
  - Inj. Calcium gluconate (10%) 10 mL IV over 3 minutes
  - May cause bradycardia and arrhythmia.

</td></tr>
</table>

<table>
<tr><td valign="top" width="30%">

Management of Recurrent Convulsion

- Convulsion occurring 30 minutes after loading dose or at any time later
- Once convulsion is ceased, administer 2 gm $MgSO_4$ (4 mL) + 6 mL distilled water (to make a total of 10 mL)
- Give slowly over 5–10 minutes

</td><td valign="top">

Obstetric Management

- Stabilize the mother
- Antihypertensives
- Anticonvulsant
- Expedite the process of delivery (regardless of gestational age)
- Other obstetric complications present, lower segment cesarean section
- No other obstetric complication:
  - *In labor*
    - ARM and oxytocin drip.

</td></tr>
</table>

- Cut short 2nd stage
- Avoid Methergin.

Not in labor
- Induction with prostaglandins
- Wait for 10–12 hours
- Progress—deliver
- No progress—LSCS.

Effect of Eclampsia on Mother and the Fetus

Effects on Mother

- Injuries during convulsions
  - Tongue bite
  - Fractures (due to fall from the bed)
  - Bed sores.
- Respiratory problems
  - Asphyxia; aspiration of vomitus
  - Pulmonary edema (due to leaky blood capillaries)
  - Bronchopneumonia (aspiration, hypostatic, infective)
  - ARDS; Embolism.
- Visual disturbances
  - Temporary blindness due to edema of the retina
  - Retinal detachment or occipital lobe ischemia.
- Hyperpyrexia
- HELLP syndrome (Hemolysis; Elevated liver enzymes; Low platelet count)
- Disseminated intravascular coagulopathy
- Effects on the brain
  - Hemorrhage, thrombosis, edema.
- Liver necrosis
- Left ventricular failure
- Acute renal failure
- Postpartum—shock, sepsis, psychosis.

Effects on Fetus

- Immediately after an eclamptic fit, fetal bradycardia occurs for 3–5 minutes
- If it occurs for more than 10 minutes, evaluate for uterine hyperstimulation or abruption
- Mortality 30–50%
- Prematurity; IUGR
- Intrauterine and postnatal asphyxia
- Effects of all the drugs used
- Admission to NICU.

Indications of Cesarean Section

(Carried out under general anesthesia after excluding coagulopathy)

- Uncontrolled fits despite therapy
- Unconscious patient
- Poor prospect of vaginal delivery (unfavorable cervix, nonreassuring FHR pattern on NST)
- Obstetric indication (malpresentation, etc.)

Chapter 47

Epileptic Fit in Pregnancy

Tania G Singh

Effects of Epilepsy on Pregnancy and Fetus

- Increased risk of IUGR/small for gestational age/oligohydramnios/still births/spontaneous abortions/anemia/preterm birth/induced labor/cesarean section/PPH
- Increased risk of fetal malformations
- Small HC at birth
- Low Apgar scores
- All anticonvulsants has adverse effects on fetus (discussed later).

Effects of Pregnancy on Epilepsy

- The condition may worsen, improve, or be unaffected by pregnancy
- Frequency of convulsions → unchanged in 50% and increases in some
- Estrogens probably activate seizure foci
- Increased plasma clearance of anticonvulsant drugs during pregnancy
- On mother → 3rd trimester bleeding and megaloblastic anemia may be related to anticonvulsant induced folate deficiency.

Dosages

- Phenobarbitone 60–180 mg daily (in 2–3 divided doses)
- Phenytoin 150–300 mg daily in 2 divided doses
- Carbamazepine 0.8–1.2 gm daily in divided doses.

During Fits

- Inj. Diazepam IV 10–20 mg
- Vitamin K 10 mg daily orally → in last 2 weeks
- Normal labor and delivery can be anticipated.

Preconceptional Counseling

- Explain the effects of epilepsy on pregnancy and fetus and vice versa
- Detailed information to the woman on risks and benefits of AEDs
- Take AED serum concentrations as reference value
- Instruct the woman to report to the obstetrician as soon as pregnancy is diagnosed
- Consultation with neurologist
- Polytherapy → changed to monotherapy (at lowest effective dose)
- Folic acid 1mg daily (for at least 1 month preconceptionally and throughout pregnancy)
- Importance of prenatal diagnosis to be discussed

Management

Antepartum

- Pregnancy unplanned—which means fetus has already been exposed to the current drug
- Pregnancy planned—change drugs at least 6 months before pregnancy to see for any change
- Monitor AED serum concentrations as soon as pregnancy is established and then monthly
- Consider increase in dose of the drug by 25% when serum concentrations fall below the patient's prepregnancy reference value or according to clinical needs
- Change in medicine may increase maternal seizures
- Any change, if done should be under the supervision of neurologist
- Folic acid 1 mg daily
- Risk of seizures is higher in 1st trimester and around delivery time
- Serum alpha-fetoprotein should be done, ideally at the end of 1st trimester though not compulsory
- NT scan at 11–13 weeks
- Anamoly scan (Level II) at 18–22 weeks
- Nonprotein bound ("free") drug levels should be obtained (remain constant)
- Total levels ↓ during pregnancy because of ↑ blood flow, ↑ hepatic and renal clearance of drug.

Intrapartum

- IV line
- Continue taking antiepileptics
- Maternal exhaustion avoided
- "Water birth" (laboring in water) → NOT recommended
- GTCS → associated with hypoxia, therefore, continuous CTG monitoring in an event of seizure
- Inj. Lorazepam/Diazepam → recommended to terminate a seizure
- Be careful, loss of baseline variability of FHR tracing expected for 1 hour after this.

Status Epilepticus

Causes

- Withdrawal of anticonvulsant drug
- Metabolic derangements (electrolyte abnormalities, hypo- or hyperglycemia, etc.)
- Eclampsia
- CVS infection, head trauma.

Management

- Correct serum hypoglycemia, if present
- Obtain blood samples for glucose, electrolytes, AED levels
- Consult neurologist
- Rest same as eclampsia management
- For continuous seizures, Inj. Lorazepam IV 2–8 mg in 2 mg increments → Drug of choice
- For intermittent seizures, use Inj. Phenytoin 20 mg/kg IV at less than 50 mg/min
- If phenytoin fails, phenobarbital 20–30 mg/kg IV
- If both phenytoin and phenobarbital fail → paraldehyde 3–5 mL deep IM.

AED Level Measurements in Pregnancy:
- Before conception (baseline)
- At beginning of each trimester
- During last 4 weeks of pregnancy
- Additional monitoring if any change in seizure frequency

Status Epilepticus
Continuous seizure activity that persists for ≥30 minutes or as recurrent seizures that occur without full recovery between attacks

Chapter 48

Preterm Labor

Tania G Singh

Risk Factors for Preterm Birth

- Past obstetric history
  - Previous spontaneous preterm birth
  - Previous second trimester abortions
  - Use of ART.
- Present pregnancy
  - Antepartum hemorrhage
  - Rupture of membranes
  - Cervical/uterine factors
    - Cervical insufficiency/uterine anomalies
    - Fibroids/excisional cervical treatment for CIN.
- Fetal/intrauterine factors
  - Multifetal gestation/IUFD/fetal anomaly
  - Polyhydramnios/maternal hypertension, diabetes, IUGR.
- Infection
  - Chorioamnionitis/bacteriuria/periodontal disease
  - Current bacterial vaginosis with a prior preterm birth
  - Gastroenteritis.
- Demographic factors
  - Low socioeconomic status
  - Low-level of education
  - Ethnicity (black women)
  - Maternal age less than 18 years or more than 35 years.
- Lifestyle issues
  - Cigarette smoking, illicit drug use, stress, physical abuse
  - Coitus late in pregnancy.
- Inadequate prenatal care, low prepregnancy weight and poor weight gain in pregnancy
- Iatrogenic
  - Indicated preterm birth
  - Induction following calculation of wrong dates.
- Idiopathic.

Management

- Gestational age less than 24 weeks and cervical length less than 25 mm: cervical cerclage preferably
- Gestational age more than 24 weeks
  - Progesterone 100–200 mg daily vaginally
  - Reduction of various day to day activities at work, travel, etc.
  - Administration of corticosteroids

Contd...

- Relocation near tertiary care centre
- Adequate antenatal visits with ultrasonographic cervical assessments at regular intervals
- Watch for signs and symptoms of preterm labor.
- Antibiotics
- Corticosteroids:
  - A single course of corticosteroids is recommended between 24^{+0} and 34^{+6} weeks of gestation who are at risk of preterm delivery within 7 days
  - Betamethasone is the steroid of choice, when available, to be given in a course of two doses of 12 mg administered intramuscularly 24 hour apart
  - An alternative regimen would be four doses of 6 mg dexamethasone intramuscularly every 12 hours
  - For multiple pregnancy, dose remains the same due to similar maternal serum and cord blood concentrations in twin and singleton pregnancies.
- Tocolysis.

Beta Agonists (Mainly Ritodrine)

- It has β_2 receptor effects, relaxing the muscles in uterus, arterioles and bronchi
- Dose: Initially 50 mcg/minute increased by 50 mcg every 10 minutes until a maximum of 350 mcg/minute for 48 hours
- Maternal side effects:
  - Tachycardia, Palpitations; Tremor
  - Nausea or vomiting, headache
  - Chest discomfort/pain, dyspnea, hypotension
  - Hypokalemia, hyperglycemia
  - Pulmonary edema though rare.
- Fetal side effects—tachycardia
- Contraindicated in tachycardia sensitive maternal cardiac disease and poorly controlled diabetes milletus.

Calcium Channel Blockers (Nifedipine)

- It has fewer side effects
- Oral administration, low-cost
- Maternal side effects:
  - Flushing, palpitations, nausea, vomiting
  - Hypotension, dizziness.
- Contraindicated in hypotension and preload-dependent cardiac lesions like aortic insufficiency
- To be used with caution in multiple pregnancy and diabetes (because of the risk of pulmonary edema)
- Suggested dosage:
  - Initial 20 mg orally followed by 10–20 mg, 3–4 times/day and adjusted according to uterine activity for up to 48 hours
  - Doses more than 60 mg—associated with serious adverse effects.

Isoxsuprine

- Oral: 10–20 mg bid/tid
- IM: 5–10 mg injection 2–3 times/day
- IV:
  - Infusion is prepared by dilution of the injection in an appropriate quantity of 5% dextrose injection

---

Contd...

- Cigarette smoking, alcohol use should be stopped or significantly reduced in pregnancy
- Serial ultrasounds to exclude any fetal abnormality or changes in liquor

Contraindications to Cervical Cerclage Insertion

- Active preterm labor (≥4 cm cervical dilatation)
- Clinical evidence of chorioamnionitis
- Continuing vaginal bleeding
- PPROM
- Gross congenital anamolies
- IUD

Risks of Cervical Cerclage Insertion

- Bleeding during insertion
- Rupture of membranes
- Premature contractions
- Use of anesthesia during removal of cerclage inserted by Shirodkar's technique
- Bucket handle tear if labor sets in, with suture in place

Absolute Contraindications to Tocolysis

- Intrauterine fetal demise
- Severe pre eclampsia/eclampsia
- Severe anemia
- Advanced cervical dilatation
- Known lethal congenital or chromosomal malformation

Contd...

- Placental abruption
- Intrauterine infection (chorioamnionitis)
- PPROM (in absence of maternal infection, consider tocolysis only in case of maternal transport or antenatal steroids administration)
- Evidence of fetal compromise or placental insufficiency

Relative Contraindications to Tocolysis

- Mild hemorrhage due to placenta previa
- Nonreassuring CTG
- IUGR
- Multiple pregnancy

Atosiban when used in women at very early gestations (<26 weeks) may lead to fetal vasopressin receptor blockade, leading to changes in amniotic fluid volume, with resultant alterations to fetal renal and lung development

Indomethacin is Contraindicated in:

- Platelet dysfunction or bleeding disorder
- Hepatic dysfunction
- Gastrointestinal ulcerative disease
- Renal dysfunction
- Asthma (in women with hypersensitivity to aspirin)

- – Do not dilute in 0.9% sodium chloride because of the risk of pulmonary edema.
- Side effects to the fetus:
  - – Tachycardia, hypoglycemia, hypocalcemia, ileus
  - – Hypotension in the neonate.
- Contraindications:
  - – Cardiac disorders, hyperthyroidism, chorioamnionitis
  - – Antepartum hemorrhage, intrauterine fetal death
  - – Eclampsia and severe pre eclampsia; pulmonary hypertension.

Nitroglycerine

- 10 mg patch releases drug at the rate of 10 mg in 24 hour
- Applied on anterior abdominal wall
- Headache—main and most important side effect.

Terbutaline (Beta mimetic)

- Initial dose is 5 mcg/minute for 20 minutes, increasing by 2.5 mcg/minute at 20 minutes intervals until contractions stop to a maximum 20 mcg/minute
- Followed by 5 mg tds orally for 48 hours.

Atosiban

- Oxytocin receptor agonist
- Nausea (main), vomiting, headache, chest pain, dyspnea
- Injection site reaction is a documented side effect
- Diabetes and cardiac disease are not contraindications
- Suggested dosage: A three step procedure
  - – An initial bolus dose of 6.75 mg over 1 minute, followed by
  - – An infusion of 18 mg/hour for 3 hours, then
  - – 6 mg/hour for up to 45 hours (to a maximum of 330 mg).

Indomethacin

- Loading Dose:
  - – Rectal suppository: Loading dose of either 50 mg or 100 mg
  - – Oral: loading dose of 50 mg.
- Maintenance dose:
  - – Oral route: Either 25 mg or 50 mg every 4–6 hours for 24–48 hours
  - – Rectal: 50 mg indomethacin every 6 hours.
- Maternal side effects:
  - – Nausea, vomiting, esophageal reflux, gastritis.
- Fetal side effects: Increased risk of constriction or premature closure of ductus arteriosus, with consequent
  - – Pulmonary hypertension; persistent PDA
  - – Oligohydramnios
  - – Necrotizing enterocolitis; intraventricular hemorrhage.

Role of Progesterone in Preventing Preterm Birth

- In women with history of preterm labor, 17-alpha-hydroxyprogesterone 250 mg IM weekly OR progesterone 100 mg daily vaginally
- In women with short cervix (<15 mm) at 22–26 weeks, progesterone 200 mg daily vaginally.

Chapter **49**

Postpartum Hemorrhage

Tania G Singh

Precautions Taken Antenatally and During Labor to Prevent PPH

Antenatal Prophylaxis

- Frequent ANCs to detect early, any complication arising in high-risk cases and timely referral to higher centres for management and delivery.

Avoidable Risk Factors

- Teenage pregnancy (<20 years)
- Pregnancy at more than 40 years
- Anemia
    - Iron and folate supplementation in pregnancy
    - Recheck Hb at 32–34 weeks
    - Hb should be ≥11 gm/dL at onset of labor
    - Hb lower than or equal to 8 gm/dL → should be referred to higher centre for delivery, where there is facility for blood transfusion.
- Prolonged labor
- Chorioamnionitis/pyrexia in labor
- Obstructed labor
- Retained placenta
- Patients in following categories should have blood cross-matched on admission for delivery
    - History of PPH in previous pregnancy
    - Antepartum hemorrhage
    - Previous cesarean section
    - Hemoglobin lower than 10 gm/dL
    - Intrauterine death
    - Fetal distress.
- At risk women, should deliver in the hospital
    - Those mentioned above and
    - Parity more than 5
    - BMI higher than 35
    - Where estimated weight of the baby is more than or equal to 4 kg.
- Monitoring 1st stage of labor with partograph (to prevent prolonged labor)
- In cases of previous cesarean section
    - Placental site should be determined before, by USG to rule out placenta percreta, accreta
    - MRI can be offered where facilities exist (to look for bladder invasion, etc.)
    - Blood and all blood products should be kept ready before surgery.

Stages of Shock or Hemorrhage

Class I
- Palpitations; dizziness; mild thirst
- SBP normal
- Blood loss ≈ 750 mL (500–1,000 mL)

Class II
- Mild form
- Tachycardia (100 beats/min)
- Minimal tachypnea and pallor
- Extremities cool (anxious/restless)
- Sweating
- Systolic BP: 80–100 mm Hg
- Blood loss: 1,000–1,500 mL
- Therapy: Crystalloids

Class III
- Moderate form
- PR: >100 <120
- Pallor ++
- Tachypnea; Oliguria
- Systolic BP: 70–80 mm Hg
- Blood loss: 1,500–2,000 mL
- Therapy: Transfusion

Class IV
- Severe form
- Collapse; Air hunger
- Marked pallor ; Anuria
- PR >120
- Systolic B.P: 50–70 mm Hg
- Blood loss: >2,000 mL
- Give massive transfusion

- Cautious use of oxytocin and misoprostol in multigravidae
- Injudicious use of oxytocin and misoprotol for induction of labor; using excessive doses and continuing these drugs in the presence of adequate uterine activity can lead to uterine rupture
- Also inappropriate use of oxytocin for augmentation when there are already signs of CPD or a malpresentation can lead to uterine rupture
- Management of 2nd stage is important:
    - Deliver baby's trunk slowly in order to allow little time for uterine retraction
    - Prefilled syringe with syntometrine or ergometrine—keep ready in 2nd stage.
- Constant watch on blood loss after 2nd stage
- Start thinking when 250 mL mark in the collecting drape is reached and be prepared to act when loss $\approx$ 450 mL (don't wait for 500 mL mark)
- In case of cesarean section, 5 IU by slow IV injection can be given to facilitate contraction of uterus
- Following this, oxytocin infusion 10 IU in one litre fluid can be commenced.

Prevention of Atonic PPH

- Oxytocin (10 IU, IV/IM) is recommended uterotonic for both vaginal and cesarean delivery
- When oxytocin is unavailable: Injectable ergometrine/methylergometrine or oral misoprostol (600 µg) is recommended
- Controlled cord traction for all vaginal as well as cesarean births
- Late cord clamping (1–3 minutes after birth) is recommended for all births while providing essential newborn care side by side for both term and preterm infants
- Postpartum abdominal uterine tonus assessment for early identification of uterine atony is recommended for all women.

PROTOCOL FOR MANAGEMENT OF PPH

Initial Assessment

- Quick history
- Check vital signs
- Brief examination
- Documentation of every move is very important
- Relatives should be kept informed of the situation, consented and possibly reassured.

Initial Intervention

Airway and Resuscitation

- Call for help
- Maintain airway and breathing
- Oxygen by mask at 10–15 litres/minute
- Endotracheal intubation, if SPO_2 is not satisfactory
- Secure two IV lines with 16/18 G (14 G – orange, preferably)
- Collect 15–20 mL blood for investigations:
    - CBC; Hemoglobin; PCV
    - Blood group and type
    - Platelet count
    - Coagulation profile

Early cord clamping (<1 minute after birth) only when the neonate is asphyxiated

Delayed Cord Clamping
Facilitates transfer of 80–100 mL blood → helps neonate receive additional blood which increases hemoglobin up to 6 months and lesser need for iron therapy

Carbetocin is associated with a reduction in the use of additional uterotonic agents but is considerably more expensive than oxytocin

Sustained uterine massage is not recommended as an intervention to prevent PPH in women who have received prophylactic oxytocin

Components of Coagulation Profile
- Fibrinogen
- Prothrombin time
- Thrombin time
- Partial thromboplastin time
- INR

- – Renal function test with electrolytes
- – Liver function test.
- Cross-matched blood (minimum 4 units)—if unavailable, 'O negative' blood can be transfused.
- Flat position
- Foot end elevation
- Infuse rapid warm fluids
  - – 2 L of Normal saline fast, followed by 200 mL/hr [3.5 litres of warm crystalloid; Hartman's solution 2L] and/or colloid 1–2 L.
- Do not infuse 5% dextrose
- Catheterize and monitor urine output
- Remove wet clothes and keep patient warm
- Arrange and transfuse blood and blood products
- Strict monitoring of PR, BP, RR, temperature every 15 minutes
- Find out the cause—atonic or traumatic and arrest bleeding by following measures.

Uterotonics

- Intravenous oxytocin alone is the 1st line of management
- If intravenous oxytocin is unavailable, or if the bleeding does not stop, give 2nd line uterotonics:
  - – IV ergometrine,
  - – Oxytocin-ergometrine fixed dose, or
  - – Sublingual misoprostol, 800 μg
- Isotonic crystalloids instead of colloids
- Tranexamic acid is given only if uterotonics fails to stop bleeding or if it is thought that the bleeding may be partly due to trauma.

Uterine Massage

Intrauterine Balloon Tamponade

Surgical Interventions

- Stepwise uterine artery devascularization
- Bilateral internal iliac artery ligation
- Peripartum hysterectomy
- Uterine artery embolization.

Temporizing Measures

- Bimanual uterine compression
- External aortic compression
- Nonpneumatic antishock garments
- Uterine packing.

Referral of the Case

- Arrange for rapid transport and refer to a centre where blood transfusion and emergency obstetric care is available
- Establish two wide bore IV cannulas (≈ ≤18 G)
- Start resuscitation with NS/RL
- Catheterize the patient and foot end elevation
- Keep patient warm
- Bimanual or aortic compression of uterus during transport

The use of ergometrine for the management of retained placenta is not recommended as this may cause tetanic uterine contractions which may delay the expulsion of the placenta

Recommended Method for Removal of Placenta

- Clamp cord close to perineum (after pulsation stops)
- Keep slight tension on cord and await a strong uterine contraction (2–3minutes)
- Place the other hand over suprapubic region and apply upward counter traction (without waiting for signs of placental separation) – discontinue CCT, if:
  - – Placenta does not descend within 30–40 seconds
  - – Wait for next uterine contraction and repeat CCT
  - – When uterus becomes rounded or cord lengthens, very gently pull downwards on the cord to deliver the placenta (turn the placenta so that membranes are twisted into a rope)

Initial Goals to be Achieved after Resuscitation

- Systolic BP >90 mm Hg
- Urine output ≥ 30 mL/hour
- Hemoglobin >8 gm/dL
- Platelet count >75,000
- Prothrombin (PT) <1.5 x mean control
- Activated prothrombin time (aPTT) <1.5 x mean control
- Fibrinogen >1.0 mg%

When the blood loss reaches about 4.5 litres (80% of blood volume) and large volumes of replacement fluids have been given, there will be clotting factor defects and blood components should be given. Up to 1 litre of fresh frozen plasma (FFP) and 10 units of cryoprecipitate (two packs) may be given empirically in the face of relentless bleeding, while awaiting the results of coagulation studies

- If possible, transfer the patient with intrauterine condom catheter which acts as uterine tamponade and arrests hemorrhage
- Ensure adequate donors and attenders accompany the patient
- Inform the case and especially blood group of patient, if known, to referral hospital.

Chapter **50**

Disseminated Intravascular Coagulopathy (DIC)

Tania G Singh

CONDITIONS ASSOCIATED WITH DIC

- Abruptio
- Amniotic fluid embolism
- Retained IUD fetus
- Puerperal sepsis and septic abortion
- Excessive blood loss
- Severe pre eclampsia/eclampsia
- Induced abortion especially using hypertonic saline
- Acute fatty liver of pregnancy
- Molar pregnancy.

CLINICAL FEATURES OF DIC

- Petechiae
- Purpura
- Ecchymosis
- Hemorrhagic bullae
- Subcutaneous hematoma
- Bleeding from wound or venepuncture sites
- Variable degrees of shock and acidosis.

DIAGNOSIS

Bed Side Tests

Whole Blood Clotting Time

- Normal 1–10 minutes
- Take 5 mL of blood in glass tube and observe for clot formation
- If prolonged, deficiency of clotting factors
- If clot is not formed → fibrinogen is <50 mg/dL.

Clot Retraction Time

- Normal 30–60 minutes
- Weak friable clot → hypofibrinogenemia
- Early dissolution → enhanced fibrinolysis.

Laboratory Tests

- Peripheral smear
  - Thrombocytopenia
  - Leukocytosis
  - Evidence of hemolysis.

DIC: A thrombo-hemorrhagic disorder occurring as a consequence of aberrant activation of coagulation cascade seen in association with well-defined clinical situations

Naturally Occurring Anticoagulants

- Antithrombin III
- Protein C and S

DIC is Characterized by

- Intravascular coagulation
- Fibrinolysis
- Consumption of coagulation factors and inhibitors
- End organ damage

Crystalloids or Colloids?

Crystalloids

- ✌ Are more readily available and are less expensive
- ✌ Are to be infused in volume boluses calculated at 3 times the estimated blood loss because they remain in intravascular circulation for short time

Colloids

- ✌ Have higher intravascular oncotic pressure with smaller amount as compared to crystalloids
- ✌ But as a disadvantage, there is delayed postresuscitation diuresis and higher incidence of post resuscitation hypertension

Why dextrans can't be used?

- ✌ It affects platelet function
- ✌ Causes pseudo agglutination
- ✌ Interfere with interpretation of subsequent blood grouping and cross matching
- ✌ They cause anaphylactic reactions

Hemaccel

- ✌ Derivative of bovine gelatin
- ✌ Shelf life of 8 years
- ✌ Can be stored at room temperature
- ✌ Isotonic and does not interfere with platelet function or blood grouping/cross matching
- ✌ Renal function is improved when given in hypovolemic shock
- ✌ Generally, nonimmunogenic
- ✌ Reactions, if they occur, are due to histamine release

- DIC profile
  - Prothrombin time (PT)
    - 10–13 seconds
    - It tests the integrity of extrinsic and common pathway
    - When fibrinogen is lower than 100 mg/dL → PT is increased.
  - INR (International normalized ratio)
    - Patient's PT: Laboratory's control PT
    - Normal → 0.9–1.2
    - Increased in deficiency of factors I, II, V, VII or X
    - Most sensitive to fall in factor VII.
  - Partial thromboplastin time (aPTT)
    - Normal 25–35 seconds
    - Tests the integrity of intrinsic and common pathway
  - Thrombin time
    - Normal is less than 18 seconds
    - Extended when functional fibrinogen is lower than 100 mg/dL
    - Increases when FDPs are increased.
  - Fibrinogen
    - Bleeding occurs when levels fall below 100–150 mg/dL.
  - D-dimer
    - Measures cross-linked fibrin derivatives
    - Fragments Y, D, E are retained to a lesser extent
    - Is a more specific FDP assay
    - Has been found to be the most useful test in diagnosing DIC
    - Normally lower than 0.5 mg/lit.
  - FDP titer
    - Normal is lower than 10 micrograms/dL
    - Increases in DIC.
  - Platelets
    - Normal is ≈1.5–4.0 lakhs
    - In DIC, platelets decrease.

Management

- Correction of underlying problem
- Fluid resuscitation to restore the circulatory system, maintain BP and electrolyte balance
- Amount of blood loss should be estimated and blood products transfused accordingly (Refer to chapter on blood transfusion)
- Coagulation studies and platelets should be urgently requested
- By the time the reports are ready, up to 4 units of FFPs and 10 units of cryoprecipitate can be transfused
- If the patient is on anticoagulant therapy (LMWH) and she bleeds, she is advised not to take any further doses unless she consults her obstetrician
- She should be managed with intravenous, unfractionated heparin until the risk factors for hemorrhage have resolved.

Chapter 51

HELLP Syndrome

Tania G Singh

Diagnostic Criteria

Tennessee Classification System by Sibai

True or complete HELLP has been proposed by:
- Abnormal peripheral blood smear
- ↑ S. bilirubin (≥1.2 mg/100 mL)
- ↑ LDH (>600 Units/L)
- ↑ Platelets (100000/mm^3)
- ↑ AST (≥70 IU/L).

The Mississippi-Triple Class System

Class 1
- Platelets less than or equal to 50,000/mm^3
- AST or ALT higher than or equal to 70 IU/L
- LDH higher than or equal to 600 IU/L.

Class 2
- Platelets less than or equal to 1,00,000 but more than or equal to 50,000/mm^3
- AST or ALT higher than or equal to 70 IU/L
- LDH higher than or equal to 600 IU/L.

Class 3
- Platelets less than or equal to 1,50,000 but ≥1,00,000/mm^3
- AST or ALT higher than or equal to 40 IU/L
- LDH higher than or equal to 600 IU/L
- This class is a clinically significant transition stage which has the ability to progress.

Clinical Symptoms

- Right upper abdominal (fluctuating, colic like), quadrant or epigastric pain
- Nausea and vomiting
- History of malaise some days before presentation
- Headache in 30–60%
- Visual symptoms in 20%
- Might have unspecific symptoms or subtle signs of pre eclampsia or nonspecific viral syndrome—like symptoms
- Also characterized by exacerbation during the night and recovery during the day.

Pathology
Blood
- Hemolysis → ↓ Hb → Microangiopathic hemolytic anemia → ↑ LDH
- Liberated hemoglobin is converted to unconjugated bilirubin in the spleen or may be bound in the plasma by haptoglobin
- The hemoglobin-haptoglobin complex is cleared quickly by the liver → low or undetectable haptoglobin levels in the blood
- Low haptoglobin concentration (<1g/L – <0.4 g/L) is the preferred marker of hemolysis and can be used for diagnosis
- Therefore, for diagnosis:
  - ↑ LDH
  - Presence of unconjugated bilirubin
  - Low or undetectable haptoglobin (more specific indicator)
- Peripheral smear:
  - Schizocytes-fragmented red cells
  - Burr cells-contracted red cells with spicula
  - Echinocytes

Contd...

Contd...

Liver
- Primary target organ
- Periportal or focal parenchymal necrosis
- ↑ AST and ALT → mark liver injury

Thrombocytopenia
- Thrombocytopenia is due to increased consumption and increased turnover with shorter lifespan

Based on Number of Abnormalities Present
- When 1 or 2 abnormalities present → partial or incomplete HELLP
- When all 3 present → full or complete HELLP

Platelet Therapy for HELLP Syndrome
- If platelet count is >50,000 and no active bleeding or platelet dysfunction, prophylactic transfusion is not recommended even prior to cesarean section
- Platelet transfusion is strongly recommended prior to delivery (vaginal or cesarean), when platelet count is <20,000
- Steroids can be administered with a platelet count <50,000
- No recommendation regarding the usefulness of plasma exchange or plasmapheresis
- Only in women who demonstrate progressive elevation of bilirubin or creatinine for >72 hours after delivery may benefit from plasma exchange with fresh frozen plasma

Treatment
- Platelet count and LDH levels → Best markers to follow disease progression
- Class I/II or Class III with symptoms of impending eclampsia:
  - Give—High dose parenteral corticosteroids
  - Arrest progression
  - Improve biochemical parameters
  - ↓ Transfusion rates.
- Mississippi protocol
  - Dexamethasone IV 10 mg BD → antepartum HELLP
  - Postpartum Dexa IV 10 mg (2 doses 12 hourly) followed by Dexa IV 5 mg (2 doses 12 hourly).
- IV fluids
- Antihypertensives
- Prophylactic anticonvulsants.

Termination
- According to:
  - Gestation
  - Favorability of cervix (Bishop score)
  - Severity of disease.
- Delivery → Definitive treatment
- HELLP per se is NOT an indication for immediate cesarean section
- <30–32 weeks and those with oligohydramnios and/or unfavorable Bishop score → Cesarean section (give GA):
  - Delay in delivery for 6 hours and give aggressive steroid therapy, if possible
  - If not possible to delay and platelet count less than 40,000 → give 6–10 units platelets before intubation.
- More than 32 weeks → Induction and vaginal delivery (continue steroid treatment)
- No DIC and absent fetal lung maturity, give 2 doses of steroids and do intense monitoring.
- Pudendal block or epidural anesthesia (platelet count <75,000) → contra-indicated because of risk of bleeding in these areas
- BP should be kept below 155/105 mm Hg.

Recurrence rate → 2–19%

Chapter 52

Acute Fatty Liver of Pregnancy

Tania G Singh

- A rare life-threatening complication of pregnancy
- More common in nulliparous and in those who have male fetus or twins
- $\approx 50\% \rightarrow$ have signs of pre eclampsia
- Liver normal or small
- Presence of hypoglycemia and increased prothrombin time (PT) differentiates it from HELLP
- Occurs in the 3rd trimester or in the immediate period after delivery
- Cause: Disordered metabolism of fatty acids by mitochondria in the mother, caused by deficiency in the LCHAD (long-chain 3-hydroxyacyl-coenzyme A dehydrogenase) enzyme
- Intravenous fluids, blood products and an early delivery has improved prognosis.

CLINICAL SIGNS AND SYMPTOMS

- Usually manifests in the 3rd trimester (34th-36th week) of pregnancy
- May occur any time in the second half of pregnancy, or in the puerperium
- Symptoms are usually nonspecific:
  - Nausea, vomiting, anorexia
  - Abdominal pain
  - Jaundice and fever may occur in as many as 70% of patients
  - Pre eclampsia occurs in more severe disease.
- Other systems may get involved and manifest as:
  - Acute renal failure
  - Hepatic encephalopathy
  - Pancreatitis
  - Diabetes insipidus (though uncommon).

Lab Abnormalities

- AST/ALT up to 1,000 IU/L (usually 300–500)
- Bilirubin $\uparrow\uparrow$; Alkaline phosphatase $\uparrow\uparrow$
- $\uparrow$ WBCs
- Hypoglycemia
- $\uparrow$ INR; $\downarrow$ fibrinogen
- Frank DIC may occur in as many as 70% of patients.

Diagnosis

- Usually made on clinical grounds
- Definitive diagnosis: Liver biopsy (but not done in pregnancy).

Understanding the Disease

Deficiency of LCHAD (3-hydroxyacyl-CoA dehydrogenase) enzyme in fetus → accumulation of unmetabolized medium and long chain fatty acids in fetus → these will re-enter the maternal circulation through the placenta → overwhelm the beta-oxidation enzymes of the mother → triglycerides accumulates within maternal hepatocytes → impaired function → liver failure in mother

Treatment

- Admission to ICU
- Intravenous fluids, intravenous glucose and blood products, including fresh frozen plasma and cryoprecipitate to correct DIC
- Fetus → NST
- Delivery anticipated after stabilizing the mother, often vaginal but in cases of severe hemorrhage → cesarean section
- Mortality is reduced to 18%.

Uterine Rupture in Previous LSCS

Tania G Singh

Signs of Uterine Rupture

- Nonreassuring FHR pattern → 1st sign of uterine rupture
  - Fetal bradycardia → most consistent finding
  - Others—prolonged and variable decelerations.
- Scar tenderness (suprapubic pain and tenderness)
- Unexplained tachycardia
- Hypotension
- Sudden onset of shortness of breath
- Suprapubic bulge
- Rarely, chest pain or shoulder tip pain.

Symptoms of Uterine Rupture

- Suprapubic pain persisting in between contractions and aggravated during contractions
- Slight fresh vaginal bleeding
- Loss of station of presenting part
- Changes in uterine contour
- Bladder tenesmus
- Development of incoordinate uterine action in active labor and complete cessation of contractions
- There can be development of frank hematuria.

Advantages of the Lower Segment over Upper Segment Cesarean Section

- Less blood loss due to less vascularity and the placental bed is away from the incision
- Easier to repair
- Though both upper and lower uterine segments heal by primary intention, forming a fibrous tissue that has 80% of the tensile strength of the surrounding tissue but lower segment being thinner, better coaptation of the edges is achieved and maintained
- Better healing as the lower segment is more 'at rest' than the upper segment in the postpartum period (However, the lower segment also undergoes dramatic cellular atrophy and diminution in size)
- Where there has been prior classical cesarean section, the placenta is likely to be found implanted over the scar (i.e. on the anterior uterine wall) in approximately 40% of pregnancies, which might account for a higher rate of rupture of classical scars (2% in upper segment versus 0.2% in lower segment)

Factors for Weakening of Scar

- Infection
- Placental site in the index pregnancy
- Imperfect apposition of cut margins
- Pressure of sepsis
- Pressure of hematoma in wound (incidence of hematoma after cesarean section → 2.4–5.6%)
- Implantation of placenta over site of old scar (anterior placenta previa)

Risk of Rupture

- 4–9%: Classical and T–shaped scar
- 1–7%: Low vertical incision
- 0.2–1.5%: Low transverse incision

Indications of Upper Segment Cesarean Section

- Dense adhesions, extensive varicosity or myoma in the lower uterine segment making it's exposure or incising through it difficult
- Impacted shoulder presentation
- Anterior placenta previa
- Defective scar in the upper segment
- Rapid delivery is indicated
- Previous successful repair of high vesicovaginal or cervicovaginal fistula
- Cancer cervix
- Postmortem hysterectomy

- Less subsequent adhesions to the bowel and omentum
- Less liability to acute gastric dilatation and paralytic ileus
- Less liability to peritonitis due to better peritonization and healing.

Types of Hematoma after Cesarean Section

Retrovesical Hematoma

- Common after lower segment operation
- (May) Cause pyrexia
- Not much troublesome.

Hematoma in Abdominal Incision

- May cause dehiscence or infection.

Rectus Sheath Hematoma

- Rare
- May present with hypovolemic shock or consumptive coagulopathy → surgery.

Technique of Repeat Cesarean Section

Does not differ much from the primary

- Peritoneum → open as high as possible with great care because
    - Bladder may be displaced upwards
    - Intestines may be adherent to original wound.
- Uterovesical pouch → much shallower than in fresh case and more adherent to uterus
- Reflecting down bladder from lower segment
    - Be extra careful because it may be adherent
    - Safer to dissect this down by sharp dissection in proper plane than by blunt dissection.

Chapter 54

Acute Manifestation of Sickle Cell Disease

Tania G Singh

Infarctive or Painful Crisis

- Severe skeletal pain but no change in Hb%.

Sequestration Crisis

- Sudden massive pooling of red cells in spleen with an acute fall in Hb concentration with the potential for hypovolemic shock
- Because of its narrow vessels and function in clearing defective red blood cells, the spleen is frequently affected → infarction of spleen
- This autosplenectomy increases the risk of infection from encapsulated organisms.

Hemolytic Crisis

- Uncommon
- Acute accelerated ↓ in Hb concentration with ↑↑ in jaundice
- This is particularly common in patients with coexistent G6PD deficiency.

Vaso-occlusive Crisis

- ↑ blood viscosity → ischemia, pain and infarction
- Following organs are affected:
  - Lung—Pulmonary hypertension due to vaso-occlusive disease in lung vessels leading to strain on the right ventricle and a risk of heart failure; typical symptoms are shortness of breath, decreased exercise tolerance and episodes of syncope
  - Bone—Osteomyelitis
  - The most common cause of osteomyelitis in sickle cell disease is Salmonella (especially the nontypical serotypes, *Salmonella typhimurium, Salmonella enteritidis, Salmonella choleraesuis and Salmonella paratyphi B*), perhaps because intravascular sickling of the bowel leads to patchy ischemic infarction
  - Avascular necrosis (aseptic bone necrosis) of the hip and other major joints, which may occur as a result of ischemia
  - Spleen—hyposplenism; autosplenectomy
  - Priaprism
  - Kidney—Acute papillary necrosis
  - Eye—Background retinopathy, proliferative retinopathy, vitreous hemorrhages and retinal detachments, resulting in blindness
  - Stroke, which can result from a progressive narrowing of blood vessels, preventing oxygen from reaching the brain. Cerebral infarction and cerebral hemorrhage can occur in adults

 – Silent stroke is probably five times as common as symptomatic stroke, predominating in the younger patient.

Aplastic Crisis

- This is an acute worsening of the patient's baseline anemia, producing pallor, tachycardia, and fatigue
- Normally triggered by parvovirus B19, directly affecting erythropoiesis by invading the red cell precursors and eventually leading to their destruction
- Parvovirus infection nearly completely prevents red blood cell production for two to three days, which in normal individuals, is of little consequence, but the shortened red cell life of sickle-cell patients results in an abrupt, life-threatening situation
- Reticulocyte counts drop dramatically during the disease, and the rapid turnover of red cells leads to the drop in hemoglobin
- This crisis takes 4 days to one week to disappear
- Overwhelming post-(auto) splenectomy infection (OPSI), which is due to functional asplenia, caused by encapsulated organisms, such as Streptococcus pneumoniae and Hemophilus influenza
- Most episodes of sickle cell crisis last between five and seven days.

Chapter 55

Acute Cholecystitis/Acute Appendicitis/ Degenerating Myoma/Rupture of Ovarian Cyst

Tania G Singh

Acute Cholecystitis

- History of previous episodes present
- Most reliable symptom → acute (moderate/severe) epigastric or right upper quadrant pain which may radiate to the back
- Pain lasts for a longer time
- Vomiting occurs in ≈ 50% of cases
- Fever only occasionally
- Jaundice is rare
- Cholecystitis can mimic appendicitis in the 3rd trimester
- Hospitalization is definitely required
- Murphy sign may not be elicited
- Aspartate transferase and alanine transferase levels—may help to distinguish cholecystitis from hepatitis
- Serum amylase levels—elevated transiently in up to 1/3rd of patients
- Initial treatment:
  - IV fluids
  - Nasogastric suction—in case of ↑ vomiting
  - Analgesia—morphine may produce spasm of the sphincter of Oddi
  - Broad spectrum antibiotics—ampicillin, cephalosporins and clindamycin.
- If cholelithiasis is present, laparoscopic cholecystectomy can be safely performed with intense fetal monitoring
- Tocolysis may be required, when operating in the 3rd trimester.

If surgery is delayed in case of gallstones, there are increased chances of:
- Hospitalization
- Spontaneous abortion
- Preterm labor
- Preterm delivery
- Prematurity
- Low birth weight
- Admission to NICU

Acute Appendicitis

- Abdominal pain is always present
- Nausea—present in nearly all cases
- Vomiting—present in 2/3rd of pregnant patients
- Anorexia—present in only 1/3rd to 2/3rd of pregnant patients
- Patients usually lie down, flex their hips, and draw their knees up to reduce movements and to avoid worsening their pain
- Fever and tachycardia may or may not be present
- Vomiting that precedes pain is suggestive of intestinal obstruction, and the diagnosis of appendicitis should be reconsidered
- Rebound tenderness—present in 55–75% of cases
- Abdominal muscle rigidity—observed in 50–65% of patients
- The Rovsing sign—observed as frequently in pregnant patients with appendicitis than in nonpregnant persons
- Psoas irritation—observed less frequently in pregnancy than it is in nonpregnant women

Location of pain in acute appendicitis varies according to different trimesters:
- 1st trimester → located in the right lower quadrant
- 2nd trimester → appendix is located at the level of the umbilicus (periumbilical pain)
- 3rd trimester → pain is diffuse or in the right upper quadrant

- Rectal tenderness—usually present, particularly in the 1st trimester
- Management
  - Surgery (Appendectomy) → definitive treatment
  - Laparoscopic appendectomy is the preferred method.

Rupture of Ovarian Cyst

- Rare condition
- There may be a history of mild trauma but may occur spontaneously
- The patient may have mild, chronic lower abdominal discomfort that suddenly intensifies
- Tenderness and guarding may be present
- Adnexal size not of much help, due to collapsed cyst
- Hemoglobin is reduced (depends upon the extent of bleed)
- Management and prognosis
  - Surgical
  - Conserve as much ovarian tissue as possible
  - In the absence of malignancy, the prognosis is excellent.

Degenerating Myoma

- Red degeneration occurs in 5–10% of pregnant women with myomas
- Often occurs between 12 and 20 weeks' gestation
- Acute onset
- Significant, localized abdominal pain
- Vomiting present
- Low-grade fever may be present
- Constipation
- Tenderness and rigidity over tumor
- Malaise or increased temperature
- Dry or furged tongue
- Rapid pulse
- Leiomyomas tend to become smaller during pregnancy, and leiomyomas initially less than 5 cm in diameter usually involute completely during pregnancy
- Earlier months: Fibroid diagnosed but pregnancy missed
- Later months: Pregnancy diagnosed but fibroid missed
- Large leiomyomas can undergo hemorrhagic infarction resulting in the painful myoma syndrome
- Ultrasonography and MRI are usually diagnostic
- Management
  - Red degeneration—a self-limited process, therefore, conservative management
  - Infection has no role to play (Vascular in origin)
  - Close monitoring of the patients
  - Analgesia with narcotic or anti-inflammatory agents
  - If narcotics are ineffective, a very short course of indomethacin can be given before 32 and 34 weeks.

Pelvic ultrasound in case of ruptured cyst:
- Complex mass appearance
- Fluid in the pouch of Douglas

Effect of Fibroid on Pregnancy
- Recurrent pregnancy loss
- Spontaneous abortion (especially with submucous fibroid)
- Uterine carceration: If placenta posteriorly and of bigger size
- Abruptio (in retroplacental fibroids)
- Malpresentation (breech) → when situated in lower part of uterus below presenting part
- Dystocia: cervical fibroids or those very low in uterine wall
- Anterior fibroids – good chances of being drawn up out of pelvis after onset of labor (give chance of vaginal delivery)
- Posterior fibroids → get trapped within pelvis
- Premature rupture of membranes
- Uterine rupture (especially after prior myomectomy)
- More frequent cesarean delivery
- Uterine torsion
- Postpartum hemorrhage
- Puerperal sepsis

Chapter 56

Cardiac Arrest in Pregnancy

Tania G Singh

Key Interventions

- Start CPR with chest compression (CAB [circulation, airway, breathing] instead of ABC [airway, breathing, circulation])
- Place the woman on hard surface in left lateral position (15°–30° tilt)
- Establish IV access and administer fluids using upper extremity veins
- Consider the possible cause of cardiac arrest.

Airway and Breathing

- Ventilate with 100% oxygen
- Apply continuous cricoid pressure during ventilation and intubation due to the risk of regurgitation
- Start with two rescue breaths of one second each
- Bag-mask ventilate at a rate of 8–10 breaths/minute, during pauses of compressions (synchronization)
- Synchronization between chest compressions and ventilation is not necessary with an advanced airway (endotracheal tube) in place.

> Hyperventilation is harmful and should be avoided

Circulation

- Chest compressions are performed higher than in nonpregnant patients, slightly above the centre of the sternum due to the elevated diaphragm and abdominal contents
- "Push fast and hard"! Place the heel of one hand on the centre of the chest. Place the other hand on top
- Interlock the fingers and compress the chest at a rate of 100/minute, a depth of 45 cm and equal compression: relaxation times
- It is recommended that the CPR operator be changed every 2 minutes
- Incorrectly applied cardiac compressions in pregnant patients may lead to:
  - Liver laceration
  - Uterine rupture
  - Hemothorax
  - Hemopericardium.
- A single dose of vasopressin 40 units is an alternative to repeated epinephrine injection
- Amiodarone 300 mg IV has replaced lidocaine for treatment of ventricular arrhythmias.

Defibrillation

- Survival rates are highest with immediate CPR and defibrillation within 3–5 minutes of a witnessed pulseless ventricular tachycardia or fibrillation
- Electric cardioversion during pregnancy appears to be safe for the fetus.

Emergency Delivery

- If cardiac arrest is not immediately (4–5 minutes) reversed by basic and advanced life support, emergency hysterotomy (or cesarean delivery, even if fetus is dead) should be performed at more than 20 pregnancy weeks
- Hysterotomy ideally should be performed no longer than 45 minutes after initiation of CPR.

Section IV:

Labor Ward Rounds

Chapter 57

Labor in Anemia Patient

Tania G Singh

Labor/Delivery in Case of Severe Iron Deficiency Anemia

- Propped up position
- O_2 inhalation
- Strict watch on volume of fluids
- Intermittent chest auscultation
- Partograph (do not allow prolonged labor)
- Blood cross matched and saved—more prone for PPH
- Antibiotics cover
- Active management of 3rd stage of labor
- Avoid IV ergometrine
- Keep other oxytocics ready
- If possible, delay blood transfusion till delivery
- Digitalization and cardiac support in cardiac failure.

Intrapartum Management in β Thalassemia Major

- IV line
- Propped up position
- O_2 inhalation
- Maintain partograph → prolonged and obstructed labor in no way is accepted
- Do not increase total blood volume; this can precipitate cardiac failure and pulmonary edema
- Oxytocics and cross-matched blood to be kept ready
- Active management of 3rd stage of labor
- Avoid IV ergometrine.

Intrapartum Care In Sickle Cell Disease

- Delivery should be in a tertiary care centre
- If growth is normal, induction of labor is offered at 37 completed weeks
- Blood should be promptly available in case of emergency
- Keep the woman warm
- IV fluids to prevent dehydration
- O_2 through mask
- Pulse oximeter to detect early hypoxia
- If oxygen saturation is less than or equal to 94% → ABG analysis
- Maternal vitals and FHR monitoring meticulously
- Avoid repeated vaginal examinations to minimize risk of infection
- Left lateral position

- Avoid prolonged and obstructed labor (avoid maternal exertion and exhaustion)
- Vaginal delivery allowed
- Cesarean section for other indications
- Avoid general anesthesia
- Regional anesthesia is recommended.

Chapter 58

Vaginal Birth after Cesarean Section

Tania G Singh

Delivery → always where facility for emergency cesarean section is present.

First Stage

- Blood group and cross-match
- Patient kept NPO or on a liquid diet
- IV line secured
- Anesthetist and neonatologist kept informed
- Monitoring done meticulously
  - FHS
    - If facilities available—CTG
    - If not, intermittent auscultation or use of Doppler.
  - Partograph for progress of labor (PR, BP, FHS, contractions and scar tenderness)
  - Oxytocin can be used for augmentation but judiciously
  - Once good uterine contractions start, cervical dilatation should be minimum 1 cm/hour
  - Amniotomy can be performed once cervix is 3–4 cm dilated
  - Slow IV fluids started (avoid dehydration)
  - Epidural analgesia is not contraindicated in VBAC
  - Watch for symptoms and signs of scar dehiscence and impending rupture.
- Scar dehiscence can be totally SILENT (detected at the time of cesarean section only)
- Impending rupture → earliest finding is fetal distress.

Second Stage

- Should not be prolonged
- Bladder should be emptied
- Patient should be allowed to bear down on her own (no fundal pressure)
- Episiotomy to cut short 2nd stage
- Vacuum and outlet forceps application is not a contraindication in VBAC, but used with caution.

Third Stage

- Exploration of the uterine scar is not warranted unless there is postpartum hemorrhage which fails to settle with appropriate medication

Chapter 59

Twin Vaginal Delivery

Tania G Singh

Optimal Time of Delivery

- Twins: 37-38 weeks; no later than 39 weeks (risk of fetal death is lowest at this gestation)
- Triplets: 36 weeks (no later than 37 weeks)
- Fetal lung maturity occurs at an earlier gestation in multiple pregnancy and, therefore, term gestation is considered earlier than singleton
- Postmaturity—uncommon with multiple gestation

Indications for Cesarean Section

Accepted indications

- Noncephalic presentation of twin 1
- IUGR in dichorionic twins
- Twin 2 significantly larger (>500 gm) than twin 1 including antepartum death of twin 1
- Placenta previa
- Fetal abnormality precluding safe vaginal delivery
- Chronic TTTS in monochorionic twin
- Monoamniotic twins

Contd...

There are nine possible combinations which can be divided into three categories:

- Vertex-vertex → 42%
- Vertex-nonvertex → 45%
- Nonvertex-nonvertex → 13%.

Before anticipating delivery, carefully consider the following:

- Gestational age
- Weight of each twin
- Chorionicity
- Lie and presentation of both twins
- Portable ultrasound machine
- CTG machine with dual probes
- IV access
- Blood-cross match and availability
- Pediatrician and anesthetist to be kept informed and that two obstetricians and two neonatologists (preferably) are required at the time of delivery
- Labor analgesia (epidural)
- Delivery bed with lithotomy stirrups
- 5 cord clamps
- All oxytocics should be kept ready for active management of 3rd stage of labor and to combat PPH, if it occurs
- Working condition of vacuum should be checked well before and forceps made available
- Provision to carry out emergency cesarean section
- Last but not the least, written and informed consent.

MANAGEMENT PROPER

Vertex-Vertex

First Twin

- Allow delivery by vaginal route
- Continuous CTG monitoring in active labor (>4 cm dilatation)
- Discuss the options and benefits of intrapartum epidural analgesia
- An epidural is recommended due to increased risk of operative delivery in twins and the possibility of intrauterine manipulation in second twin
- Patient should be kept on soft diet in latent phase and on liquid diet once active labor begins
- Main problems in first stage:
  - Over distension of uterus
  - Uterine inertia

- Prolonged active phase
- Increased frequency of contractions with lesser intensity.
- First twin delivered as in singleton pregnancy
- After delivery of first twin, clamp it's umbilical cord with two clamps and do not deliver the placenta
- Withhold IM oxytocin after the delivery of first twin
- In case of fetal distress, expedite delivery using vacuum or forceps
- Cesarean section is indicated in cases of:
    - Cord prolapse
    - Premature separation of placenta
    - Malpresentation.

Second Twin

- Repeat abdominal and per vaginal examination and reconfirm the presentation of second twin by USG (as it may change)
- External version, if necessary
- After the delivery of the first twin, uterine contractions may cease for sometime, therefore start oxytocin drip after 10 minutes and wait for contractions
- Continuous FHR monitoring
- Amniotomy of the 2nd sac once the head is engaged
- Time interval between deliveries of both fetuses is important
- Longer the interval between delivery, greater is the risk of hypoxia
- Umbilical cord blood gas deteriorate with increasing time interval— maximum time limit of 30 minutes with documentation of reassuring FHR pattern (but should deliver within 10–15 minutes)
- But adverse outcome is not expected as long as FHR is continuously being monitored
- Use three clamps, leaving a double clamp on placental side for identification
- Give IM oxytocin.

Vertex-Nonvertex

- There are ongoing controversies to which mode of delivery should be opted, as rates of morbidity and mortality are the same for both vaginal delivery as well as cesarean section
- If vaginal delivery is anticipated, recheck the weight especially of the second twin.

Estimated Fetal Weight more than 1500 gm

Second Twin is Breech

- Vaginal delivery of twin 1
- Twin 2 → attempt ECV → failed → breech extraction → failed → cesarean section.

Second Twin is Transverse

- ECV
- Internal podalic version (the only accepted indication of internal podalic version is breech extraction in case of second twin when cervix is fully dilated)

Contd...

Contentious indications

- Maternal request
- Unfavorable cervix at 39 weeks in nullipara
- Death of twin 2
- Uncomplicated monochorionic twins
- Previous cesarean section

Prerequisites for Internal Podalic Version

- Skilled operator, well-versed with the procedure
- EFW >1500 gms
- Adequate liquor
- Available anesthesia for effective uterine relaxation
- Simultaneous preparation for emergency cesarean section

<table>
<tr><td style="vertical-align:top; width:30%">

Third Stage: Most Dangerous

Increased risk of PPH because of:

- Large placenta, which may take longer time for complete separation
- Larger placental site → capable of more profuse bleeding
- Uterine inertia due to over distension
- As blood loss is more after twin deliveries, this blood may accumulate within the uterine cavity, hampering it's further contraction
- Placenta may occupy lower segment
- Employ the following:
  - AMTSL
  - Oxytocics
  - Scrupulous monitoring of vitals for a period of minimum 4 hours after delivery
  - Oxytocin drip should be continued

</td><td style="vertical-align:top">

Estimated Fetal Weight less than <1500 gm

- Perinatal outcomes same for both—cesarean section and vaginal delivery
- So, any mode can be selected.

Nonvertex-Nonvertex

- Cesarean section would be a better option
- Risk factors:
  - Twin 1 breech/twin 2 vertex
  - IUGR or fetal demise of one fetus.
- Monoamniotic—elective cesarean section. Cord of twin 2 may be inadvertently clamped during delivery of twin 1 in case of vaginal delivery.

Special Situations

Twins with Previous Scar

- Trial of labor is not an absolute contraindication if first twin has a vertex presentation
- Better to perform cesarean section in case of first nonvertex twin
- Success rate 30–75%
- Risk of uterine rupture is the same as VBAC in a singleton pregnancy.

Twin Entrapment

- Here, the after coming head of twin1 (presenting as breech) is prevented from entering the pelvis by presenting part (head) of twin 2 → immediately induce anesthesia
- Push second head out of the way so that first head can enter the brim (difficult manoeuvre) → mostly twin 1 dies of asphyxia
  - Decapitate twin 1
  - Deliver body
  - Retrieve head after delivery of twin 2.
- Therefore, better to go for elective cesarean section in case of MCMA twins.

Triplets or Higher Order

- Elective cesarean section
- Vaginal delivery can be planned, if following criteria is fulfilled:
  - Noncontracted pelvis
  - Cephalic presentation of first triplet
  - Unscarred uterus
  - Gestation more than 32 weeks
  - No fetal compromise.

</td></tr>
</table>

Chapter 60

Vaginal Breech Delivery

Tania G Singh

Precautions Before Anticipating Delivery

- It should be a frank breech and near full-term. Any other type will not dilate the birth canal adequately
- Head of the fetus should be flexed, with the baby's chin on his or her chest
- Mother pelvis is adequate for the weight/size of the baby
- The doctor and other medical personnel should be experienced in attending breech births
- Spontaneous and normally progressing labor
- A healthy and well, mother and fetus
- Should take place in a hospital setting where there is well-maintained operation theatre for emergency cesarean section
- Epidural analgesia is not routinely recommended.

General Considerations

- Continuous electronic fetal heart monitoring is preferable in the 1st stage and mandatory in the 2nd stage of labor
- Fetal membranes should be left intact as long as possible which helps in dilatation and prevent cord prolapse
- If there is inadequate progress, proceed for cesarean section
- Induction of labor:
  - Not recommended for breech presentation
  - Oxytocin augmentation is acceptable in cases of uterine dystocia due to epidural analgesia.
- Assessing full dilatation in breech presentation is more difficult than in cephalic presentation because the fully dilated cervix does not disappear behind the cephalic crown. Instead, the cervix remains palpable as the fetal trunk descends through it
- Avoid pushing before full dilatation
- Assess for and perform episiotomy, if required in between contractions
- Hands off until there is reason to assist
- Anesthetist and pediatrician should be available.

Thick meconium passage is common as the breech is squeezed through the birth canal. This is usually not associated with meconium aspiration because the meconium passes out of the vagina and does not mix with the amniotic fluid

Assisted Breech Delivery

- Once the buttocks have crowned, maximize maternal bearing down efforts, upright posture and suprapubic pressure
- After crowning, an assistant should exert gentle suprapubic pressure from above to keep the fetal head flexed and facilitate it's engagement.

Pinard's Manoeuvre
Flex the knee by applying gentle pressure on the popliteal fossa by index and middle fingers and then hook it down by movement of abduction

Delivery of Legs

- Do per vaginal examination and check for the position of legs
- If legs are flexed, they will deliver spontaneously with the next contraction
- If legs are extended, they are delivered by Pinard's manoeuvre
- Use a dry towel to wrap around the hips (not the abdomen) to help with gentle downward and outward traction which is applied in conjunction with maternal expulsive efforts until the scapula and axilla are visible.

Delivery of Arms

- After spontaneous delivery to the fetal umbilicus, once the scapula is visible, rotate the infant 90° and gently sweep the anterior arm out of the vagina by pressing on the inner aspect of the arm or elbow
- Rotate the infant 180° in the reverse direction, and sweep the other arm out of the vagina
- Once the arms are delivered, rotate the infant back 90° so that the back is anterior.

Delivery of the Fetal Head—The Most Decisive and Fundamental Step

- Should not take more than 10–15 minutes
- Various manoeuvres can be followed in practice.

I. Burns-Marshall Technique

- Allow baby's body to hang, until you can see the hair at the back of the neck
- Hold both feet
- Swing the feet upwards over to mother's abdomen
- Free baby's mouth and pause while you clean it
- Finish delivery by swinging the baby over mother's abdomen.

II. Mauriceau–Smellie–Veit Manoeuvre

- It is done by an assistant and an obstetrician to maintain the head in a flexed position to allow it's smallest diameter to pass
- Assistant applies suprapubic pressure
- Obstetrician inserts left hand in vagina
- The index and middle finger are kept on either side of maxilla and gentle pressure is applied on it, which flexes the neck moderately
- Left hand's palm should rest against the fetal chest
- Right hand:
  - Ring and little fingers are placed on baby's right shoulder
  - Middle finger in suboccipital region
  - Index finger on left shoulder
  - This helps in flexion of the neck.
- Suprapubic pressure to allow for delivery of the fetal head.

Advantages of Piper's Forceps:
- Controlled delivery of head
- Flexion is well-maintained
- Pull is directly applied over fetal head contrary to other manual methods, where it is applied via vertebral column

Precaution:
- During delivery of the head, avoid extreme elevation of the body, which may result in hyperextension of the cervical spine and potential neurologic injury

III. Piper Forceps can also be Used for Head Flexion

- Piper forceps are specialized forceps used only for the after-coming head of a breech presentation
- The after-coming head must have descended to fill the pelvis and must be in direct occipito anterior position
- Assistant holds trunk of fetus upwards horizontally, so that it may be out of way as much as possible

- Forceps blades are introduced at 4 o'clock and 8 o'clock position and made to lie against the sides of the head through a short arc
- Handles then lie along ventral aspect of fetus, so as to promote flexion
- Traction first made downwards and backwards till chin appears, then forceps and fetus are carried upwards towards mother's abdomen
- Very little or no traction is needed for delivery with Piper's forceps.

Chapter **61**

Labor Management in Hypertensive Disorders

Tania G Singh

Ergometrine or syntometrine should NOT be given as it may produce an acute rise in BP

- Written and informed consent (explaining all complications and associated risks) is very important in all hypertensive cases (as complications may occur at low BP readings)
- Vaginal delivery unless cesarean section is indicated for other reasons
- Steroids should be given
- Cervix unfavorable—cervical ripening is done using prostaglandins and augmentation with oxytocin and amniotomy
- Antihypertensive treatment should be continued throughout labor and birth to maintain systolic BP at less than 160 mm Hg and diastolic BP less than 110 mm Hg

If oxytocin is indicated, it should be concentrated and this fluid should be considered as intake

- Much lower values of BP are not recommended due to risk of placental abruption and hypoperfusion
- IV access
- Attention to administration of fluids
- Epidural can be given
- Vitals charting (every 2 hourly in latent phase and 1/2 hourly in active phase)
- For all cases of severe pre eclampsia, blood should be kept arranged
- Strict vigilance on signs of impending eclampsia
- Anesthetist and pediatrician to be informed beforehand
- Assistance with 2nd stage is *not routinely* required
- Active management of 3rd stage is recommended due to the increased risk of postpartum hemorrhage.

Assistance in 2nd Stage is Required if:

- BP is poorly controlled
- Progress is inadequate
- There are premonitory signs of eclampsia

Chapter 62

Monitoring Labor in a Diabetic Mother

Tania G Singh

- Wait for spontaneous onset of labor
  - Till 40 weeks in cases of GDM, well-controlled diet
  - Till 38–39 weeks in cases of GDM on insulin
  - Till 38 weeks in case of well-controlled pre-existing diabetes
  - Uncontrolled pre-existing diabetes, can be terminated earlier, when indicated
  - If glucocorticoid is given for lung maturity, caution is advised with close glycemic control during three days after the 1st dose
  - The steroid effect begins approximately 12 hours after the first dose and lasts for five days.
- Risks at the time of vaginal delivery
  - Shoulder dystocia
  - Brachial plexus injury
  - Clavicle fracture
  - Need for Roberts manoeuvre
  - Birth asphyxia
  - Need for interventional delivery.

LABOR

Spontaneous Labor

- Patient to be kept NPO
- GDM patients well-controlled on diet do not require insulin or sugar monitoring during labor
- Secure 2 IV lines.

First IV Line

- Insulin infusion with 1 unit/mL (50 units Insulin + 50 L of Normal saline)
- Infusion rate 1 mL/hr
- 2 hourly sugar monitoring and titrate infusion as per Table below.

Table 1: Insulin titration in Labor

Blood glucose levels (mg/dL)	Insulin (unit/hour)	Infusion rate (mL/hour)
≤ 100	No insulin	
101–140	1	1
141–180	1.5	1.5
181–220	2	2
>250→5% Dextrose changed to Normal saline		

Cesarean section is done in case where EFW is ≥4 kg or for other obstetric indications

Factors Associated with Shoulder Dystocia

- Previous shoulder dystocia
- Prolonged first stage of labor
- Macrosomia >4.5 kg
- Secondary arrest
- Diabetes mellitus
- Prolonged second stage of labor
- Maternal body mass index >30 kg/m^2
- Oxytocin augmentation
- Induction of labor
- Assisted vaginal delivery

Signs of Shoulder Dystocia

- Difficulty with delivery of the face and chin
- The head remaining tightly applied to the vulva or even retracting (turtle-neck sign)
- Failure of restitution of the fetal head
- Failure of the shoulders to descend

Second IV Line
- Start 5% dextrose @ 100–125 mL/hr (to meet the calorie demands).

Induced Labor
- With prostaglandins (after assessing Bishop's score)
- To be started early morning
- Give night dose of insulin and omit the morning dose
- Monitoring as mentioned above
- Strict FHS monitoring
- Partograph (to avoid obstructed labor) which is even more worse in a diabetic patient.

Chapter 63

Management in Molar Pregnancy

Tania G Singh

Suspicion of Molar Pregnancy

- Take complete history/physical examination/check vitals
- Send basic investigations (CBC, urine routine, ABO Rh, HIV, UPT, β hCG)
- Perform USG
- Review all reports
- Molar pregnancy confirmed → send additional investigations
- Ask the patient whether she desires future fertility
- If yes, evacuate the uterus (if hemodynamically stable)
- If no, can proceed with hysterectomy
- Blood availability should be confirmed prior to evacuation (especially when uterine size is >16 weeks).

Evacuation of Molar Pregnancy

- Suction curettage is done irrespective of the uterine size
- Only when fetal parts are large enough (as in case of partial mole) making suction evacuation impossible, then medical evacuation is done (very rarely)
- Cervical preparation immediately before the procedure
- After giving anesthesia, a 12–14 mm suction cannula is passed into lower uterine segment, rotated and contents sucked
- Gentle sharp curettage is done after that
- Oxytocin infusion (saline drip with 30 units of syntocinon running at 30 drops/minute) is started at the onset of evacuation and is continued for several hours after
- There is no need to send the POCs for histological examination in confirmed cases of molar pregnancy
- Prophylactic administration of single chemotherapeutic agent at the time of evacuation or immediately after, reduces the risk of postmolar GTN from 15–20% to 3–8%.

Various Agents and Doses

- Methotrexate 50 mg IV drip lasting for 3–4 hours during evacuation
- Actinomycin D IV 12 μg/kg daily (3 days prior and 2 days after)
- Methotrexate 15 mg orally daily (3 days prior and 2 days after).

Follow-up

- Repeat hCG after 1–2 weeks of evacuation (within 6–8 weeks) to see for regression, till three consecutive tests show normal levels

Additional Investigations

- LFT, RFT, Thyroid function tests
- CXR (lungs are a primary site of metastasis for malignant trophoblastic tumors)
- ECG, if appropriate
- Head CT/MRI (in case of choriocarcinoma or central nervous system signs)
- ECHO, only in suspected cases of acute left ventricular failure due to anemia, thyrotoxicosis, pulmonary embolization, etc.

Anesthesia

If hemodynamically stable patient, give spinal anesthesia (preferable). If hemodynamically unstable or have a coagulation defect, give general anesthesia

Reassuring Signs of Complete Evacuation:

- Prompt uterine involution
- Cessation of bleeding
- Ovarian cyst regression

- If normal, follow-up for 6 months from the day of evacuation (hCG at 3 month interval)
- If it is not normal, follow-up for 6 months from the day of normalization of hCG (hCG at 3 month interval)
- Hysterectomy—alternative to suction evacuation, if family is completed
- Metastasis can occur even after hysterectomy.

C h a p t e r **64**

Management of Cardiac Patient in Labor

Tania G Singh

Treatment Proper

First Stage of Labor

- Accurate assessment of pelvis because trial of labor is absolutely contraindicated
- Patients with cardiac disease of restrictive variety (e.g. mitral stenosis) are at increased risk of developing failure, therefore, extra caution is required
- Labor is fairly easy in majority of cases as inertia is rare and cervix dilates easily because it is softer and more vascular than usual because of venous congestion
- Antibiotics—recommended only for high and moderate risk patients
- Sedation: IV morphine (2–4 mg) → liberal use
- Pain relief: If patient is not anticoagulated, anesthesia of choice is epidural
- An epidural can be given for more than 12 hours after prophylactic thromboprophylaxis dose or for more than 24 hours after therapeutic dose or earlier at the discretion of the anesthetist
- IV fluids— less than or equal to 75 mL/hr
- Pulse oximeter, propped up position, oxygen and IV frusemide for class III and IV
- Class I and II—no serious problem
- Duration of 1st stage should not be more than 8 hours
- Onset of failure in 1st stage is a contraindication for interventions like cesarean section.

Second Stage of Labor

- Episiotomy (for easy delivery)
- Vacuum (better than forceps).

Third Stage of Labor

- Routine use of ergometrine is not allowed as it will increase the cardiac load
- Give oxytocin IV in drip and give frusemide 40 mg IV (to relieve heart of it's volumetric load)
- Ergometrine should not be used until 400 mL blood have been lost
- Immediately after delivery and episiotomy suturing:
  - Patient should be propped up
  - Give morphine
  - O_2 by mask
  - Pulse oximeter.
- Patient should be brought out from delivery room in trolley with propped up position only
- In case of PPH, misoprostol 600 mcg/rectally is preferred.

General Measures

- Labor and delivery in lateral decubitus position
- Pulse oximeter
- Adequate pain relief
- Restrict IV fluids to 75 mL/hour
- Antibiotic prophylaxis
- Invasive monitoring, if needed
- Medical therapy, optimization of loading conditions
- Cesarean section as per obstetric conditions
- Oxygen by mask
- Avoid bolus oxytocin and ergot compounds
- Thrombosis prophylaxis
- Prevention of pulmonary edema after delivery

Place of Cesarean Section

- Mortality higher 2 or 3 times
- Vaginal delivery is preferred as chances of infection, bleeding, clotting complications, acute shift in blood volume decreases in vaginal delivery
- In class IV and sicker patients, opt for elective cesarean section

Chapter 65

Preinduction Score or Modified Bishop Score or Prelabor Scoring

Tania G Singh

Components of Original Bishop's Score

- Cervical dilatation
- Cervical effacement
- Cervical consistency
- Cervical position
- Fetal station

- Bishop score is a prelabor scoring system to assist in predicting whether induction of labor will be required
- According to the Modified Bishop's preinduction cervical scoring system, *effacement* has been replaced by *cervical length in cm.*

Score	0	1	2	3
Dilatation	Closed	1–2	3–4	5
Length	>4	3–4	1–2	0
Consistency	Firm	Medium	Soft	-
Position	Posterior	Midline	Anterior	-
Station	–3	–2	–1/0	+1, +2

Interpretation

- Total score = 13
- Favorable score = 6–13
- Unfavorable score = 0–5
- A score of less than or equal to 5 suggests that labor is unlikely to start without induction
- A score of more than or equal to 9 indicates that labor will most likely commence spontaneously.

C h a p t e r **66**

Induction of Labor

Tania G Singh

RISKS

- Increased risk of operative vaginal delivery
- Cesarean section
- Excessive uterine activity
- Abnormal FHR pattern
- Uterine rupture
- Prolonged labor due to abnormal uterine action
- Possibly cord prolapse with AROM
- Failed induction (prolongation of latent phase beyond 12–18 hours)
- Prematurity
- Maternal water intoxication
- Partial placental detachment and bloody tap
- Fetal pneumonia (in case of PROM >18 hour without antibiotics).

Definition
Artificial initiation of uterine contractions prior to their spontaneous onset, any time after fetal viability, with or without ruptured membranes by a method that aims at vaginal delivery

Prerequisites for Induction

- Determine the appropriate indication/any contraindication
- Confirm gestational age
- Determine Bishop score
- Assess for CPD
- Membrane status (intact or ruptured)
- Assess fetal health—NST for minimum 20 minutes (facilities should be available)
- Informed consent
- During induction obstetrician must be present.

Factors for Successful Induction
- Term or post-term
- Bishop score ≥6
- Positive oxytocin sensitivity test
- Parous woman
- PROM

METHODS OF INDUCTION

Surgical Methods

Sweeping/Stripping of Membranes

- Releases phospholipase A_2 and $\uparrow$ production of $PGF_{2\alpha}$
- Finger inserted in internal os is moved circumferentially, when cervix is sufficiently dilated or try to open the cervix or cervical massage, when closed
- Concerns:
  - Patient discomfort
  - Bleeding
  - Accidental rupture of membranes
  - Initiation of irregular uterine contractions.

Common Side Effects with Prostaglandins
- Nausea
- Vomiting
- Diarrhea
- Pyrexia
- Bronchospasm
- Shivering

Amniotomy

- Artificial rupture of membranes
- Works well, when amniotomy is followed by oxytocin.

Pharmacological Methods

Prostaglandins

- PGE_2 (Dinoprostone)
- PGE_1 (Misoprostol)

DINOPROSTONE (PGE₂)

Gel (Intracervical/Intravaginal)

Intracervical Gel

- Bring gel to room temperature before application
- Monitor FHR and uterine activity continuously starting 15–30 minutes before gel introduction and continuing for 30–120 minutes after gel insertion
- Each prefilled syringe contains 0.5 mg of PGE_2 gel
- Gel is inserted under direct vision using a vaginal speculum into endocervix just below the level of internal os
- Patient to remain recumbent for 30 minutes
- Maximum recommended dosage 1.5 mg of dinoprostone (3 doses) in 24 hours
- May be repeated every 6–8 hours, depending upon the response
- Do not start oxytocin for 6 (intracervical)–12 (intravaginal) hours after placement of last dose, to allow for spontaneous onset of labor and to protect the uterus from hyperstimulation
- Drawback: Expensive drug.

Intravaginal Gel

- Available in prefilled syringes containing 1 mg and 2 mg
- 2 mg (per vaginally) → nulliparous woman with unfavorable cervix
- 1 mg (per vaginally) → for multiparous woman
- Second dose → 1–2 mg PGE_2 may be administered 6 hours later
- Maximum dose in a 12 hour period.

Intravaginal Tablets

- Recommended dosage: 3 mg into posterior fornix
- Available as 3.0 mg tablet form
- Dose can be repeated 6-8 hours after the first dose
- Maximum total dose → 6 mg for all women.

Dinoprostone Vaginal Inserts/Controlled Release Prostaglandin

- Consists of a polymer base containing 10 mg of dinoprostone with a polyester retrieval string
- Insert releases 0.3 mg/hour of PGE_2 over a 12 hour period
- Is placed in posterior fornix of vagina
- Removed after 12 hours or with:
    - Onset of labor
    - Spontaneous rupture of membranes
    - Excessive uterine activity.
- Oxytocin can be used 30 minutes after it's removal.

Contraindications to Prostaglandins

- Hypersensitivity to drug
- Glaucoma
- Asthma

Oral Misoprostol Solution

- A single misoprostol tablet is dissolved in drinking water so that 1 mL contains 1 µg (e.g. 100 µg tablet in 100 mL water), rather than breaking the tablet into 4 or 8 pieces
- 25 mL of misoprostol solution is then given every 2 hours
- Solution is stable for up to 24 hours at room temperature but should then be discarded

MISOPROSTOL (PGE$_1$)

- Vaginal Misoprostol: 25 µg per vaginally every 4–6 hourly (maximum of 6 doses)
- Oral Misoprostol Solution
- Oral Misoprostol Tablets: 50 µg every 4 hourly (maximum of 6 doses) OR 25 µg 2 hourly.

Monitoring

- Before starting induction, NST for 30 minutes
- Once started, woman must be monitored closely
- FHR, uterine activity and maternal vitals are continuously monitored for 30 minutes after each dose of misoprostol and every 30 minutes from the onset of uterine contractions
- Oxytocin infusion should not to be started
  - Less than 4 hours after last dose of vaginal misoprostol and
  - 2 hour after last dose of oral misoprostol.

> If there are ≥3 clinically adequate contractions in every 10 minutes after misoprostol, dose can be withheld till further needed

Side Effects of Misoprostol

- Rapid onset
- Prolonged action
- Shivering, pyrexia, diarrhea
- Total bioavailability >> oral route, therefore, not to be used for induction of labor
- Not recommended for women with previous cesarean section.

Benefits of Misoprostol

- Inexpensive
- Stored at room temperature
- No refrigeration required, therefore, easily transported
- Shorter induction to delivery interval
- Lower cesarean section rates

Pain Relief after Induction of Labor

- Simple analgesics by oral route
- Epidural analgesia can be offered.

Oxytocin

- In 1st trimester, uterus is almost refractory to oxytocin
- As pregnancy advances, number of oxytocin receptors in uterus increases and, therefore uterus becomes responsive to it
- Onset of action starts 3–5 minutes after starting the infusion.

Side Effects

- Uterine tachysystole or changes in CTG tracings
- Water intoxication can occur at higher concentrations of oxytocin
- Hypotension may occur following a rapid IV oxytocin injection.

Uterine Tachysystole

- >5 contractions in 10 minutes
- Contractions lasting 2 minutes or more

Dose

- Commence oxytocin @ 1–2 mU/minute (i.e. 6–12 mL/hour of 10 units oxytocin diluted in 1000 mL of an isotonic solution for an oxytocin concentration of 10 mIU/mL
- Use minimum dose possible and aim for a maximum of 3–4 contractions in 10 minutes
- Maximum dose → 20 mIU/minute.

Chapter **67**

First Stage of Labor

Tania G Singh

Latent First Stage of Labor

- Painful contractions present
- There is some cervical effacement
- Cervical dilatation up to 4 cm.

Established First Stage of Labor

- Regular painful contractions
- There is progressive cervical dilatation more than 4 cm.

Duration

- In primigravida: Last on an average 8 hours and rarely more than 18 hours
- Multigravida: Last on an average 5 hours and rarely more than 12 hours.

Observations during the Established First Stage

- Use of partogram once labor is established
- Record the following:
    - Half hourly documentation of frequency of contractions
    - Hourly pulse
    - Four hourly temperature and blood pressure
    - Frequency of passing urine
    - Vaginal examination 4 hourly.
- Try to give one to one support or be very humble to the patient
- Give her the option of labor analgesia.

> In normally progressing labor, do not perform amniotomy and/ or oxytocin use routinely

Delay in the First Stage

Delay suspected:

- Amniotomy should be considered for all women with intact membranes
    - It will shorten the labor by about an hour and
    - It may increase the strength of contractions.
- Perform 2 hourly vaginal examination
- Oxytocin can be started
- Offer the woman an epidural before oxytocin is started
- If oxytocin is used, increase the dose only after every 30 minutes until there are 4–5 contractions in 10 minutes
- A vaginal examination 4 hours after starting oxytocin
- If cervical dilatation has increased by less than 2 cm after 4 hours of oxytocin, case is to be reviewed to assess the need for cesarean section
- If cervical dilatation has increased by more than or equal to 2 cm, advise 4 hourly vaginal examinations.

> For a multiparous woman with confirmed delay in the established first stage of labor, obstetrician should perform a full assessment, including abdominal palpation and vaginal examination, before a decision is made about using oxytocin

Chapter 68

Second Stage of Labor

Tania G Singh

Passive Second Stage of Labor

- Full dilatation of the cervix before or in the absence of involuntary expulsive contractions.

Active Second Stage of Labor

- Baby is visible
- Expulsive contractions present
- Cervix fully dilated.

Observations during the Second Stage

- Station at the onset of the second stage
- Frequency of contractions
- Expulsive efforts of the mother
- Intermittent auscultation of the fetal heart rate immediately after a contraction for at least 1 minute, at least every 5 minutes
- Palpate the woman's pulse every 15 minutes to differentiate it from fetal heart rate
- Adequate hydration
- Comfortable position to the woman (avoid lying supine or in semisupine position).

Preventive Measures

- Empty the bladder
- Start oxytocin, if not started earlier
- If already started, increase the dose to get adequate contractions
- Artificial rupture of membranes, if still intact
- Assess the need to undertake an operative vaginal birth
- Advise the woman to have a cesarean section if vaginal birth is not possible

Delay in the Second Stage

For a Nulliparous Woman

- Birth would be expected to take place within 3 hours of the start of the active second stage
- Suspect delay and start preventive measures, if birth has not lasted for 2 hours or there is inadequate rotation or descent of the presenting part after 1 hour of the active second stage

For a Multiparous Woman

- Birth would be expected to take place within 2 hours of the start of the active second stage in most women
- Suspect delay and start preventive measures
  - If birth has not lasted for 1 hour or
  - If rotation and/or descent of the presenting part is inadequate after 30 minutes of active second stage.

Interventions to Reduce Perineal Trauma

- Do not perform perineal massage in the second stage of labor
- Assist in spontaneous birth by guarding the perineum and flexing the baby's head ('hands on')
- Lidocaine spray should not be used
- Do not carry out a routine episiotomy during spontaneous vaginal birth
- If an episiotomy is performed, it should be a right mediolateral episiotomy (preferably) originating at the vaginal fourchette
- The angle to the vertical axis should be between 45 and 60°.

Chapter 69

Labor Analgesia and Anesthesia

Tania G Singh and Gagandeep Anand

Nonregional Methods

- Breathing and relaxation techniques
- Massage
- Labor in water.

Nonpharmacological Analgesia

Inhalational Analgesia

Entonox (a 50:50 mixture of oxygen and nitrous oxide)

- Side effects: Nausea and lightheadedness.

Intravenous and Intramuscular Opioids

Pethidine, diamorphine

- Side effects for mother: drowsiness, nausea and vomiting
- Administer an antiemetic at the same time
- Baby: Short-term respiratory depression and drowsiness which may last several days
- They may interfere with breastfeeding.

Regional Analgesia

Epidural Analgesia

- Provides more effective pain relief than opioids
- Not associated with long-term backache
- Not associated with a prolonged first stage of labor or an increased chance of a cesarean birth
- It is associated with a longer second stage of labor and an increased chance of vaginal instrumental birth
- Patient's mobility may be reduced as intensive monitoring and intravenous access is required with it
- Timing of regional analgesia: latent first stage of labor
- During establishment of epidural analgesia or after further boluses (≥10 mL of low-dose solutions), measure blood pressure every 5 minutes for 15 minutes
- Continuous CTG for at least 30 minutes during establishment of regional analgesia and after administration of each further bolus of more than or equal to 10 mL
- Assess the level of the sensory block hourly

For women laboring in water, monitor the temperature of the woman and the water hourly to ensure that the woman is comfortable and not becoming pyrexial. The temperature of the water should be <37.5°C

Do not offer transcutaneous electrical nerve stimulation (TENS) to women in established labor

Preloading and maintenance fluid infusion need not be administered routinely before establishing low-dose epidural analgesia and combined spinal–epidural analgesia

- Patient can adopt any upright positions they find comfortable throughout labor
- Continue epidural until after completion of the third stage of labor and any necessary perineal repair
- Even with complete cervical dilatation, in a woman with regional analgesia, pushing can be delayed for an hour or so if the woman has no urge to push, after which she should be actively encouraged to push during contractions
- Do not routinely use oxytocin in the second stage of labor for women with regional analgesia.

Combined Spinal-epidural Analgesia

- Bupivacaine and fentanyl is used for combined analgesia
- Initial dose: 10–15 mL of 0.0625–0.1% bupivacaine with 1–2 mcg/mL fentanyl which is a test dose, and therefore, administer cautiously to avoid inadvertent intrathecal injection
- For maintenance: 0.0625–0.1% bupivacaine or equivalent combined with 2.0 mcg/mL fentanyl.

> If the woman is not pain-free 30 minutes after each administration of local anesthetic/opioid solution, recall the anesthetist

Chapter 70

Use of a Partograph

Tania G Singh

Observations Charted on the Partograph

- Progress of labor
  - Cervical dilatation
  - Uterine contractions.
- Fetal condition
  - Fetal heart rate
  - Membranes and liquor
  - Moulding of the fetal skull.
- Maternal condition
  - Pulse: Measured half hourly
  - BP, Temp: Measured every 4 hourly
  - Urine
  - Drugs; IV fluids
  - Oxytocin regimen.

The Graph Sections of the Partograph

- On the top: Patient's identification details
- Below that: Recordings of the Fetal Heart Rate, at the beginning and then every 30 minutes
- Below the fetal heart rate, there are two rows close together:
  - The first is to record liquor—if the fetal membranes have ruptured, mention the color of the amniotic fluid initially and then 4 hourly
  - The row below 'liquor' is labeled moulding—assess the degree of moulding initially and every 4 hours.
- Below 'Moulding' there is an area of the partograph labeled cervix (cm) (Plot X) for recording cervical dilatation
  - This area of the partograph is also where you record descent of head (Plot O), which is how far down the birth canal the baby's head has progressed
  - These are measured every 4 hourly
  - There are two rows at the bottom of this section of the partograph to write the number of hours since you began monitoring the labor and the time on the clock.
- The next section of the partograph is for recording contractions per 10 minutes initially and then every 30 minutes
- Below that are two rows for recording administration of oxytocin during labor and the amount given
- The next area is labeled Drugs given and IV fluids given to the mother
- Near the bottom of the partograph, record the mother's vital signs

Partograph is to be started when it is sure that the woman is getting adequate contractions:

In latent phase: ≥2 contractions in 10 minutes each lasting ≥20 sec

In the active phase: contractions must be ≥1 in 20 minutes each lasting ≥20 seconds

Cervical Dilatation

- **Latent Phase:** 0–3 cm
- **Active Phase:** 4–10 cm (full cervical dilatation)

Descent of Head

- Should always be assessed by abdominal examination immediately before doing a vaginal examination
- It is expressed in terms of fifths above the pelvic brim, where the width of the five fingers act as a guide
- A head that is freely mobile will accommodate the full width of five fingers
- It is found to be a more reliable way of estimating the descent than vaginal examination where large caput formation often leads to confusion

- Below that you record the mother's temp °C
- At the very bottom, record the characteristics of the mother's Urine—protein, acetone, volume.

Alert and Action Lines

- In the section for cervical dilatation and fetal head descent, there are two diagonal lines labeled Alert and Action
- The Alert line starts at 4 cm of cervical dilatation and travels diagonally upwards till 10 cm at the rate of 1 cm/hour
- The Action line is parallel to the Alert line, and 4 hours to its right
- These two lines warn us to take action quickly, if the labor is not progressing normally.

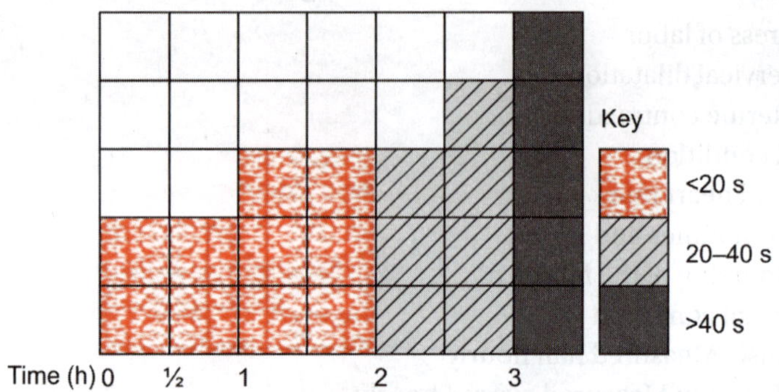

Fig. 1: Three ways of shading shows the duration of contractions

Moulding

- If bones are separated and the sutures can be felt easily: "O"
- If bones are just touching each other: record as "+"
- If bones are overlapping: record as "++"
- If bones are overlapping severely: record as "+++".

Four Different Ways to Record State of Liquor on Partograph

- If the membranes are intact—record as letter "I" for Intact
- If the membranes are ruptured and liquor is clear: "C"
- If the membranes are ruptured and liquor is meconium stained: letter "M"
- If the membranes are ruptured and the liquor is absent—letter "A" is written

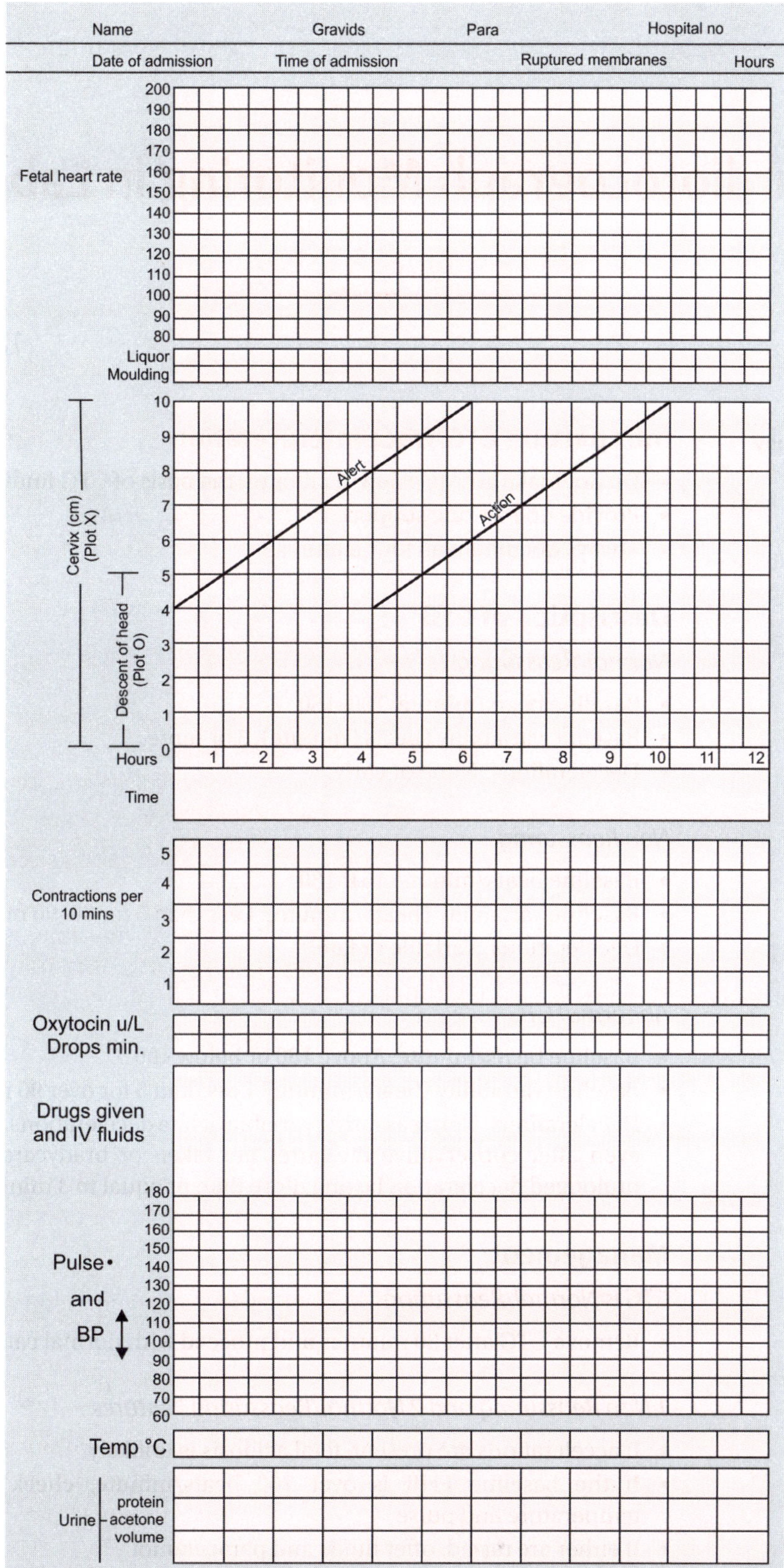

Fig. 2: Simplified partograph

Chapter 71

Cardiotocograph Monitoring in Labor

Tania G Singh

Cardiotocography Features
- Baseline fetal heart rate
- Baseline variability
- Presence or absence of decelerations
- Presence of accelerations

Intrapartum CTG Trace Interpretation

- Do not make any decision in labor on the basis of CTG findings alone
- Provide one-to-one support
- Always document all four features.

Description of CTG

Normal/Reassuring

- Baseline beats/minute: 100–160
- Baseline variability (beats/ minute): 5 or more
- Decelerations: None or early.

Non Reassuring

- Baseline beats/minute: 161–180
- Baseline variability (beats/minute): Less than 5 for 30–90 minutes
- Decelerations: Variable or late.

Abnormal CTG

- Baseline beats/minute: Above 180 or below 100
- Baseline variability (beats/minute): Less than 5 for over 90 minutes
- Decelerations: Non reassuring variable or late decelerations, not improving even after conservative measures are taken or bradycardia or a single prolonged deceleration lasting more than or equal to 3 minutes.

Management

CTG is Normal/Reassuring

- Remove CTG after 20 minutes and proceed with normal care.

1 Non Reassuring and 2 Normal/Reassuring Features

- If accelerations are present, fetal acidosis is unlikely
- If the baseline FHR is over 160 beats/minute, check the woman's temperature and pulse
- If either are raised, offer fluids and paracetamol
- Encourage her to mobilise or adopt a left-lateral position
- Avoid being in supine position
- Give oral or intravenous fluids
- Stop oxytocin and offer tocolysis, if required
- Inform the obstetrician.

1 Abnormal Feature or 2 Non Reassuring Features

- Fetal acidosis is very likely to happen
- Offer all the measures mentioned above
- Scalp stimulation
- Take fetal blood sampling or expedite birth, if an FBS cannot be obtained and no accelerations are seen as a result of scalp stimulation
- Take action within half an hour, if late decelerations are accompanied by tachycardia and/or reduced baseline variability.

CTG is Abnormal and Indicates Need for Urgent Intervention

- Bradycardia or a single prolonged deceleration with baseline less than 100 beats/minute, persisting for more than or equal to 3 minutes or more
- Associated with current fetal acidosis or imminent rapid development of fetal acidosis
- Make preparations for urgent birth especially if it persists for 9 minutes.

Chapter 72

Fetal Blood Sampling

Tania G Singh

Keep a close watch on CTG tracings and repeat the test, only if required Try to expedite delivery

AN OVERVIEW

- The blood sample will be used to measure the level of acid in the baby's blood, to see how well the baby is coping with labor
- A small instrument similar to speculum will be inserted in vagina
- Sample of blood will be taken from the baby's head by making a small scratch on the baby's scalp
- This will heal quickly after birth
- Risk of infection is small
- The procedure can help to reduce the need for further, more serious interventions
- If a sample cannot be obtained (especially if the cervix is <4 cm dilated), a cesarean section or instrumental birth (forceps or ventouse) may be needed
- First exclude all the contraindications to it
- Sample is to be taken with the woman in the left-lateral position
- Measure either lactate or pH when performing fetal blood sampling
- Measure lactate if the necessary equipment and suitably trained staff are available; otherwise measure pH.

CLASSIFICATION OF FETAL BLOOD SAMPLE RESULTS

Lactate (mmol/L)	*pH*	*Interpretation*
≤4.1	≥7.25	Normal
4.2–4.8	7.21–7.24	Borderline
≥4.9	≤7.20	Abnormal

Chapter 73

Meconium-stained Liquor

Tania G Singh

CAUSES

Under Normal Circumstances

- MSAF may be a natural phenomenon that simply reflects a post-term fetus with a mature gastrointestinal tract in which motilin levels have risen
- Vagal stimulation produced by cord or head compression also may be associated with the passage of meconium in the absence of fetal distress.

In Conditions of Stress

- Fetal hypoxia and acidosis producing relaxation of the anal sphincter
- It increases the risk of intra-amniotic infection and subsequent meconium aspiration syndrome
- Early ARM may help in such cases.

MECHANISMS OF MECONIUM INJURY

- Mechanical obstruction of airways
- Chemical pneumonitis
- Vasoconstriction of pulmonary vessels
- Inactivation of surfactant.

An Overview

- Meconium usually appears from 20th week
- At term: Uniformly distributed throughout gut up to rectum → presence of intestinal peristalsis
- Composition: Lanugo, hair, epithelial cells, mucus, intestinal epithelial cells (exfoliated), intestinal juices
- Color: Greenish black due to bile pigments especially biliverdin

Recent studies contradict the use of saline amnioinfusion and aggressive naso/oropharyngeal suctioning at perineum to decrease the risk of meconium aspiration

Chapter 74

Third Stage of Labor

Tania G Singh

For active management, administer 10 IU of oxytocin by intramuscular injection with the birth of the anterior shoulder or immediately after the birth of the baby and before the cord is clamped and cut. Use oxytocin as it is associated with fewer side effects than oxytocin plus ergometrine

DEFINITION

The time from the birth of the baby to the expulsion of the placenta and membranes.

Active Management of the Third Stage (AMTSL) Components

- Routine use of uterotonic drugs
- Delayed clamping and cutting of the cord
- Controlled cord traction after signs of separation of the placenta.

Physiological Management of the Third Stage Components

- No routine use of uterotonic drugs
- No clamping of the cord until pulsation has stopped
- Delivery of the placenta by maternal effort.

Prolonged Third Stage

- If it is not completed within 30 minutes of the birth with active management OR
- Within 60 minutes of the birth with physiological management.

Observations in the Third Stage

- Make a note of the general physical condition of the woman (as shown by her color, respiration and her own report of how she feels)
- Vaginal blood loss
- Do not clamp the cord earlier than 1 minute from the birth of the baby unless there is concern about the integrity of the cord or the baby has a heartbeat less than 60 beats/minute
- Clamp the cord before 5 minutes in order to perform controlled cord traction as part of active management
- Record the timing of cord clamping in both active and physiological management.

AMSTL is associated with a lower risk of a postpartum hemorrhage and/or blood transfusion and also shortens the third stage. But there is a little more risk of nausea and vomiting as compared to physiological management

Do not use either umbilical oxytocin infusion or prostaglandin routinely in the third stage of labor

Chapter 75

Perineal Care after Birth

Tania G Singh

Perineal Care

- First degree—injury to skin only
- Second degree—injury to the perineal muscles but not the anal sphincter
- Third degree—injury to the perineum involving the anal sphincter complex:
  - 3a—less than 50% of external anal sphincter thickness
  - 3b—more than 50% of external anal sphincter thickness
  - 3c—internal anal sphincter injury
- Fourth degree—injury to the perineum involving the anal sphincter complex (external and internal anal sphincter) and anal epithelium.

Assessing the Genital Trauma

Make arrangements for:
- Local (infiltration with up to 20 mL of 1% lidocaine) or regional analgesia
- Comfortable position to the woman
- Ensure good lighting for visual assessment of the extent of perineal trauma, the apex of the injury and assessment of bleeding
- Initial examination should be performed very gently
- Perform a rectal examination as well to assess whether there has been any damage to the external or internal anal sphincter.

Repairing the Trauma

- Use aseptic techniques
- First degree trauma: Suture the wound in order to improve healing, unless the skin edges are well-opposed
- Second-degree trauma: The muscle should be sutured
  - If the skin is well-opposed after suturing of the muscle, there is no need to suture it
  - If the skin does require suturing, use a continuous subcuticular technique
- Perineal repair: Use a continuous nonlocked suturing technique for the vaginal wall and muscle layer
- An absorbable synthetic suture material should be used to suture the perineum
- Instruments, mop and swab count should be checked before and after the procedure
- Insert an indwelling catheter for 24 hours to prevent urinary retention in cases of third and fourth degree trauma or paraurethral tears
- Carry out rectal examination after completing the repair
- Pelvic floor exercises should be taught before discharge.

Initial Assessment after Birth
- Record her temperature, pulse and blood pressure
- Uterine contraction and lochia
- Examine the placenta for completeness
- Early assessment of the woman's emotional and psychological condition
- Encourage voiding
- Inform immediately if even 6 hours after, the bladder is palpable and patient is unable to pass urine

Give rectal nonsteroidal anti-inflammatory drugs routinely after perineal repair of first- and second-degree trauma provided these drugs are not contraindicated

Section V:

Postnatal Ward Rounds

General Postnatal Care

Tania G Singh

Hospital Care

First 24 Hours after Vaginal Delivery

- Vitals/Blood loss
  - Every 15 minutes in first hour, at 2 hours, then after 6 hours of birth.
- Voiding—within first 6 hours
- Abdominal and vaginal examination
  - Due each time with vitals
  - Fundus firm, central, +/– 1 finger above/below umbilicus
  - Perineal heating.
- Oral Intake
  - Ensure adequate hydration within half an hour after delivery of placenta.
- Ambulation
  - Immediately after delivery.
- Breastfeeding
  - Immediately after delivery
  - Then × 2 hourly.

First 24 Hours after Cesarean Section

- Vitals/Blood loss:
  - Every 15 minutes in first hour, at 2 hours, then 4 hourly × 24 hours.
- Voiding
  - Catheter for first 24 hours (urine should not be concentrated and should not be < min 30 mL/hour).
- Abdominal and vaginal examination
  - Due each time with vitals
  - Rest same as above.
- Oral intake
  - Sips of water after 6 hours and subsequent feeds depending on that.
- Ambulation
  - Encourage ambulation within 12–24 hours
  - Start leg movements after 6 hours of surgery.
- Breastfeeding
  - In the first hour after surgery
  - Then × 2 hourly.

Immediately after labor, the woman is in a state of physical fatigue in many cases, slight shivering, muscular tremors and chattering of teeth occur for about 10–15 minutes

- Breasts should be soft and colostrum can be expressed
- Nipples intact, may appear flat or inverted but protrude well on latching, with minimal tenderness

Dressing should be changed at 24–48 hours and waterproof dressing should be provided so as to encourage the patient to take bath

Subsequently (In the Hospital)

Abdomen/Fundus

- Fundus firm/central, descending ≈ 1–1.5 cm/day
- Not palpable after 7–10 days
- Prepregnant state at 6 weeks.

Abdominal Wound

- Fundus may be tender but improving
- Scar should be well approximated and free of inflammation
- Little or no drainage
- Dressing should be clean, dry and intact
- Incision swelling decreases
- No signs of gaping
- No signs of infection
- Patient may experience numbness around incision after a week
- Patient should take a lateral position while getting up from bed.

General Assessment
- Fundal height
- Uterine contraction and retraction
- Vaginal bleeding, including per vaginal examination to look for any hematoma development
- Blood loss measurement for first 2 hours

Breasts and Feeds

- After 24–48 hours, breasts feel firmer, colostrum more easily expressed
- Frequent breastfeeding prevents engorgement
- Well-supported brassiere should be worn (not restricting the feed)
- Teach the mother signs of proper latching.

In Nonbreastfeeding Women

- Breasts soft, colostrum may be present
- Wear supportive bra within 6 hours of birth
- To be worn continuously until lactation is suppressed, about 5–10 days
- Use of anti-inflammatory agents
- Application of cold treatments, such as gel packs, cold packs or cold cabbage leaves for comfort
- Avoid stimulation of the breasts, such as heat, pumping, etc. until lactation is suppressed
- Medication to aid suppression
- Small amounts of milk may be produced for up to a month postpartum
- Breasts will start to become softer as lactation is suppressed
- Resumption of menstrual periods — as soon as 6–8 weeks
- Use contraception.

If patient is not able to void urine, use the following measures to help void:
- Ambulation, oral analgesia
- Squeeze bottle with warm water
- Running water
- Hands in water
- Blow bubbles through a straw
- Sitz bath
- Shower
- Teach contraction and relaxation of pelvic floor

Other Measures

Mother

- Adequate rest for mother
- General assessment
- Keep the mother warm
- Breathing and pelvic floor exercises should be taught before discharge
- Ensure extra care, if woman had any antepartum or intrapartum complications
- Assess lochia
- Change pad every 4 hourly

Assessment of Lochia
- Amount
- Clots
- Color
- Odour
- Stage of involution
- Usually subsides by 4 weeks (changes from lochia rubra to lochia serosa, then to alba)
- It should not be foul smelling

- Perineal care
  - Wipe the perineum and remove the pad from front to back. This avoids dragging infection from the anal area to the vaginal area
  - Do not use tampons after delivery → cause of infection
  - Sitz bath ideally after every bowel movement.
- Avoid constipation by eating foods rich in fibre and drinking plenty of oral fluids
- Kegels exercises: No one can tell that you are doing Kegels and you can do them anywhere
- Analgesics.

Care of Baby

- Ensure thermal protection immediately after the birth and subsequently, educate the mother the importance of burping after each feed—method, its clinical relevance, the risks of not doing it
- Teach mother to observe for danger signs in the baby
- Skin-to-skin contact, massaging a baby's feet or tickling behind baby's ears should be used to wake the baby while feeding
- Assessment of baby by pediatrician before discharge
- Pediatrician should be informed, if baby doesn't pass meconium in first 24 hours
- Neonates developing jaundice within first 24 hours should be urgently evaluated
- Anti-D to the mother, if mother Rh negative and baby's blood group is positive
- Baby vaccination (MMR)
- A hearing screen of the neonate should be completed prior to discharge.

Sitz Bath

Sitting in shallow water, only deep enough to cover the hips and buttocks

Take at least three sitz baths every day for 20 minutes for the first 7 days.

Cold sitz bath can decrease swelling at the perineum

After the first 2–3 days, warm sitz baths will improve blood flow to the perineum, which eases urination and relieves pain

Kegel's Exercises

- Squeeze the perineal muscles as if you are trying to stop the flow of urine
- Hold for 5–10 sec and then relax
- Do this exercise 10 times/day in sets of 10 repetitions
- Do at least 10 Kegel exercises every time you urinate and at least 100 Kegels each day

Chapter 77

Breastfeeding Advice

Tania G Singh

Attachment and Position

Indicator of Good Position and Attachment

- Less areola visible underneath the chin than above the nipple
- Chin touching the breast, with both the upper and lower lip turned out (everted)
- With the nose free and at the level of the nipple
- Mouth is wide open
- The baby is swallowing
- Baby's head and body in straight line and supported.

Signs of Successful Milk Transfer

The baby has:
- Audible swallowing
- Sustained rhythmic suck and swallowing with occasional pauses
- Relaxed arms and hands
- Moist mouth
- Satisfaction after feeding
- Regular soaked/heavy nappies.

Mother
- Feels no breast or nipple pain
- Experiences her breast softening
- May experience uterine discomfort
- Experiences no compression of the nipple at the end of the feed
- Feels relaxed and sleepy
- Feels thirsty (due to release of oxytocin with suckling).

Various Positions

Sitting Position

- Baby's head on her forearm on same side
- Neck slightly extended
- Baby's ear, shoulder and hip in one line.

Lateral Position

- On her side between trunk and arm.

Factors Influencing Breastfeeding/Milk Production

- Hormones
- Suckling helps in triggering a rise in prolactin, which usually falls after delivery

Factors having Positive Impact

Those Influenced by Prolactin (Milk Secretion Reflex)

- The first feed
- Feeding according to need (night feeds, demand feeds)
- Baby behavioral states
- Proper attachment.

Those Influenced by Oxytocin (Milk Ejection Reflex)

- Rooming in—Thought, sight and sound of baby
- Skin-to-skin contact (SSC).

Factors which may Negatively Impact

- Use of dummies/pacifiers.

The First Feed

- Putting the baby to breasts within the first one to two hours
- Baby will usually demonstrate the following sequentially:
  - Opens eyes, quietly looks around and searches for mother's nipple
  - Uncurls fists and makes grasping movements toward nipple
  - Makes small 'licking' movements
  - Demonstrates 'rooting' behavior which may include:
    - Opening mouth
    - Turning head towards the nipple
    - Rubbing chin into breast
    - Attempting to self-attach.
- It is important that the breastfeed should not be interrupted until baby indicates satiety by:
  - Spontaneously detaching from the nipple without further rooting behavior
  - Falling asleep at the breast.

Advantages of Feeding According to Need

Mother

- Increases the rate of successfully establishing lactation
- Reduces the incidence of breast engorgement
- Establishes a supply and demand pattern.

Baby

- Increases breastfeeding duration
- Decreases the incidence and severity of physiological jaundice.

Milk Ejection Reflex

- Stimulates neurohypophysis to liberate oxytocin
- Contraction of myoepithelial cells in the alveoli $\rightarrow$ expulsion of milk into milk ducts $\rightarrow$ milk expression from lactating breast
- Occurs a number of times during a feed
- Different mothers will react differently to this reflex
  - May experience a sensation of warmth or tingling in their breasts
  - May experience 'afterbirth'/abdominal pain or discomfort during MER
  - May be unaware of the milk letdown.

Rooming-in
Kangaroo Mother Care, where mother and baby remain together 24 hours a day, helps in Milk Ejection ('letdown') Reflex (MER)

Dummy (Pacifier) Use
- Associated with shortened breastfeeding duration
- May contribute to breastfeeding difficulty
- Not recommended in the healthy, term-breastfed baby until breastfeeding is well-established
- At sleeping time, their use has been associated with a reduced incidence of SIDS in both breastfed infants and those fed with infant formula
- Frequent use may negatively impact upon breastfeeding which may reduce milk supply and slow baby's weight gain

Drugs Compatible with Breastfeeding
- Penicillins
- Many topical agents
- Analgesics
- Antihypertensives
- Antiepileptics
- Anxiolytics
- Antidepressant drugs

- Changes in the baby's sucking pattern throughout the feed will indicate that MER is occurring.

Benefits of Rooming-in

- Unrestricted breastfeeding access
- Increases breastfeeding duration
- Mother becomes familiar with their baby's feeding patterns
- Promotes relaxation and sleep
- Reduces the risk of SIDS.

Skin-to-Skin Contact

Mother

- Stimulates release of oxytocin which:
  - Minimizes blood loss
  - Decreases anxiety
  - Promotes mother baby emotional attachment
- May prevent or alleviate breastfeeding problems (engorgement, sore nipples).

Baby

- Maintains body temperature
- Decreases length of crying time
- Increases interaction with mother
- Promotes innate behaviors that assist in establishing breastfeeding
- Increases the duration of breastfeeding
- Maintains normal blood glucose levels.

Feeding Frequency

- The initiation of lactation is hormonally driven
- Storage capacity of breasts impacts upon the length and frequency of breast feeds
  - Range from 80 mL to as much as 600 mL but this cannot be determined by visual assessment
  - Large breasts may contain increased adipose tissue, rather than mammary tissue
  - The baby of a mother with a smaller storage capacity should feed more frequently than the baby of a mother with a larger storage capacity to receive the same amount of milk in a day.
- Most healthy babies will feed between 8 and 12 times in a 24-hour period
- Total length of time at each breast does not correlate with amount of milk transferred.

Sucking Patterns

Nonnutritive Sucking

- Rapid and shallow
- 2 sucks/seconds
- Infrequent swallows

Nutritive Sucking

- Deeper and slower
- Approximately 1 suck/second
- Swallows after every 1 or 2 sucks

Chapter **78**

Complications after Cesarean Section

Tania G Singh

OPERATIVE

- Maternal mortality
- Injuries to the bladder or ureter
- Transient tachypnea of the newborn is more common after cesarean section
- Fetal injuries.

POSTOPERATIVE

Early

- Thrombosis and pulmonary embolism
- Acute dilatation of the stomach and paralytic ileus
- Wound infection, puerperal sepsis and burst abdomen
- Chest infection.

Late

- Rupture of the uterine scar
- Incisional hernia
- An increased risk of placenta previa, placental abruption and placenta accreta (in subsequent pregnancies).

POSTOPERATIVE INFECTIONS

Fever

- Presence of temperature more than or equal to 100.4°F (38°C) on two occasions at least 4 hours apart during postoperative period, excluding first 24 hours OR two consecutive temperature elevations more than 101°F (38.3°C)
- In early postoperative period, it is often self-limited, resolves without therapy and is usually noninfectious in origin
- Over zealous evaluations of early postoperative fever are time consuming, expensive and uncomfortable for the patient.

NONOPERATIVE SITE INFECTIONS

UTI

- *E. Coli* — most common organism
- Catheterization of urinary tract → main cause of contamination
- Treatment—hydration and antibiotics.

Primary maternal mortality is 4 times that of vaginal delivery which may be due to:

- Shock
- Anesthetic complications particularly Mendelson's syndrome
- Hemorrhage usually due to extension of the uterine incision to the uterine vessels, atony of the uterus or DIC

The most common fetal injury is laceration to the skin

Difficult cesarean birth may result in:

- Fractures
- Peripheral nerve damage
- Spinal cord injury
- Subdural hematoma

Postoperative Care

- Strict monitoring of vital signs, urine output, signs of uterine relaxation and hemorrhage
- Restricting oral intake for a minimum of 6 hours, though Cochrane does not support this
- Early ambulation
- Skin-to-skin contact with the baby and breastfeeding are encouraged

Risk Factors for Infection

- Altered immunocompetence
- Obesity
- Absence of perioperative antibiotics
- Excessive intra-operative blood loss
- Prolonged operative time
- Low socioeconomic status
- Diabetes Milletus
- Poor nutrition
- Surgery in an infected operative site
- Poor surgical technique

Vascular

Phlebitis

- IV line to be inspected daily
- Catheter to be removed if, associated fever, pain, redness or induration or a palpable venous cord
- Incidence increases after 72 hours
- Therefore, should be changed every 3 days
- Usually resolves within 3–4 days
- Treatment—warm, moist compresses and removal of catheter from infected vein.

Respiratory

- Not a very common site for infection after cesarean section
- Basilar atelectasis → most common pulmonary complication
- Adversely affected by inhalational anesthetics
- Retention of pulmonary secretions → alveolar collapse → atelectasis → possibly pneumonia
- Early ambulation and aggressive management of atelectasis are most important preventive measures
- Pneumonia (rare) → may be hospital acquired caused by gram negative organisms.

OPERATIVE SITE INFECTIONS

Wound Complications

Superficial Wound Separation

- Separation of skin and subcutaneous tissue
- Fascia is intact
- Is a consequence of:
  - Hematoma
  - Premature removal of skin clip
  - Excessive distracting forces on the wound edges
  - Infection.

Factors Increasing the Risk of Dehiscence

- Wound infection
- Obesity
- Hypoproteinemia
- Hypertension
- Excessive tension on suture line
- Sutures placed within 0.5 cm of cut fascial edge
- Elderly
- Pulmonary disease
- Ascites

Dehiscence

- Separation of fascia with variable separation of superficial tissues
- Sentinel warning sign → serosanguinous drainage from the wound after 1st postoperative day

Infection

- Most common complication
- Diagnosis: erythema, purulent drainage, leucocytosis, fever
- Bacteriodes—most common anaerobes that infect necrotic wounds

Bowel Obstruction

- Stomach remains atonic for 18–24 hours after surgery
- Small bowel exhibits return of normal peristaltic activity within hours of lower abdominal surgery
- Colon regains function, based on passage of flatus, ≈ 48 hours after abdominal surgery.

Paralytic Ileus

- Most patients experience some degree of ileus
- Exact mechanism—not known
- Associated with opening of peritoneal cavity and aggravated by manipulation of intestinal tract and prolonged surgical procedures
- Features: Abdominal distension, absence of bowel sounds and flatus, abdominal tenderness, nausea, vomiting
- Abdominal radiography in flat (supine) position and in upright position—useful in diagnosis
- Most common finding—dilated loops of small and large bowel as well as air-fluid levels while the patient is in upright position
- Fluid and electrolyte replacement
- Treatment—nasogastric tube to evacuate stomach of it's fluids and gaseous contents
- If no improvement within first 48–72 hours—other causes of ileus should be sought.

Adhesion Formation

- Prevention by good surgical technique and use of antiadhesive barriers
- The ideal adhesion barrier should meet the following criteria:
  - Achieves effective tissue separation
  - Has a long half-life within the peritoneal cavity so that it can remain active during the critical 7-day peritoneal healing period
  - Is absorbed or metabolized without initiating a marked pro inflammatory tissue response
  - Remains active and effective in the presence of blood
  - Does not compromise wound healing
  - Does not promote bacterial growth.

Antiadhesive Barriers

- Expanded Polytetrafluorethylene (Gore-Tex Surgical Membrane)
- Oxidized-regenerated cellulose (Interceed)
- Modified sodium hyaluronate/carboxymethylcellulose (Seprafilm)

Chapter 79

Postpartum Advice in High-risk Patients

Tania G Singh

Diabetes

- If patient has delivered by cesarean section, give insulin according to sliding scale for first 24 hours, checking sugars every 4–6 hourly
- If delivered vaginally:
  - Type I DM—Reduce dose of insulin by 1/3rd to 1/2. Start oral meals
  - Type II DM—May not require any medications
  - GDM—check FBS
  - If FBS <126 mg/dL—they can continue with diet therapy and exercise with regular check on sugar levels.
- GDM patients should be screened for diabetes at 6–12 weeks postpartum, using nonpregnant OGTT (100% sensitivity) criteria or by using FBS (67% sensitivity)
- If postpartum blood sugar is normal, then rescreen with OGTT every 3 years
- GDM found to have IFG or IGT or both (prediabetes)
  - Lifestyle interventions or metformin to prevent diabetes
  - OGTT at 1 year postpartum
  - FBS yearly
  - OGTT at 3 years.
- HbA_1C is not recommended postpartum
- Recurrence in subsequent pregnancies from 30 to 84%.

Iron Deficiency Anemia

- Breastfeeding
- Treatment of infections
- Contraception for atleast 2 years
- Continue iron and folic acid for minimum 3 months postpartum.

Beta Thalassemia Major

- Continue breastfeeding
- Desferrioxamine restarted within a week in the postpartum period
- Contraceptive counseling
- OCPs avoided because of the risk of thrombosis especially if splenectomy done.

Sickle-Cell Anemia

- Antibiotics
- Thromboprophylaxis should be administered:
  - While in hospital

Contraception in Diabetic Patient

- **Intrauterine devices:** ideal contraceptive for women with prior GDM
- Very effective; reversible; no metabolic disturbances
- No increased risk of pelvic inflammatory disease (with copper or LNG IUDs) or bleeding disturbances
- Failure rate: <1%
- No restriction in any type of diabetes
- No influence on blood glucose, HbA_1C or insulin levels
- Sterilization: Best in diabetics with completed families or not desiring more children
- **Barrier methods** are also accepted well

Tuberculosis Postpartum

- Breastfeeding should not be discouraged for women being treated with the first-line anti-TB drugs because the concentrations of these drugs in breast milk are too small to produce toxicity in the nursing newborn
- Congenital TB (though rare) has morbidity and mortality approaching 50%

- 7 days postdischarge following vaginal delivery or
- For a period of 6 weeks following cesarean section.
- Antithrombotic stockings
- Family planning:
    - Permanent sterilization
    - Progesterone only pills
    - Injectable progesterone (Depo provera)
    - LNG IUD
    - Estrogen containing contraceptives can also be used
    - Avoid OCPs and IUCD.

Postnatal Management in Severe Pre Eclampsia

- Measure BP 4 times/day till patient in hospital, then every 1–2 days till 2 weeks and antihypertensives according to BP
- Physician reference after 2 weeks of delivery and at 6–8 weeks, if required
- Investigations:
    - Platelet count, transaminases and serum creatinine at 48–72 hours after birth
    - If normal–do not repeat
    - If reducing but still abnormal—measure at 6–8 weeks or as clinically indicated
    - If not improving—measure as clinically indicated.

Postnatal Gestational Hypertension

- BP measurement
    - Daily × 2 days
    - At least once between day 3 and day 5
    - As clinically indicated, if antihypertensive drugs are changed after birth.
- Antihypertensives to be continued ($\uparrow$ or $\downarrow$ according to BP)
- Stop methyldopa within 2 days of birth
- Physician reference—after 2 weeks of delivery and at 6–8 weeks, if required.

Postpartum in Eclamptic Fit

- Close observation for 24–48 hours (convulsion can recur)
- Continue antihypertensives, if diastolic BP is higher than 100 mm Hg
- Continue anticonvulsant for 24 hours (after delivery or convulsion, whichever is last)
- Monitor urine output carefully for at least first 24 hours (Do not give extra fluids during this period)
- Allow breastfeeding
- Do not give methyldopa postpartum
- Can give labetalol, nifedepine
- Reassess after 1 week and again at 6 weeks (12 weeks will be too late in a complicated case)
- Contraceptives (barrier, progesterone only pills)
- Recurrence in subsequent pregnancies in 2% of cases
- Eclampsia will recur to daughters of these patients in 3% of cases.

Postpartum in Epilepsy Patient

- Monitor maternal serum concentrations
- Consider restricted breastfeeding, if necessary

Contraception and Breastfeeding in Hypertensive Patients

- Low dose progesterone only pills
- Puerperal tubal ligation avoided especially in cases of severe hypertension because of:
    - Anesthetic complications
    - Thromboembolic disorder
    - Pulmonary embolism
- Allow breastfeeding
- Avoid diuretics
- Labetalol, nifedipine, enalapril, captopril, atenolol, metoprolol have no adverse effects on baby

Postpartum Rx of HELLP Syndrome

- Maternal platelet counts continue to decrease immediately postpartum but start increasing on the 3rd day
- Risk of renal failure and pulmonary edema is significantly increased
- 1/3rd ($\approx$ 30%) cases develop postpartum mainly within 48 hours (up to 6 days)

Contraception in Epilepsy

- Mirena (LNG releasing IUCD) – highly effective and reversible. Failure rate 1% (1st line contraceptive for patients on enzyme inducing drugs or on lamotrigine)
- COCP: when COCP is necessary, increase both estrogen and progesterone, (>50 mcg of estrogen) e.g. microgynon 30, 2 tabs daily
- Barrier methods
- DMPA 3 monthly

HIV Postpartum

- Support her in her breastfeeding choice
- Proper care of episiotomy wound to prevent infection
- Watch for puerperal sepsis, mastitis and UTI
- Persistence of lochia >15 days, heavy bleeding, foul smelling lochia are abnormal and should be watched for
- Safe disposal of soiled napkins
- Effective contraception should be started early
- Assess eligibility (WHO clinical stage 3 or 4 or CD4 $\leq$500 cells/mm^3) for treatment for her own health
- If eligible, continue ART
- If not eligible but breastfeeding
  - Stop ART after 1 week of complete cessation of breastfeeding and refer to care for reassessment
- If not breastfeeding
  - Stop ART after delivery

- Maternal plasma levels of AEDs may fluctuate until 8th postpartum week, therefore, monitoring is required
- Gradually reduce the dose if it has been increased during pregnancy, to avoid overdosing
- Breastfeeding—not contraindicated but feeds may be given before female takes her AED doses
- Seizures can occur because of sleep deprivation, therefore, adequate sleep is necessary (express breast milk so that partner can give night feeds)
- Feeding the baby on floor is recommended (in case seizures occurs during feeding)
- Bathing the baby when alone should be avoided
- Proper medicines at regular time
- Neurologist consultation → must.

Advice after Evacuation of Molar Pregnancy

- Less than 50% patients will show regression within 2 months of evacuation
- Effective contraception is important
- OCPs and barrier methods during entire hormonal follow-up period
- IUCD should not be used until hCG levels are normal to reduce the risk of uterine perforation
- Further continuation of contraception should be for 6 months after the first normal hCG.

Puerperium in a Cardiac Patient

- First 12 hours—most crucial (because right side of heart suffers some overload with diversion of blood that normally would have gone to placenta and uterus)
- Look for signs of pulmonary congestion and edema
- Sedatives for 1st few days—to relieve anxiety and tachycardia
- Bed rest—out of bed in reclining chair
- Any infection—taken seriously
- Visitors restricted to minimum—they interfere with rest, bring respiratory tract infection
- Breastfeeding—contraindicated in class IV and in most cases of class III
- Treat anemia, if present
- Resumption of anticoagulants
- Patients on warfarin are allowed breastfeeding (as less drug is secreted in milk)
- These patients are very fertile, therefore:
  - Permanent sterilization
  - Barrier methods
  - Inj. Depot Medroxyprogesterone acetate 150 mg IM 3 monthly
  - Low-dose OCPs—in stable patients after 6 months.
- Proper counseling—explain the need for valve replacement, if required.

Section VI:

Ward Rounds in Antenatal and Postnatal Infections

Chapter 80

Septic Abortion

Tania G Singh

Indications of Unsafe Abortion

Presence of:
- Vaginal laceration
- Cervical injury
- Uterine enlargement equivalent to a pregnancy of more than 12 weeks of gestation
- Products of conception visible at the cervix.

Clinical Features Suggestive of Infection

- Temperature above 37.5°C
- Localized or general abdominal tenderness, guarding and rebound
- Foul odor or pus visible in the cervical os
- Uterine tenderness.

Features Suggestive of Sepsis

The features suggestive of sepsis indicating the need for urgent intervention are as follows:
- Hypotension
- Tachycardia
- Increased respiratory rate
- Decreased urine output.

Minimum Required Investigations

CBC; Urine routine; Blood group; KFT; LFT; Urine culture; Cervical swab; High vaginal swab and other investigations as per need and facility available

Management

- Evacuate the uterus urgently (preferably surgical evacuation)
- If facility for urgent surgical uterine evacuation is not available, misoprostol can be used:
  - 14–28 weeks: 200 micrograms administered vaginally, sublingually or buccally 6 hourly
  - 28+ weeks: 25 micrograms vaginally 6 hourly or 25 micrograms orally every 2 hourly.
- Start broad-spectrum antibiotics immediately intravenously
  - Ampicillin 0.5–1 g 6 hourly
  - Metronidazole 500 mg 8 hourly and
  - Gentamicin 120 mg daily.
- Management of shock
  - IV fluids, blood and blood products
  - Oxygen by mask
  - Pulse oximeter
  - Insert Foley's catheter and measure urine output after evacuation
  - Send investigations.

Chapter 81

TORCH Infection in Pregnancy

Tania G Singh

RUBELLA

Clinical Presentation

- Nonspecific, maculopapular, transient, generalized or diffuse punctate rash
- Characteristically begins on the face, becoming generalized and spreads to the trunk and extremities
- Resolve within 3 days in the same order in which it appeared (face first and then body)
- Lymphadenopathy
- Polyarthralgia/polyarthritis
  - Transient
  - Involves fingers, hands, wrists, knees, ankles
  - Occurs symmetrically
  - Pain will last for 1–4 weeks.

Diagnosis

- Positive serologic test for rubella-specific IgM (most commonly used) by ELISA
- 4-fold increase in rubella-specific IgG titers between acute and convalescent serum specimens by ELISA
- Detection of virus either through virus culture or PCR.

Serologic Testing

- Performed within 7–10 days after the onset of the rash
- Repeated after 2–3 weeks.

Viral Cultures

- Drawn from nose, blood, throat, urine or cerebrospinal fluid
- May be positive from 1 week before to 2 weeks after the onset of rash.

Treatment

- No specific antibiotic required
- Risk of transmission is highest in 1st trimester, termination of pregnancy can to offered to a nonimmune mother
- Counseling is very important

Incubation Period

- ≈ 14–17 days (range of 12–23 days from exposure to clinical illness)
- Period of infection begins from 1 week before and lasts 4 days after the onset of rash

Lymphadenopathy in Rubella

Generalized, particularly of the

- Posterior auricular
- Suboccipital
- Posterior cervical lymph nodes
- Precedes the rash by 5–10 days

Transmission

- 80–85% in 1st trimester
- 25% in late 2nd trimester
- 35% in early 3rd trimester
- 100% at term

- If mother is already vaccinated for rubella and there occurs a reinfection in the 1st trimester, she should be informed that the fetal risk for congenital infection in such a case is estimated at 8%
- In infections occurring after 12 weeks, congenital rubella syndrome in the infant is rare.

TOXOPLASMOSIS

Symptoms

- More than 90% cases are asymptomatic and self-limited
- Recover very quickly
- Symptoms:
  - Low-grade fever, malaise
  - Myalgia, lymphadenopathy.

Lymph Nodes Afftected
- Cervical
- Suboccipital
- Supraclavicular
- Axillary
- Inguinal

Diagnosis

I. Serological Testing (IgM Antibodies and IgG Antibodies)

Interpretations

- Both IgG and IgM are –ve: Absence of infection or very recent acute infection
- When IgG +ve but IgM is –ve: Old infection (>1 year)
- If both are +ve: Either a recent infection or a false-positive test result
- If acute infection is suspected: Repeat the test within 2–3 weeks
- A 4-fold rise in IgG antibody titers between tests indicates a recent infection.

Confirmation of Toxoplasmosis
- Sabin-Feldman dye test → maximum levels after 2 months of infection (>300 IU/mL)
- IgM indirect fluorescent antibody test

II. Ultrasonography

- Intracranial calcifications
- Ventricular dilatation
- Hepatomegaly
- Ascites
- Placental enlargement.

III. Amniocentesis

- Organism identified in amniotic fluid by polymerase chain reaction
- Should be offered at more than or equal to 18 weeks gestation.

Transmission to Fetus

Overall risk of congenital infection without treatment ranges from 20 to 50%
- 3rd trimester → 60–81% (milder or asymptomatic disease)
- 2nd trimester → 25% (Intermediate severity)
- 1st trimester → 6–17% (severe disease; results in miscarriage/congenital abnormalities).

Treatment

Only Maternal Infection

- Spiramycin→ 1 g (3 million U) orally every 8 hours.

<table>
<tr><td>

Serious Complications of Cytomegalovirus (Though not Common)
- Interstitial pneumonitis
- Hepatitis
- Meningoencephalitis
- Myocarditis
- Thrombocytopenia

</td><td>

When Both are Infected

- Give combination of pyrimethamine and sulfadiazine
- Pyrimethamine 25–100 mg/day + Sulphadiazine 1 gm qid × 3–4 weeks until term
- Started after 14 weeks of gestation (to avoid teratogenicity)
- Folinic acid 5 mg twice weekly (as both are folate antagonists).

</td></tr>
</table>

CYTOMEGALOVIRUS

Clinical Manifestations

- Most pregnant women have either no symptoms or have only flu like symptoms
- Malaise
- Persistent fever
- Myalgia
- Cervical lymphadenopathy.

Prevention

- Use of latex condoms helps
- Hygiene especially at centers of infection
  - Avoiding contact with salivary secretions and urine from young children
  - Careful hand washing after changing diapers and wiping secretions.

Prenatal Diagnosis

Maternal

- When before pregnancy IgG was negative but now it has become positive or
- Detection of IgM antibodies
- IgG avidity assay.

Fetal

- USG is helpful but not diagnostic
- Amniocentesis is the test of choice
- Must be done after 21 weeks of gestation and at least 5–6 weeks after seroconversion in order to reliably detect CMV
- Viral culture and DNA by PCR in amniotic fluid (to confirm fetal infection).

Management

- There is no effective therapy
- Pregnancy termination can be offered once fetal infection is confirmed after weighing the risks and benefits.

HERPES SIMPLEX VIRUS

Modes of Transmission

- Direct contact through broken skin or mucosal surface or infected body fluids, during close physical contact, most commonly sexual
- Mother to child transmission
- Recurrent: Genital herpes has a tendency to show recurrent infection as viral particles reside in nerve ganglia and gets reactivated in the same patient, but is less severe

IgG Avidity Assay
- It can help clear the confusion between primary infection acquired before pregnancy or recurrent infection
- Also determines when the infection has occurred
- Avidity levels are reported in terms of avidity index
- An avidity index of >60% is highly suggestive of past or secondary infection
- An index of <30% suggests a recent primary infection (duration <3 months)

HSV 2 Strains:
- Genital herpes is a chronic, life-long viral infection
- HSV-1: causes oropharyngeal infection
- HSV-2: genital tract infections

Risk of Transmission to the Neonate

- If genital herpes is acquired near the time of delivery, risk is 30–50%
- Genital herpes acquired during 1st half of pregnancy or in women with history of recurrent herpes → less than 1%.

Disease Manifestations

- Prodromal Stage
  - Paresthesias, tingling sensations
  - Neuralgia (pain where lumbosacral nerves innervate the skin)
  - Flu like symptoms.
- This is followed by eruption of painful vesicles over external genitalia → these when rupture → forms small ulcers which coalesce together and form encrustations and heal without scarring
- Entire duration: 2–4 weeks.

Diagnosis

- Clinical (as mentioned above but should be confirmed with laboratory testing)
- HSV, DNA, PCR is the test of choice
- Culture (less sensitive)
- Type specific serology testing:
  - Type-specific antibodies to HSV develop during the first several weeks after infection and persist indefinitely
  - Distinguish HSV 1 infection from HSV 2 infection.

Management

Mother

- Analgesics and topical anesthetics
- If there is urinary retention: Indwelling catheter
- 1st clinical episode or severe recurrent herpes:
  - Oral acyclovir 200 mg 5 times/day × 5 days OR
  - Oral acyclovir 400 mg 3 times/day × 5 days
  - Safe in 1st trimester.
- In systemic infection (severe HSV infection):
  - Inj. Acyclovir 5–10 mg/kg body weight 8th hourly × 7 days.
- Valcyclovir
  - 1000 mg Bid × 7–14 days (category B drug)
  - Advantages: Higher levels of acyclovir with less frequent dosing.
- Famciclovir
  - 250 mg tid × 7–14 days.

Mode of Delivery

- Vaginal delivery is best avoided in patient with active genital herpes
- Women without symptoms or signs of genital herpes or it's prodrome can deliver vaginally.

Facts

- Failure to detect HSV by culture or PCR does not indicate an absence of HSV infection because viral shedding is intermittent
- IgM testing for HSV is not useful because the IgM tests are not type-specific and might be positive during recurrent episodes of herpes
- Although cesarean section does not completely eliminate the risk for HSV transmission to the infant, women with recurrent genital herpetic lesions at the onset of labor should be delivered by cesarean section to prevent neonatal HSV infection

Chapter 82

Malaria in Pregnancy

Tania G Singh

COMPLICATED MALARIA

Generally caused by P. Falciparum. May manifest as:

- Fever (>104° F): intermittent or continuous
- Chills/rigors, headache, myalgia, arthralgia
- Nausea/vomiting, diarrhea, cough
- Jaundice, perspiration, pallor
- Splenomegaly
- Respiratory distress, impaired consciousness/coma
- Repeated generalized convulsions
- Renal failure (s. creatinine >3 mg/dL)
- Jaundice (serum bilirubin >3 mg/dL)
- Severe anemia (Hb <5 g/dL)
- Pulmonary edema /acute respiratory distress syndrome
- Hypoglycemia (plasma glucose <40 mg/dL)
- Metabolic acidosis
- Circulatory collapse/shock (Systolic BP <80 mm Hg)
- Abnormal bleeding and DIC
- Hemoglobinuria.

UNCOMPLICATED MALARIA

- Less than 2% of RBCs are infected with no signs of severity or complications
- It has two stages:
    - Cold stage: Cold sensation, shivering
    - Hot stage: Fever, headache, sweating, seizures (occasionally)
    - Symptoms in hot stage generally last for 6–10 hours and occur every 2–3 days, depending on the infecting species.

Treatment

- Admit in hospital
- Avoid starting treatment on an empty stomach
- The first dose should be given under observation
- Dose should be repeated if vomiting occurs within 30 minutes
- For vomiting, metoclopramide can be given even in 1st trimester
- If persistent vomiting, stop oral therapy
- Do not give primaquine in pregnancy.

P. Falciparum Malaria

- Oral quinine 600 mg tid + Oral clindamycin 450 mg tid, together for 7 days
- In case of persistent vomiting:
  - Quinine 10 mg/kg IV in 5% dextrose over 4 hours × 8 hourly +
  - Inj. Clindamycin 450 mg IV × 8 hourly.
- When vomiting stops, therapy including quinine and clindamycin to be given orally for complete 7 days.

For All Other Species

- Tab. Chloroquine 25 mg/kg divided over 3 days.

Diagnosis of Malaria

- Microscopy of thick and thin blood smears (Gold standard)
- In a febrile patient, three negative malaria smears 12–24 hours apart rules out the diagnosis of malaria.

Treatment

- Admit in ICU
- Give Inj. Artesunate 2.4 mg/kg IV or IM (after diluting the powder in 5% sodium bicarbonate provided in the pack) 12 hourly for the 1st day and then give OD dose from next day
- Adverse reactions are not common
- If not available, give quinine:
  - Loading dose: 20 mg/kg IV infusion in 5% dextrose/dextrose saline over a period of 4 hours
  - Maintenance dose: 10 mg/kg 8 hourly.

Obstetric Management

- Maintain airway, breathing, circulation
- Prompt management and a strict close watch to avoid complications
- Treat pyrexia with paracetamol, tepid sponging and antimalarials
- Frequent checks on blood sugars to avoid hypoglycemia
- Maintain hydration
- Even acute malaria is not an indication for induction
- Tocolysis and steroid therapy can be considered, if no contraindications
- Ultrasound for fetal growth. Doppler in cases of IUGR
- Explain the patient and relatives the risks associated
- NST may show changes like decelerations, fetal tachycardia or bradycardia
- Pediatrician to be kept informed
- Blood should be sent for grouping/cross-match/platelet count in severe cases
- Intrapartum malaria can lead to infection of the neonate, therefore, send placenta for histology, cord and baby's blood group analysis to detect congenital malaria in neonate.

Recurrence in Malaria

- Mostly seen with uncomplicated *P. falciparum*
- Recurrence usually occurs between 4 and 6 weeks.

If there is no provision for diagnostic tests but the signs and symptoms are suggestive of malaria, start treatment with chloroquine in full therapeutic dose. It should be considered as **'clinical malaria'**

Note

- Never give bolus injection of quinine
- Maximum quinine dose—1.4 gm
- Recommended treatment in the 1st trimester of pregnancy
- To be avoided in the 2nd and 3rd trimesters as it is associated with recurrent hypoglycemia

Artemisinin Combination Therapy (ACT)

- Consists of an artemisinin derivative + Long acting antimalarial
- National programme in India → artesunate + sulfadoxine-pyrimethamine
- Presently, Artemether + Lumefantrine fixed dose combination and blister pack of artesunate + mefloquine are also available in India
- ACTs can be given in the 2nd and 3rd trimester of pregnancy

Chapter 83

Tuberculosis in Pregnancy

Tania G Singh

SIGNS AND SYMPTOMS

Pulmonary TB

Classic Symptoms

- Chronic cough with blood-tinged sputum
- Fever, chills, night sweats
- Loss of appetite, weight loss, fatigue
- Chest pain
- About 25% of people may remain 'asymptomatic'
- Upper lung lobes → more frequently affected than the lower ones either due to better airflow or due to poor lymph drainage within the upper lungs.

DIAGNOSIS OF ACTIVE TUBERCULOSIS

Sputum Examination

- Any patient presenting with cough for less than 2 weeks is a pulmonary TB suspect and is to be referred to the RNTCP Designated Microscopy Center
- All TB suspects undergo 2 sputum smear examination (spot and morning) over two consecutive days.

Definitive Diagnosis

- By identifying *M. tuberculosis* in a clinical sample (e.g. sputum, pus, or a tissue biopsy) but it may take 2–6 weeks for blood or sputum culture
- Thus, treatment is often begun before cultures are confirmed.

LATENT TUBERCULOSIS

Mantoux test/Tuberculin test/PPD test is a screening test.

- It consists of an intradermal injection of one-tenth of a millilitre of PPD tuberculin
- The size of induration is measured 48–72 hours later
- A person who has been exposed to the bacteria is expected to mount an immune response in the skin containing the bacterial proteins
- The reaction is read by measuring the diameter of induration (palpable raised, hardened area) across the forearm (perpendicular to the long-axis) in millimetres
- If there is no induration, the result should be recorded as "0 mm"
- Erythema (redness) should not be measured.

PREGNANCY AND TB

- Pregnancy itself is not a risk factor for TB
- Untreated TB in pregnancy is associated with an increased risk of:
  - Miscarriage, low birth weight
  - Major fetal abnormality (rare)
  - Neonatal TB (rare).
- High doses of rifampicin (much higher than used in humans) causes neural tube defects in animals, but no such effect has ever been found in humans
- There may be an increased risk of hepatitis in pregnancy and during the puerperium
- It is important to advise all women of child-bearing age to avoid getting pregnant until TB treatment is completed
- Aminoglycosides (STM, capreomycin, amikacin) should be used with caution in pregnancy, because they may cause deafness in the unborn child.

Difficulties in Diagnosing Tuberculosis in Pregnancy
Because of the vague, nonspecific nature of the symptoms, common to both TB and pregnancy, such as fatigue, shortness of breath, sweating, tiredness most physicians are reluctant to order a chest X-ray for fear of harming the fetus

MANAGEMENT (CDC)

Active Disease

First 2 Months (Daily)

- Isoniazid (along with pyridoxal phosphate to obviate peripheral neuropathy caused by isoniazid)
- Rifampicin
- Ethambutol.

Note
Streptomycin should not be used because it has been shown to have harmful effects on the fetus. In most cases, pyrazinamide (PZA) is not recommended to be used because its effect on the fetus is unknown

For Next 7 Months

- Isoniazid and rifampicin alone, daily or twice weekly.

Latent Tuberculosis

- The standard treatment is 9 months of isoniazid (300 mg) alone, administered either daily or twice weekly
- Women taking isoniazid should also take pyridoxine (vitamin B6) supplementation.

Chapter 84

Acute Pyelonephritis in Pregnancy

Tania G Singh

AN OVERVIEW

- Acute pyelonephritis is the infection of kidney and the pelvic ureter
- A serious systemic illness affecting 1–2% of all pregnancies and the most common nonobstetric cause of hospital admission during pregnancy.

PRESENTATION

- Occurs beyond 16 weeks
- Usually bilateral, if unilateral, present more on right side
- Lower urinary tract symptoms (e.g., frequency, urgency, dysuria)
- Upper urinary tract symptoms (e.g., flank pain)
- Constitutional symptoms (e.g., fever, chills, malaise)
- Gastrointestinal symptoms (e.g., nausea, vomiting, anorexia, abdominal pain).

ON EXAMINATION

- Fever (temperature >100.4°F [38.0°C])
- Tachycardia
- Hypotension
- Costovertebral angle tenderness
- Possible abdominal or suprapubic tenderness.

INVESTIGATIONS

- Urine analysis
  - Leukocyte esterase positive
  - Nitrite positive
  - Pyuria
  - Bacteriuria
  - Hematuria.
- Urine culture and sensitivity: Urine culture growing $\geq 10^5$ colony—forming units/mL of urine.

MANAGEMENT

- Hospitalization
- IV Hydration
- Vitals charting (PR, BP, temperature, urine output)
- Antibiotics
  - Ampicillin
  - Gentamycin
  - Cefazolin or ceftriaxone.

Consequences

- Without treatment it can cause preterm labor and maternal septicemia
- Recurrent pyelonephritis is a cause of IUGR and IUD
- Recurrence → ≈ 2–3% and it can recur during the same pregnancy

Indications for Admissions Include:

- Severe distress (septicemia)
- Dehydration
- Poor oral food tolerance
- Maternal and fetal complications
- Where intravenous antibiotic is necessary

Chapter 85

Acute Gastroenteritis in Pregnancy

Tania G Singh

RISK FACTORS

- Drinking water from unknown or potentially contaminated sources
- Visiting developing countries (or areas with poor sanitation)
- Eating undercooked seafood
- Eating reheated meat dishes
- Poor hygiene
- Ingesting certain antibiotics and other drugs.

SYMPTOMS

- Diarrhea, abdominal cramps
- Fever/chills
- Nausea, loss of appetite.

DIAGNOSIS

- Look for signs of dehydration: Dry mouth or mucous membranes
- Lab tests to be done:
    - Complete blood count
    - Stool sample
    - Serum electrolyte tests
    - Blood cultures (if associated with fever).

MANAGEMENT

Prevention

- Wash your hands frequently and thoroughly
- If possible, use an antibacterial soap
- Eat properly cooked especially home-made food
- Use of a sanitizer, if possible.

Self Care at Home

- Drink more fluids: Start with water but diarrhea associated with gastroenteritis depletes the body of fluids and electrolytes (sodium and potassium). Therefore, replace it with WHO ORS solution
- Avoid coffee, tea, and sodas which make matters worse
- Pre- and Probiotics are very essential, to be taken twice a day.

Causes

- Rotavirus (especially in children) and Norwalk virus: commonly found in drinking water and food
- Bacteria, such as *E. coli, salmonella, shigella, staphylococcus* typically found in improperly prepared foods
- Cytomegalovirus: Found in people with impaired immune systems

Conditions that may be Mistaken for Gastroenteritis

- Crohn's disease
- Appendicitis
- Peptic ulcer disease
- Gastritis
- Colitis
- Gallbladder disease
- Diverticulitis
- Pancreatitis

Diarrhea may start preterm labor pains, therefore, treat as soon as possible

Treatment Proper

- Loperamide is antidiarrheal agent of choice during pregnancy
- It is a category B drug
- Take 2–4 mg daily or after each unformed stool
- Start antibiotics, if above measures do not help
- Hospitalization in severe cases
- Start IV antibiotics and IV fluids
- Ciprofloxacin and metronidazole can be given from 2nd trimester onwards
- Give antacid along with antibiotics
- Start antiemetics, if associated vomiting.

Chapter 86

Typhoid in Pregnancy

Tania G Singh

CLINICAL FEATURES

Acute Noncomplicated Disease

- Prolonged fever
- Disturbances of bowel function (constipation in adults)
- Headache, malaise, anorexia
- Bronchitic cough is common in the early stage of the illness
- During the period of fever, up to 25% of patients show a rash or rose spots, on the chest, abdomen and back.

Complicated Disease

- Only up to 10% of patients develop serious complications
- Complications include:
    - Intestinal perforation
    - Abdominal discomfort
    - Symptoms and signs of intestinal perforation and peritonitis
    - Altered mental status.

CLASSIFICATION OF TYPHOID FEVER

- ***Confirmed case:*** A patient with persistent fever (≥38°C) lasting more than or equal to 3 days, with laboratory-confirmed *S. typhi* organisms (blood, bone marrow, bowel fluid)
- ***Probable case:*** A patient with persistent fever (38°C or more) lasting 3 or more days, with a positive sero-diagnosis or antigen detection test but no *S. typhi* isolation
- ***Chronic Carrier:*** An individual excreting *S. typhi* in the stool or urine for longer than one year after the onset of acute typhoid fever.

ADVERSE EFFECTS IN PREGNANCY

- *Salmonella typhi* can cross the placenta and cause miscarriage, stillbirths and preterm labor
- Incidence of fetal loss in untreated typhoid can be as high as 80%
- Transplacental transmission usually presents as spontaneous second trimester abortion without premature rupture of membranes
- Neonates born to mother with Salmonellosis are more prone to severe complications like septicemia and meningitis.

Route of Transmission

Feco-oral route (most common)

Vertical transmission can occur

- Via transplacental spread or
- Because of the bacteremia during labor or
- Due to inadvertent fecal contamination of birth canal

10–15 mL of blood should be taken in order to achieve optimal isolation rates in blood culture

Preventive Measures

- Eat thoroughly cooked foods
- Ensure that cooked food is covered to protect it from flies
- Avoid raw vegetables and fruits that cannot be peeled
- When you eat raw fruits or vegetables that can be peeled, try to peel them yourself after washing your hands with soap
- Do not eat the peelings
- Avoid foods and beverages from street vendors
- Treat all drinking water by boiling it for 1 minute
- Ask for drinks without ice unless the ice is made from boiled or chlorine treated water
- Avoid flavored ice and juice because they may have been made with contaminated water

DIAGNOSIS

- The definitive diagnosis of typhoid fever depends on the isolation of *S. typhi* organisms from the blood or stool culture (from acutely ill patients)
- The classical Widal test measuring agglutinating antibody titres against *S. typhi* in serum has only moderate sensitivity and specificity which can be negative in up to 30% of culture proven cases of typhoid fever and can be falsely positive in many circumstances.

TREATMENT

- Ampicillin or amoxicillin are considered as first line drugs during pregnancy
- Ciprofloxacin/Ofloxacin can be given in fully sensitive cases
- Cefexime can be given, if there is multidrug resistance
- Ceftriaxone is the preferred drug in nalidixic acid resistant *Salmonella typhi* (NARST), also resistant to ciprofloxacin
- Typhoid vaccines (both polysaccharide and live vaccine) are category C drugs during pregnancy.

Chapter 87

Chorioamnionitis in Pregnancy

Tania G Singh

RISK FACTORS

- Prolonged rupture of membranes
- Prolonged labor
- Nulliparity
- Multiple and repeated vaginal examinations
- Meconium-stained amniotic fluid
- Colonization with group B streptococcus
- Bacterial vaginosis
- Sexually transmissible genital infections
- Vaginal colonization with ureaplasma
- Immunocompromised states.

CLINICAL SIGNS AND SYMPTOMS

- Maternal fever
  - Most important clinical sign
  - More than 100.4°F persisting more than 1 hour or any fever ≥101°F
  - Present in 95–100% of cases.
- Maternal tachycardia (>100/minute)
- Fetal tachycardia (>160/minute)
- Uterine fundal tenderness
- Purulent or foul amniotic fluid.

DIAGNOSIS

Clinically

- Presence of fever more than 100.4°F along with two any other signs (mentioned above).

Laboratory Tests

- Maternal leucocytosis (WBC >12,000/mm^3 or >15,000/mm^3) in presence of clinical chorioamnionitis
- Increased levels of C-reactive protein.

Amniotic Fluid Testing

- Obtained by amniocentesis
- Culture of amniotic fluid: Gold standard.

Routes of Spread

- Ascending polymicrobial bacterial infection secondary to membrane rupture (most common route)
- With intact membranes, in case of infection with genital mycoplasmas

Maternal fever, tachycardia and fetal tachycardia should be measured every 4 hourly

Chorioamnionitis is misdiagnosed in presence of epidural anesthesia. How?

- Fundal tenderness may not be appreciable in presence of epidural anesthesia
- May induce maternal and/or fetal tachycardia
- Epidural fever (fever in presence of epidural analgesia) creates a dilemma in the diagnosis

Drawbacks of Amniotic Fluid Testing

- Invasive procedure, therefore cannot be done when patient is in labor, hence limited value
- Results may not be available for up to 3 days

Rare Maternal Complications

- Septic shock; DIC
- Adult respiratory distress syndrome
- Maternal death

Amoxicillin/Co-amoxiclav should not be used as it may lead to increase in incidence of necrotizing enterocolitis

COMPLICATIONS

Maternal

- Cesarean delivery
- Endomyometritis; wound infection
- Pelvic abscess; bacteremia
- Postpartum hemorrhage.

Fetal

Fetal Inflammatory Response Syndrome (FIRS) may cause the following:
- Preterm labor; Prematurity; IUD.

NEONATAL AND LONG-TERM SEQUELAE

- Perinatal death
- Respiratory distress
- Early onset neonatal sepsis
- Septic shock
- Pneumonia
- Intraventricular hemorrhage
- Cerebral white matter damage
- Cerebral palsy.

MANAGEMENT

Antibiotics

- Ampicillin 2g IV (or Erythromycin 250 mg orally) 6th hourly
- Gentamicin IV every 8th hourly
- In cases of cesarean section:
  - Clindamycin OR metronidazole IV every 8 hourly
  - Single IV additional dose of antibiotics after delivery has a less than 5% failure rate.

Antipyretics

- Acetaminophen.

Chapter 88

HIV in Pregnancy

Tania G Singh

MANAGEMENT

Medical Management

General Overview

Nucleoside Reverse-Transcriptase Inhibitors (NRTIs)

- Emtricitabine (FTC) 200 mg once daily
- Lamivudine (3TC) 150 mg twice daily or 300 mg once daily
- Zidovudine (AZT) 250–300 mg twice daily.

Nucleotide Reverse-Transcriptase Inhibitors (NtRTIs)

- Tenofovir (TDF) 300 mg once daily.

Nonnucleoside Reverse-Transcriptase Inhibitors (NNRTIs)

- Efavirenz (EFV) 600 mg once daily
- Nevirapine (NVP) 200 mg once daily for 14 days, followed by 200 mg twice daily.

Protease Inhibitors (PIs)

- Atazanavir + ritonavir (ATV/r) 300 mg + 100 mg once daily
- Lopinavir/ritonavir (LPV/r) 400 mg/100 mg twice daily.

Integrase Strand Transfer Inhibitors (INSTIs)

- Raltegravir (RAL) 400 mg twice daily.

Antepartum and Intrapartum Management

First Line ART

Preferred Regimen
- A once-daily fixed-dose combination of TDF + 3TC (or FTC) + EFV (Tenofovirdisoproxil fumarate + Lamivudine/Emtricitabine + Efavirenz)
- Recommended as first-line ART in pregnant and breastfeeding women, including pregnant women in the 1st trimester of pregnancy and women of childbearing age, irrespective of viral load, CD4 count or WHO clinical staging
- The recommendation applies both to lifelong treatment for the own health of the mother and to ART initiated only for PMTCT which is then eventually stopped
- TDF is the preferred NRTI and EFV is the preferred NNRTI
- 3TC and FTC are pharmacologically comparable.

HIV Testing

Screening Tests
- ELISA
- Rapid tests
- Chemiluminescent immunoassays (CIA)

Confirmatory Tests
- Western blot
- Immunofluorescence assay
- NAAT (PCR)
- Antigen detection

Monitoring Tests
- Lymphocyte analysis (CD4 count)
- Viral load assays
- Drug resistance tests
- Human leucocyte antigen assays

Second Line ART?

Preferred regimens
- AZT + 3TC + LPV/r (Zidovudine + Lamivudine + lopinavir /ritonavir)
- AZT + 3TC + ATV/r (Zidovudine + Lamivudine + Atazanavir /ritonavir)

Alternative Regimens (If the above regimen is contraindicated or is unavailable):

- AZT + 3TC + EFV (or NVP) (Zidovudine + Lamivudine + Efavirenz/ Nepirapine)
- TDF + 3TC (or FTC) + NVP (Tenofovirdisoproxil fumarate + Lamivudine / Emtricitabine + Nevirapine).

Pregnancy Management

- All pregnant women should be offered HIV counseling and testing at booking visit and again retest in 3rd trimester or peripartum
- Offer partner testing
- If a woman declines an HIV test
  - Document this in her ANC card
  - Explore the reasons for decline
  - Try screening again at around 28 weeks.
- If testing shows HIV positive results:
  - Team approach [Obstetrician, Pediatrician, Counselor and a Physician (preferably)]
  - The result should be highly confidential
  - Testing of the partner is extremely important
  - If patient desires termination and is less than 20 weeks pregnancy, offer safe MTP services.
- If patient wishes to continue pregnancy—Triple line therapy is started in the 1st trimester and continues throughout pregnancy
- If patient is already on ART:
  - Tolerating the drugs well—she should continue with the same drugs
  - Not tolerating ART well and/or Virological failure—can start 1st line Alternative therapy
- Multivitamin, folic acid, iron and calcium supplementation is given
- Hepatitis B and pneumococcal vaccination, can be offered in pregnancy
- Bed nests should be used for prevention of malaria.

INVESTIGATIONS

- CBC, absolute lymphocyte count, blood sugar, urine analysis, blood group and type, LFT, RFT
- Viral load (HIV RNA copies)
- Dating and anamoly scans as and when required.

MODE OF DELIVERY

- Although cesarean section has been shown to protect against HIV transmission, especially in the absence of ARV drugs or in the case of high-viral load, WHO does not recommend it in resource-limited settings specifically for HIV infection
- In these settings, cesarean section is recommended for obstetric and other medical indications
- But if cesarean section is taken electively at 38 weeks, it reduces the MTCT risk by 50% (especially when viral load is >1000 copies/mL).

General Measures to be Taken in Case of Vaginal Delivery

- Reinforcing recommended antenatal visits and care, especially high-risk management in the late 3rd trimester

- Promoting facility-based delivery by trained skilled birth attendants
- Continue ARV drugs intrapartum
- Use prophylactic antibiotics
- Use standard precautions (for both patient and healthcare providers) → hand/eye/protection from sharp instruments
- Avoiding unnecessary instrumentation and premature rupture of membranes (indicated only at ≥7 cm dilatation)
- Use of a partograph to monitor stages of labor
- Pelvic examination to be done with full asepsis and only when essential
- Pediatrician should be present for newborn resuscitation
- Noninvasive suction of nasogastric secretions
- Washing away blood in the newborn
- Clamp the cord early, do not milk the cord
- Active management of 3rd stage of labor.

- If there is prolonged rupture of membranes, augment with oxytocin to avoid increased exposure of fetus to maternal blood and infected secretions and give broad spectrum antibiotics
- Avoid invasive procedures (fetal scalp electrodes, blood sampling), avoid routine episiotomy and forceps/vacuum delivery
- If instrumental delivery is indicated, outlet forceps are preferable to ventouse

Chapter 89

Hepatitis B Infection in Pregnancy

Tania G Singh

An Overview:
- ❧ Incubation period: 30–180
- ❧ Age: Young adults
- ❧ Transmission: percutaneous, perinatal and sexual
- ❧ Severity:
  – Mild/severe
  – Fulminant: 0.1%–1%
  – Becomes chronic: In 1–10%
  – Carrier: 0.1–30%
  – Cancer: Present
- ❧ Prognosis: Worse with age
- ❧ Prophylaxis: HBIG; Recombinant vaccine

VIRAL MARKERS IN HEPATITIS B INFECTION

- Sequence in which they appear: HbsAg → HbeAg → anti-HbcAg (IgM) → anti-HbeAg → disappearance of HbsAg → Appearance of anti-HbsAg.

HbsAg

- Comes before ↑ in transaminases and clinical symptoms
- Remain till end of icteric phase (from 2 to 6 months)
- Indicates that the person is infected. It may be acute disease or chronic disease or carrier state.

HbcAg: Hidden component of viral core, not detectable at all.

HbeAg: Denotes high infectivity; active disease.

Anti-HbeAg: Denotes low infectivity.

Anti-HbcAg

- 1st antibody to appear after an acute (or recent) infection
- Persists in serum even during recovery phase
  - When acute, antibody is of IgM type → remains for 6 months
  - When chronic, antibody is of IgG type → lifelong.

Window period: Period during recovery phase when both of these are negative and diagnosis may be missed if test includes only HbsAg and anti-HbsAg

Anti-HbsAg

- With it's appearance, HbsAg antigen disappears from serum
- There is a gap of several weeks
- It means patient is immune (with immunization antibody develops and HbsAg disappears)
- Patient is protected
  - Anti-HbsAg means → good immunity and protection against Hepatitis B.

Hepatitis B Viral DNA

- Refers to a test to detect the presence of Hepatitis B virus DNA in a person's blood
- A positive test means:
  - The virus is multiplying in a person's body and he or she is highly contagious and can pass the virus to others
  - If a person has a chronic Hepatitis B virus infection, the presence of viral DNA means that a person is possibly at increased risk for liver damage
  - This test is also used to monitor the effectiveness of drug therapy for chronic Hepatitis B virus infection.

Risk of Transmission in Different Trimesters

- Maximum risk of exposure is when baby comes in contact with the infected maternal blood during delivery
- In utero infection is uncommon, (no more than 5% of perinatal HBV infections)
- The following factors may be associated with antepartum infection:
  - HBeAg positive
  - Preterm labor
  - High HBsAg and HBV DNA titers.
- Risk of transmission is same for both vaginal and cesarean delivery
- Course and prognosis is not altered by pregnancy.

Response to Vaccination

- Give primary course of three doses at 0, 1 and 6 months intramuscularly
- Check anti-Hbs antibody levels in blood after 1–4 months
- Interpretation:
  - Less than 100 mIU/mL → full response (seen in 85–90% of cases)
  - Between 10 and 100 mIU/mL → poor response → give single booster dose now and no further testing is required
  - Levels less than 10 mIU/mL → no response → check whether having acute or chronic infection → again repeat the 3 doses and test levels after 1–4 months → if still no response, either give higher dose of the vaccine or give intradermal injection
- Duration of protection is indefinite.

MANAGEMENT

Mother

- Routine prenatal screening of all pregnant women is recommended regardless of previous hepatitis B vaccination or previous negative HBsAg test results, at the 1st prenatal visit
- Vaccination, if mother at risk, regardless of HBsAg status
- Dose: 3 doses total → at 0, 1 and 6 months.

Management of Chronic HBV Infection

- Telbivudine and tenofovir are pregnancy category B medications, approved by FDA
- Entecavir, lamivudine and adefovir as category C medications
- Interferon has been classified as category X.

Acute Infection

- Hospitalization, if signs of liver decompensation are present
- For HBsAg positive carriers who develop active liver disease during pregnancy, early treatment (starting in the 1st trimester) may be considered
- Tenofovir would be preferable due to overall safety and it's very low-risk of antiviral resistance.

Chronic Infection

- Ideally, HBV DNA levels and ALT should be measured in all HbsAg positive women at the end of 2nd trimester (28–30 weeks)
- If ALT and HBV DNA (titers < 10^7 IU/mL) are not high

- Vaccination and Immunoglobulin at birth to the baby → monitor maternal postpartum flares (HBV DNA and ALT every 1–2 months × 3 times) → Check baby for HbsAg and HBs Ab at 9–18 months.
- If high ALT and HBV DNA (titers $>10^7$ IU/mL)
  - Consider early treatment with antiviral drugs starting at 32 weeks → discontinue treatment at the time of delivery → vaccination and IG at birth to the baby → monitor maternal flare up postpartum → Check baby for HbsAg and HBs Ab at 9–18 months.

BABY

CDC Vaccination Schedule for HBV

Maternal Status—Positive

- Hepatitis B immunoglobulin (HBIG) and HBV vaccine within 12 hours of birth (WHO recommends the 1st dose be given within 24 hours)
- All 3 doses should be completed by 6 months of age
- Between 9 and 18 months of age, child should be tested for anti-Hbs and HbsAg to look for response and to exclude perinatal infection
- Infants with anti-HBs levels less than 10 mIU/mL should be revaccinated with a 2nd three-dose vaccine series and then retested for anti-HBs 1–2 months after completion of the series
- When birth weight of the baby is less than 2000 gm, give birth dose, but do not count as part of the three-dose series, and give next dose at one month of age (will receive four total doses).

Maternal Status—Negative

- First HBV vaccine should be given before hospital discharge in full-term infants, and one month after birth or at hospital discharge in preterm infants.

Unknown Maternal Status

- Infants should receive hepatitis B vaccine within 12 hours of birth, followed by hepatitis B immunoglobulin as soon as possible (but not later than 7 days after birth) if the mother tests positive for HbsAg.

✎ Breastfeeding is not contraindicated in those chronically infected with hepatitis B if the infant receives HBIG passive prophylaxis and vaccine active prophylaxis, as per AAP

✎ But as per WHO guidelines, breastfeeding can be continued even in infants in endemic areas where vaccination may not be readily available, owing to high antiviral properties and other benefits of breast milk

Chapter **90**

Puerperal Sepsis

Tania G Singh

CAUSES OF FEVER IN POSTPARTUM PERIOD

Infectious Causes

Puerperal sepsis, depending on how far it has spread, may present as:
- Localized infection of a wound (cesarean section scar), laceration or episiotomy
- Spread of this infection to the underlying soft tissues
- Breast infection, such as mastitis or, at a later stage, breast abscess
- Urinary tract infection
- Respiratory tract infections:
  - Pneumonia; Bronchitis; Malaria
  - Typhoid; Pharyngitis.
- Thromboembolic disorders (superficial thrombophlebitis and/or deep vein thrombosis)
- Gastroenteritis/Hepatitis
- Any skin infection.

Noninfectious Causes

- Low-grade temperature elevations are very common in the early postpartum period, particularly in the first 24 hours
- Causes: dehydration, tissue trauma, breast engorgement.

SIGNS AND SYMPTOMS

- Pyrexia more than or equal to 38°C
- Chills
- General malaise
- Lower abdominal pain
- Uterine tenderness
- Subinvolution of the uterus
- Purulent, foul-smelling lochia
- Light vaginal bleeding
- Shock.

SITES OF INFECTION

- Placental site (most common site)
- Abdominal and perineal wounds following surgery
- Lacerations of the genital tract, e.g. cervix, vagina and perineum.

Any bacterial infection of the genital tract occurring after the birth of the baby with the signs and symptoms presenting usually after the first 24 hours except in cases where the woman had prolonged rupture of membranes or a prolonged labor without prophylactic antibiotics

Spread of infection from a wound can present as any of the following:
- Metritis
- Salpingitis
- Parametritis
- Generalized peritonitis
- Septic thrombophlebitis
- Tubo-ovarian abscess
- Broad ligament abscess
- Abscess in pouch of Douglas
- Abscesses in other sites in the abdomen or chest
- Septicemia
- Septic shock may complicate septicemia

Although fever occurring in the first 24 hours after delivery has generally been regarded as unrelated to infection, a temperature of 38°C or higher within the first 24 hours, should alert to the possibility of puerperal sepsis

Management

- IV fluids
- Send investigations
- Bed rest
- Preliminary medications until culture report is available
  - Ampicillin 2 g IV every 6 hours
  - Gentamicin 5 mg/kg body weight IV every 24 hours
  - Metronidazole 500 mg IV every 8 hours.
- Antipyretics/tepid sponging
- Perineal care
- Vitals, intake output charting meticulously
- Tetanus toxoid → if possibility that woman was exposed to tetanus and no evidence of vaccination
- Suspect retained placental bits if:
  - Uterus is soft and bulky
  - Excessive lochia
  - Foul-smelling
  - Contain blood clots.
- Digital exploration of the uterus to remove clots and large pieces of placental tissue
- Ovum forceps or a large curette may be used, if required
- Kind, sensitive approach towards patient and relatives.

MASTITIS

History

- Rapid onset in a breastfeeding infant
- Breast engorgement
- Cracked nipple which has allowed bacteria to enter through the broken skin
- Difficulty in fixing the baby to the breast, leading to nipple damage
- Bruising of the breast tissues due to rough handling
- Baby may have signs of skin or eye infections.

Symptoms and Signs

- Breast pain and tenderness
- Reddened, wedge-shaped area visible on breast
- Can occur at any time but typically 3–4 weeks after delivery
- There may be inflammation preceded by engorgement
- Usually only one breast is affected.

Tests/Investigations

- Send breast milk for culture and sensitivity, by collection of hand expressed midstream clean catch sample in sterile container
- Mothers should continue breastfeeding
- It is best to begin suckling on uninvolved breast→ this will allow let down to commence before moving to tender breast
- Correct attachment and positioning
- Start broad spectrum antibiotics without delay:
  - Cloxacillin 500 mg qid for 1–3 days
  - When symptoms subside, 250 mg qid

- Total for 10–14 days
- Erythromycin is given to women who are penicillin sensitive
- MRSA—vancomycin.

URINARY TRACT INFECTION

Cystitis

- Increased frequency of micturition
- Dysuria (i.e. pain or burning on micturition)
- Slight rise in temperature.

Pyelonephritis

More serious condition
- Dysuria
- Spiking fever
- Chills and general malaise
- Increased frequency and urgency of micturition
- Abdominal pain
- Obtain a clean-catch, midstream specimen of urine and send for culture and sensitivity.

Management

- Cephalosporins and co-amoxiclav
- Resistant stains, carbapenems may be required
- If severe, intravenous antimicrobials.

THROMBOEMBOLIC DISORDERS

Includes superficial and deep vein thrombosis.

Superficial Thrombophlebitis

More common in:
- Older
- Obese
- High parity
- History of varicose veins
- Veins used for IV infusion.

Symptoms and Signs

- May have fever
- Red, inflamed, tender area over the vein
- Vein feels firm on palpation from the clot lying within it
- Obvious on clinical examination
- Real-time ultrasound
- Ascending phlebography/Isotope venography.

Deep Vein Thrombosis

More common in:
- More than 35 years
- High parity
- Obesity

- Cesarean section
- Trauma to the legs
- Immobility
- Dehydration and exhaustion
- Smoking
- Use of estrogen
- Previous h/o thromboembolism
- Spiking fever, despite antibiotics
- Calf pain may be present, or thigh or abdominal pain
- Edema and changes in leg color and temperature may also occur
- Pain in leg increased on walking
- Tender mass extending from uterine cornua on either side may be palpable
- More difficult to diagnose clinically
- Pain in the calf of the leg, especially when walking, is a suspicious symptom of deep vein thrombosis, in particular when accompanied by the above risk factors
- DVT can lead to pulmonary embolism.

Management of DVT or SVT

Prophylactic Treatment

- Early ambulation
- Avoidance of pressure on the thighs and calves
- Sitting position with knee flexed
- Encouragement of circulatory exercises, leg and deep breathing exercises.

If the Condition has Already Occurred

- Antibiotic is the mainstay of treatment in cases of septic pelvic thrombophlebitis, secondary to infection from placental site
- Fever may persist even after antibiotics
- Use of anticoagulants not indicated.

RESPIRATORY TRACT INFECTIONS

Acute

- Bronchitis, pneumonia, pleurisy.

Chronic

- Pulmonary tuberculosis, chronic bronchitis.

Investigations

- Complete blood count
- Peripheral smear for malarial parasite
- Widal test (if fever for > 5 days)
- Blood culture
- Chest X-ray
- Sputum for culture, Mantoux or Heaf test, if required.

Treatment

- β-lactam antibiotic
- Macrolides.

SKIN AND SOFT TISSUE INFECTIONS

Source of Infection

- Site of insertion of IV cannula
- Injection sites
- Cesarean or episiotomy wound site
- Drain, if used during cesarean section.

Management

- IV cannula sites should be examined twice daily for any signs of infection
- Daily dressing of abdominal wound
- Swab for culture/sensitivity from wound site
- Patient should be advised to lie flat on abdomen several times a day (to expel any accumulated collection)
- Soaked dressing should be changed without delay
- Appropriate IV antibiotics after culture report.

SUBINVOLUTION OF UTERUS

- An arrest or retardation of involution
- Cause: Retention of placental fragments, pelvic infection
- Accompanied by prolongation of lochial discharge and irregular or excessive uterine bleeding
- Bimanual examination: Uterus is larger and softer than normal for the particular period of puerperium.

Treatment

- Ergonovine or methylergonovine (Methergin)
- Oral antibiotics usually effective in metritis.

Chapter 91

Breast Infections in Puerperium

Tania G Singh

Breast Engorgement

- Tenderness, warmth, throbbing (May extend to armpits)
- Skin on breast may be taut, shiny, and transparent
- May look red
- Milk not flowing
- Bilateral nipples may be flat
- Breast(s) hard, edematous, painful
- Fever may occur
- May be areolar or peripheral
- Can occur at any time during breastfeeding
- Due to exaggerated normal venous and lymphatic engorgement of breasts.

Flat Nipple

Nipple embedded in the breast. Treatment includes:

- Compress the breast and the areola between 2 fingers to provide as much nipple to infant as possible
- Breast shell

Interventions

- Gentle massage
- Manual expression of breast milk to soften the areola before each feed
- Anti-inflammatory agents and analgesics
- Application of warm compresses, shower or breast soak before breastfeeding
- Application of cold treatments, such as gel packs, cold packs or ice application after breastfeeding
- Review of positioning and attachment
- Evaluation for ankyloglossia (tongue tie) should be made if breastfeeding problems persist even after this.

Management of Inverted Nipple

- Nipple shield
- Manual expression
- Daily attempts should be made during the last few months of pregnancy to draw the nipple out, using traction with fingers

NIPPLE PAIN (BLEEDING/CRACKED/BRUISED NIPPLES)

Cracks can be:
- Straight across the tip of nipple (caused by excessive dryness)
- Star-shaped cracks
- Cracks at the base of the nipple (caused by biting).

Interventions

- Assess infant feeding (especially for position and latch)
- Apply expressed breast milk to nipple
- Start feeding with least affected nipple (if nipple pain)
  - Only interrupt breastfeeding if feeding intolerable
  - If baby unable to feed effectively, initiate regular hand expression in the first 24 hours and expression and pumping thereafter

– Every effort should be made to heal the cracks as they are portal of entry for pyogenic bacteria—apply topical medication or nipple shield.

PLUGGED DUCT

- Usually one breast
- Localized hot, tender spot
- May be white spot on nipple
- May be a palpable lump (plugged duct).

Interventions

- Shower or warm compress to breast before breastfeeding
- Frequent feeding
- Massage behind the plug toward the nipple, prior to and during feeding
- Vary positions for feeding
- Ice and anti-inflammatory agents
- Avoid missing feeds.

Lump in Axilla
- Extra breast tissue in the axilla
- Normal variation, medical intervention not required

MASTITIS

- Parenchymatous infection of mammary glands, leading to cellulitis
- Almost always from nursing infant's nose and throat, the organism enters the breast through the nipple at the site of a fissure or abrasion
- Can occur at any time but usually 1 week postpartum
- Sudden onset of intense pain
- Usually in one breast (may be both)
- Most common organism — *staph. aureus*
- Breast may feel hot, appear red or have red streaks and/or swollen, hard, tender
- Marked engorgement → inflammation → chills or actual rigor (the first sign of inflammation), fever, tachycardia → FLU like symptoms.

Interventions

- Support/rest/adequate fluids
- Continue frequent breastfeeding—milk from affected breast is safe for infant
- Correct attachment and positioning
- If too tender, manual expression or breast pump
- Gentle massage on any firm area
- Shower or warm compresses to affected area prior to feeds
- After feeds—cool compresses
- Analgesic
- Antibiotics may be indicated, if not resolved in 24 hours
- Penicillin or cephalosporin
- Cloxacillin 500 mg qid for 1–3 days
- When symptoms subside 250 mg qid for a total of 10–14 days.

Engorgement in Axillary Region
Anti-inflammatory agents and application of cold

NIPPLE INFECTION (CANDIDA)

- Sore burning nipples
- Sore all the time but worse when feeding
- Deep burning/shooting pain

- Itchy, flaky nipples
- Tiny blisters
- Deep pink/bright red nipples/areola
- Mother may have recently been on antibiotics or has a yeast infection (infant may have signs of Candida in mouth or perineal area).

Interventions

- Differentiate from poor latch
- Frequent hand washing and washing of all items that touch breast and infants mouth
- Antifungal treatment for both mother and infant may be prescribed
- If using breast pads change when they become wet
- Avoid use of soother.

BREAST ABSCESS

- Localized collection of pus within the breast
- Usually occurs as a complication of mastitis
- Caused by group B *streptococcus.*

Treatment

- Incision and drainage under general anesthesia followed by postoperative dressing
- Small/central abscess—circumareolar skin incision at areolar border
- Large/peripheral abscess—radial incision
- Incision should be made corresponding to skin lines for a good cosmetic result
- USG-guided needle aspiration (less invasive) under local anesthesia (80–90% success rate)
- Multiple abscesses require several incisions and a finger should be inserted to break up the walls of the locules
- Resulting cavity is loosely packed with gauze, which should be replaced at the end of 24 hours by a smaller pack
- Breastfeeding through uninvolved breast.

---

3 Types of Breast Abscess

Subareolar
- Unilocular cavities located superficially near the nipples
- Favorable prognosis

Intramammary unilocular
- Solitary locus of pus deep inside the tissue and distant from nipple

Intramammary multilocular
- Require a longer treatment
- High recurrence

Chapter **92**

Operative Site Infections

Tania G Singh and Gagandeep Anand

FACTORS THAT INCREASE THE LIKELIHOOD OF WOUND INFECTION

Systemic Factors

- Obesity; Anemia
- Infection
- Malnutrition
  - Vitamin C—Maintains capillary wall integrity
  - Vitamin A—counteracts the effects of corticosteroids in wound healing
  - Vitamin B complex—permits effective cross-linking of collagen fibers required for progressive increase of tensile strength of healing incision
    - Iron supports O_2 transport and is a cofactor for collagen synthesis
    - Zinc, which can be quickly depleted by stress, small bowel fistula drainage and weight loss, is a cofactor for collagen formation and protein synthesis
  - Infection.

Surgical Factors

- Excessive use of cautery → results in thermal injury of normal tissue
- Tissue trauma
- Excessive suture tension → should be avoided
- Suture to incision length ratio >4
  - Ratio <4 → 2.5 fold higher incidence of hernia.

Postoperative Factors

- Abdominal distension
- Vomiting
- Coughing
- Straining
- Hematoma
- Wound infection.

POSTOPERATIVE WOUND COMPLICATIONS

Superficial Wound Separation

- Separation of skin and subcutaneous tissue
- Fascia is intact
- Consequence of:
  - Hematoma
  - Premature removal of skin clip

Scar Maturation
- Continues for up to 1 year or even longer
- Collagen maturation and remodeling occurs
- During this, breakdown of old disordered collagen slightly exceeds production of new organized collagen
- However, if collagen production exceeds breakdown, then keloid or hypertrophied scar results

- Excessive distracting forces on the wound edges
- Infection.
- Studies reported that use of s/c sutures for wounds more than 5 cm in depth decrease the occurrence of superficial separation.

Dehiscence

- Separation of fascia with variable separation of superficial tissues
- Sentinel warning sign → serosanguinous drainage from the wound after 1st postoperative day
- Factors increasing the risk:
  - Wound infection, obesity
  - Hypoproteinemia, hypertension
  - Excessive tension on suture line
  - Sutures placed within 0.5 cm of cut fascial edge
  - Elderly; Pulmonary disease; Ascites.

Infection

- Most common complication
- Diagnosis: Erythema; purulent drainage; leucocytosis; fever
- Bacteriodes—most common anaerobes that infect necrotic wounds
- Pseudomonas and *S. aureus*—most common pathogens in absence of nonviable tissue
- More than 10,000 organisms/gm of tissue are necessary for clinical diagnosis of wound infection.

SURGICAL WOUND HEALING

Depending on the manner of wound closure, three types of surgical wound healing are recognized.

Primary Intention

- Healing occurs by primary intention, if wound layers are reapproximated following injury
- Healing occurs in a minute of time, with no separation of wound edges and with minimal scar formation.

Secondary Intention

- Surgical wounds when left unapproximated and allowed to close spontaneously
- More complicated and prolonged than primary
- Wound heals by combination of contraction and formation of granulation tissue
- Slow and characterized by formation of excessive scar tissue.

Third Intention

- Also known as delayed primary closure
- Refers to technique of wound closure after a period of delay
- Often used after postoperative wound breakdown or as an alternative to healing by secondary intention of wounds that should not be closed primarily (infected or contaminated)
- Closure on or after 4th day is ideal
- After 7–8 days → approximation is difficult
- Between 3 and 6 days → lowest infection rates.

Section VII:

Blood Transfusion and Blood Components

Chapter 93

Blood Transfusion and Blood Components

Tania G Singh and Gagandeep Anand

Blood and blood products has a great demand in obstetrics. It is very important to get the right blood for the right patient at the right time. Proper documentation is of utmost importance while transfusing blood.

If the particular blood group or blood product is available:

- Obtain blood sample of the patient for compatibility testing in the tube with no anticoagulant
- Then label the tube correctly with patient's complete name, hospital registration number, ward, and date
    - If patient is conscious, as the patient to reveal her identity
    - If patient is unconscious, enquire the same from her relatives.
- Send the blood sample along with the blood request form to the blood bank.

Storage of Blood Products Prior to Transfusion

Whole Blood and Red Cells

- To be issued from the blood bank in a cold box or insulated carrier (temp between 2° and 6°C)
- In the ward, store it in the refrigerator at 2°–6°C until required for transfusion
- The upper limit of 6°C is essential to minimize the risk of any bacterial contamination
- The lower limit of 2°C is essential to prevent hemolysis, which can cause fatal bleeding problems or renal failure.

Platelet Concentrates

- To be issued from the blood bank in a cold box or insulated carrier (temp. between 20° and 24°C)
- At lower temperatures, they lose their blood clotting capability; therefore, should never be placed in a refrigerator.

Fresh Frozen Plasma

- Temperature in the blood transport box or in refrigerator should be maintained between 2° and 6°C

Time Limits for Infusion

Whole Blood

- Start—within 30 minutes of removing from refrigerator
- Finish—within 4 hours.

Preliminaries Before Requesting for Blood

- It's clinical need
- When it is required
- Indication for transfusion
- Inform the patient's relatives and document the same
- Select the blood product and the quantity required
- Complete the blood requisition form accurately and legibly
- Mention the reason for transfusion
- If the blood is needed urgently, contact the bloodbank by telephone

If Required Blood Group is not Available

Patient's BG	Alternative BG
O	None
A	O
B	O
AB	A; B; O

Alternative blood is given as packed cells

Platelet Concentrates

- Start—as soon as possible after pooling, generally within 4 hours
- Finish—over a period of 30 minutes.

FFP and Cryoprecipitate

- Labile coagulation factors rapidly degrade, therefore, start transfusion as soon as possible
- Complete infusion within 20 minutes.

Administration of Blood Products

Correct IV Set Up

- Only 0.9% sodium chloride can be infused in the same line as the blood
- No medications should be infused in this line
- If using a pre-existing IV site, assess the quality of the line by checking for swelling, redness or pain at the infusion site and adequate infusion rates
- The size of peripheral IV access should be 18–20 Gauge preferably.

Needle Size

- The largest possible catheter should be used
- The smaller the gauge, the slower the flow rate
- While using a smaller gauge catheter, care should be taken to avoid excess pressure.

Compatible Solutions with Blood Products

- Only 0.9% sodium chloride
- 5% dextrose in water will cause clumping of red cells and hemolysis
- Lactated Ringer's may cause clotting due to calcium content
- 5% dextrose in water (D5W) must be used only when administering IV immunoglobulin
- 0.9% sodium chloride is not compatible with IV immunoglobulin.

Warmed Blood is Commonly Required in:

- 'Large volume rapid transfusion'
- 50 mL/kg/hour
- Exchange transfusion in infants
- Patients with clinically significant cold agglutinins

Filter (For Whole Blood/Red Cells)

- Use a new sterile blood administration set containing an integral 170–200 micron filter
- Change the set at least 12 hourly during blood component infusion
- In a very warm climate, change the set more frequently and usually after every four units of blood, if given within a 12 hour period.

Blood Warming

- There is no evidence that warming blood is beneficial to the patient when infusion is slow
- Keeping the patient warm is more important than warming the infused blood
- Blood should only be warmed in a blood warmer
- Blood should never be warmed in a bowl/oven, as this can result in hemolysis of red cells which can prove fatal.

Receiving the Blood Bag from Blood Bank

- Check the compatibility label on the blood bag
- Blood pack number

- Patient's name
- Patient's hospital reference number
- Ward number
- Patient's ABO and Rh D group
- Date of compatibility test
- Expiry date
- Blood group of blood pack
- Return blood promptly to blood bank, if not used.

Checking the Blood Pack

Check for:
- Any sign of hemolysis in the plasma (Does it appear pink?) indicating that the blood has been contaminated, allowed to freeze or had become too warm
- Look for hemolysis on the line between the red cells and plasma
- Any sign of contamination, such as a change of color in the red cells, which often looks darker or purple/black when contaminated
- Any clots, which may mean that:
    - The blood was not mixed properly with the anticoagulant when it was collected or
    - There may be bacterial contamination due to the utilization of citrate by proliferating bacteria.
- Any signs that there is a leak in the pack or that it has already been opened.

BLOOD TRANSFUSION NOTES

General Information

- Patient's name
- Patient's hospital reference number
- Patient's ward
- Patient's ABO and Rh D group
- Date of compatibility test
- Expiry date
- Blood group of blood pack
- Blood bag number.

Do not administer the transfusion if the blood pack appears abnormal or damaged or it has been (or may have been) out of the refrigerator for >30 minutes. Inform the blood bank immediately

Monitoring

When?

- Before starting the transfusion
- As soon as the transfusion is started
- 15 minutes after starting the transfusion
- Afterwards hourly monitoring
- On completion of the transfusion
- 4 hours after completing the transfusion.

How?

- Measure PR, BP, RR, temperature, fluid intake.

Record

- Time when the transfusion is started
- Time when the transfusion is completed

- Volume and type of all products transfused
- Any adverse effects.

BLOOD TRANSFUSION REACTIONS

Mild Reactions

Signs and symptoms

- Urticaria/rash/pruritis/hypersensitivity.

Management

- Slow down the transfusion
- Administer antihistamine IM.

Moderate Reactions

Signs and symptoms

- Fever/rigors/urticaria/tachycardia/pruritis/headache/mild dyspnea/palpitations.

Management

- Stop the transfusion
- Replace the infusion set and keep IV line open with normal saline
- Administer antihistamine IM
- Antipyretic
- Give IV glucocorticoids and bronchodilators, if there are anaphylactic reactions like bronchospasm, stridor
- When there is clinical improvement, restart infusion with a new blood bag and monitor closely.

Severe Reactions

Signs and Symptoms

- Fever/rigors/headache/hypotension (fall in systolic BP by >20%) tachycardia (rise in heart rate by >20%)/respiratory distress/chest pain/severe dyspnea/loin/back pain/hemoglobinuria/unexplained bleeding (DIC).

Management

In case of transfusion reaction, send to the blood bank, the following:

- ➤ Blood bag with infusion set
- ➤ Fresh blood sample from a different vein
- ➤ Request form to investigate the bag
- ➤ Request form to release 1 unit of blood again

- Stop the transfusion immediately
- Start normal saline
- Elevate patient's legs
- High-flow oxygen by mask
- Attach pulse oximeter
- Administer:
    - Inj. Adrenaline 0.01mg/kg body weight slowly IM
    - IV corticosteroids and bronchodilators
    - Diuretic (Frusemide 1mg/kg body weight)
    - Antipyretic (paracetamol).
- Send urine sample for analysis
- Assess for bleeding from puncture sites. If there is clinical or laboratory evidence of DIC, manage with platelets, FFPs, cryoprecipitate
- Inotropes can be started, if hypotension continues even with fluids.

Blood Components

Packed RBCs

- Volume—300 mL
- Contain mostly red cells mixed with preservatives and anticoagulants Hematocrit of 70% (very viscous)
- For rapid transfusion, can be diluted with 100 mL normal saline
- RL should not be mixed with RBCs because it's calcium content may precipitate when it interacts with citrate preservatives
- 1 unit of RBCs increases PCV by 3% points
- Packed RBCs have no platelets and only ≈ 10–15 mL of residual plasma
- Improves oxygen carrying capacity
- Increases hemoglobin by 1 gm/dL and PCV by 3% points
- For 4 units of PRBCs → give 1 unit FFP.

> Preservatives and anticoagulants in packed RBCs are citrate, phosphate, dextrose, adenosine

Fresh Frozen Plasma (FFP)

- Is a component of whole blood that remain once platelets and cellular elements are removed
- Prepared either from single unit of whole blood (Random donor FFP) or from plasma collected by apheresis technique (Jumbo FFP)
- Frozen at -18 to -30°C
- Contents: All coagulation factors + other proteins present in original blood
- FFPs should not be used as a source of albumin or other nutrients or as a volume expander
- It should be ABO compatible, not necessary Rh specific
- Hemostasis can be achieved when the activity of coagulation factors is at least 25% of normal because 1 unit random donor FFP will increase clotting protein levels by 8%, 2 units FFP is a good starting number to transfuse
- Plasma volume in adults is ≈ 40 mL/kg, this requires a dose of FFP of ≈ 15 mL/kg, therefore, 2 units should be given at a time
- It should be transfused when PT and/or aPTT is higher than 1.5 times normal
- Can be preserved for 1 year at given temperature
- 1 unit FFP → increases fibrinogen by 10 mg/dL.

> Random donor FFP has a volume of ≈ 250 mL
> Jumbo FFP has a volume of ≈ 800 mL

Cryoprecipitate

- Prepared by thawing 1 unit of FFP at 4°C and collecting the formed precipitate in a concentrated volume of 10–15 mL/bag
- Indication for transfusion:
  - Fibrinogen lower than 75–100 mg/dL
  - 1U/10 kg of body weight with fibrinogen lower than 75 mg/dL.
- Each unit increases fibrinogen by 10 mg/dL.

> Each bag of cryo-precipitate contains:
> - 200–300 mg/dL fibrinogen
> - 100 units of factor VIII
> - vWF, factor XIII and
> - 55 mg fibronectin in equal volume of 15–20 mL/bag

Platelets

- Obtained from whole blood from multiple donors or by apheresis collection (60–90 single unit equivalents)
- ABO typing is not essential but Rh typing is necessary
- In case Rh negative is required and is not available, transfuse Rh positive platelets with a cover of Anti-D immunoglobulin
- Indication: Lower than 50,000/mm^3 platelets
  - Goal: Minimum 1 lakh/mm^3
  - In nonbleeding patients, a platelet number of 20,000/mm^3 is usually taken but can be taken as 10,000/mm^3 as the difference between the two is clinically not significant.

> One Random Donor Platelet increases platelets by 5,000–10,000
> One Single Donor Platelet increases platelets by 50,000

Section VIII:

Fluid Management

Chapter 94

Fluid Management

Tania G Singh and Gagandeep Anand

IV FLUIDS

- Daily fluid requirement = U.O. + 700 mL
- 700 mL = insensible loss.

Ringer's Lactate

- 1 litre of fluid supplies:

Na^+	130 mEq
K^+	4 mEq
Cl^-	109 mEq
Ca^{2+}	3 mEq
HCO_3	28 mEq

- Most physiological fluid
- As sodium concentration is high, it expands intravascular volume very effectively
- Useful in correction of metabolic acidosis.

Isotonic Saline (0.9% NaCl-Normal Saline)

- 1 litre of fluid contain:

Na^+	154 mEq
Cl^-	154 mEq

- Provides major EC electrolytes
- Increases intravascular volume substantially.

Dextrose Saline (DNS)

- 1 liter of fluid contains:

Glucose	50 gm
Na^+	154 mEq
Cl^-	154 mEq

- Has advantage of both 5% dextrose (to provide energy) and isotonic saline (to provide salt)
- Increases only ECF volume.

5% Dextrose

- 1 litre of fluid contains—glucose 50 gms
- Corrects dehydration and supplies energy
- After consumption of glucose, remaining water is distributed in all compartments proportionately
- Therefore, best agent to correct intracellular dehydration
- Selected when there is a need of water but not electrolytes.

- Total body water content in females = 50% of body wt.
- Total body fluid is mainly divided into 2 compartments
- ICF: 2/3 of body wt.
- ECF: 1/3 of body wt. Interstitial fluid (3/4 of ECF) Plasma or intravascular vol. (1/4 of ECF)
- Transcellular fluid— includes synovial, peritoneal, pericardial, cerebrospinal and intraocular spaces (1–2 liters)

Electrolytes	ECF	ICF
Sodium	142	10
Potassium	4.3	150
Chloride	104	2.0
Bicarbonate	24	6.0
Calcium	5.0	0.01
Magnesium	3.0	40
Phosphate and sulphate	8.0	150

FLUID AND ELECTROLYTE THERAPY

- Standard "cookbook" approach for every patient should be avoided
- Postoperative fluid administration is based on
  - Estimated blood loss
  - Urine output
  - Vitals.
- 24-hour maintenance therapy include:
  - 1 litre of NS or RL (to provide for renal solute excretion)
  - 600–900 mL 5% dextrose (to replace insensible losses).

Complications with Fluid and Electrolytes

- Most common fluid and electrolyte disorder—fluid overload
- Over enthusiastic excessive infusion of intraoperative fluid or blood transfusion or large volume of blood loss replaced exclusively with 3 times volume of crystalloid can cause volume excess
- Volume excess due to blood—pulmonary congestion
- Excessive saline—weight gain, periorbital puffiness
- Excess of hypotonic saline like 5% dextrose—hyponatremia like mental confusion, drowsiness
- Oliguria:
  - Urine output lower than 0.5 mL/kg/hour rather than urine output lower than 30 mL/hour
  - Reflects intravascular volume depletion
  - Dry tongue, ↓ skin turgor, sunken eyeballs, low volume pulse with tachycardia, postural hypotension and concentrated urine
  - Rapid infusion of 250 mL of NS or RL results in prompt ↑ in urine production
  - Diuretic therapy to be given in patient who has normal intravascular volume and ↓ output secondary to ↑ ADH or in a hypertensive patient who is diuretic dependent.

Hypokalemia

- Most common electrolyte abnormality
- Important causes:
  - Gastrointestinal loss (diarrhea, vomiting)
  - Prolonged administration of K^+ free fluids
  - Postoperative infusion of diuretics.
- Consequences:
  - Extreme weakness (muscular hypotonia)
  - Ileus
  - Arrhythmias (especially on digitalis therapy).
- Symptomatic hypokalemia occurs at serum levels lower than 2.5 mEq/L.

Hyponatremia

- Mild hyponatremia—common observation
- Stress of surgery→↑ADH + ↑aldosterone
- ↓ Free water clearance with retention of water relative to sodium
- Patient drowsy, weak, confused or gets convulsions, always rule out hyponatremia
- Na^+ lower than 130 mEq/L—treated with water restriction and diuretics.

How to calculate rate of fluid infusion?

- ➤ 15 drops = 1 mL
- ➤ RULE OF TEN (24 HRS)
  - From fluid volume, how to calculate drop rate?
  - IV fluid in liter/ 24 hours x 10 = Drop rate/min
  - Drop rate/min ÷ 10 = IV fluid in liter/ 24 hours
- ➤ RULE OF FOUR (1 hour)
  - Volume in mL/hour ÷ 4 = drop rate/min
  - Drop rate/min x 4 = vol. in mL/hour

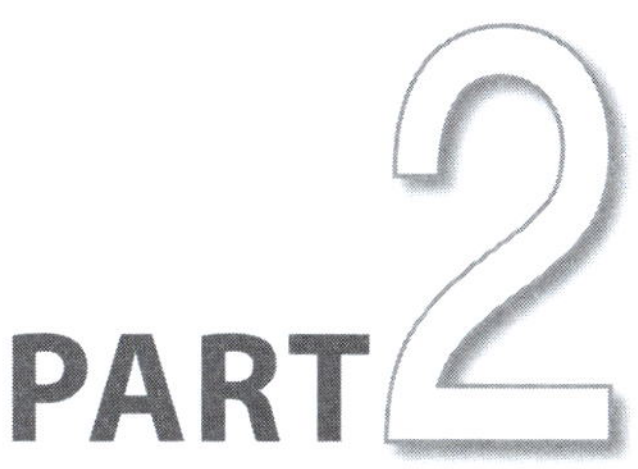

NEONATOLOGY

Section Outline

IX.   Essential Newborn Care

Section IX:

Essential Newborn Care

Chapter 95

Normal Newborn

Earl Jaspal

- Average birth weight — 2500–4000 gm
  - Indian babies average weight ranges from 2.5 to 3.2 kg
- Babies below 2.5 kg at birth are considered to be low birth weight
- Babies lose less than or equal to 10% of birth weight during the 1st 3–4 days of life.
- Regain birth weight within the first 2 weeks
- Average Length at birth — 45–52 cm
- Average OFC (occipital-frontal circumference) at birth — 32–37 cm
- Average Chest circumference at birth — 30–35 cm.

CAPPUT SUCCEDANEUM

- Odema of the scalp at newborn's presenting part of the head
- Often appears over vertex of the newborn's head
- Results from pressure against the mother's cervix during labor
- Crosses the suture lines.

Causes

- Mechanical trauma of the initial portion of scalp pushing through a narrowed cervix
- Vacuum extraction
- Prolonged or difficult delivery.

Signs and Symptoms

- Soft and puffy swelling of part of a scalp in a newborn's head
- Scalp swelling extends across the midline and over suture lines
- May have some degree of discoloration or bruising
- May be associated with increased molding of the head.

Treatment

- Resolves by itself in a few days. No treatment is required.

Complication

- Jaundice—results as the bruise breaks down into bilirubin.

CEPHALHEMATOMA

- Collection of blood between the periosteum of a skull bone and the bone itself.

- Occurs in one or both sides of the head
- Occasionally forms over the occipital bone
- Swelling is not present at birth
- It develops within the first 24–48 hours after birth
- Does not crosses suture lines.

Causes

- Rupture of a periostal capillary due to the pressure of birth
- Instrumental delivery.

Signs and Symptoms

- Swelling of the infant's head 24–48 hours after birth
- Discoloration of the swollen site due to presence of coagulated blood
- Has clear edges that end at the suture lines.

Treatment

- Observation and reassurance of parents.

Complication

- Jaundice.

Breasts in a Newborn

Size—1 cm in diameter in term newborns

Breast Engorgement

- Occurs secondary to the effects of maternal estrogens
- Subsides as maternal hormones are eliminated
- Symptoms may last for one week

MILIA

- A rash of pin-head size papules
- Occurs in 40–50% of newborns
- Location—upper cheeks, nose, or chin
- Caused by obstruction of hair follicles and eccrine glands
- Typically appear on 1st or 2nd day in term babies
- In preterm babies, may present after few days or weeks
- Usually disappears by 2nd week of life
- No treatment is required.

ERYTHEMA TOXICUM NEONATORUM

- Harmless skin rash that affects healthy newborn babies
- Appears in about 50% of newborn infants
- Cause—exact cause is unknown
- More common in term babies as compared with preterm babies
- Rash generally appear on day 1 or 2 after birth and increase in number over next few days
- Can appear up to14 days of age
- Classically, the rash appears as small, yellow-to-white-colored papules surrounded by red skin. There may be a few or several papules
- Location—face and in the middle of the body, can also be seen on upper arms and thighs
- Rash can change rapidly, appearing and disappearing in different areas over hours to days
- No treatment is needed
- Rash usually clears within 2 weeks. It is usually completely gone by age 4 months.

MONGOLIAN BLUE SPOTS

- Most common type of birthmark
- Large flat lesions
- Typically appear on buttocks and lower back
- Lesions present at birth or soon after birth
- Color—blue-gray spots ranges from deep brown to slate gray or blue-black
- Common in people with dark skin, e.g. African, East Indian or Asian descent
- Caused by collections of pigment-producing cells (melanocytes) located in a deeper layer in the skin
- Blue-gray spots may be single or multiple
- Size—range from a few millimeters to 10 centimeters or more in diameter
- Treatment—No treatment required. Reassurance of parents
- Lesions naturally fade within the first year of life
- In very rare cases, they persist into school age years and even into adulthood.

STOOL PATTERN IN NEWBORNS

Normally, healthy newborn babies should pass first stool or meconium within first 24 hours after birth.
- 60% of newborns pass stool by 8 hours of life
- 91% by—16 hours of life
- 98.5% by—24 hours of life

Stool Pattern

- 1st two days—baby passes meconium
- 2nd to 5th day of life—baby passes loose green brown to yellow brown seedy stools
- After 5th day of life—breast fed baby passes golden yellow stools, often after each feed.

Inability to Pass Stools by First 24 hours after Birth Consider-
- Meconium plug syndrome
- Hirschsprung disease
- Imperforate anus
- Hypothyroidism
- Sepsis

Urine Pattern

- First void within 24 hours (most babies) to 48 hours (all babies) of birth
- Urine has mild odor.

NEONATAL REFLEXES

Moro Reflex

Triggers that turn on the reflex
- Loud noise
- Bright light
- Sudden rough touch
- Dropping
- Tilting.

How to Elicit this Reflex?

- Gently positioning the baby in a near-seated stance few inches above the mattress with the head supported
- Drop baby's head backwards slightly
- Catch the head before he/she hits a pillow or mattress.

Asymmetry Moro's Reflex Indicates

❧ Fractured clavicle

❧ Hemiparesis

❧ Brachial plexus injury

Response

Four components:

- Startle
- Abduction of the upper limbs (spreading out arms)
- Adduction of the upper limbs (unspreading the arms) and closing of the fists
- Crying (usually, may be absent).

Disappears by — 4–6 months.

Babinski Reflex

- Stroke underside of baby's foot, from the top of the sole toward the heel
- Response—Baby's toes will fan out and big toe will move upward
- Duration: 6-24 months.

Grasp Reflex (or Palmar Grasp)

- Place finger in baby's open palm
- Response—baby will grasp the finger and can even maintain a firm grip on the finger
- Duration: 3-4 months.

Tonic Neck Reflex

- When infant is lying down and the head is turned gently to one side
- Arm on that side stretches out and the opposite arm bends up at the elbow
- This is known as "fencing" position
- Disappears by 6–7 months.

Rooting Reflex

- Stroke/touch the infant's cheek and corner of the mouth
- Response—baby turns toward the touch and mouth opens
- Disappears by 3–4 months.

Sucking Reflex

- Touch or stroke the baby's lips
- Mouth opens and sucking movements begin
- Duration—12 months.

Walking (or Stepping) Reflex

- Hold baby upright with his feet on a flat surface
- Response—baby lifts one foot, then the other, as if walking
- Duration—About two months.

Glabellar Reflex (Blink Reflex)

- Tap gently over the forehead and the eyes will blink.

Bulging Anterior Fontanelle

❧ Increased intracranial pressure

❧ Meningitis

❧ Hydrocephalus

Anterior and Posterior Fontanelles

Anterior fontanelle

- Diamond in shape (3 cm × 2 cm)
- Closes by 9–12 months.

Posterior fontanelle
- Triangular in shape (1 cm × 2 cm)
- Closes by 2–4 months.

Large anterior fontanelle
- Hypothyroidism
- Hypophosphatasia
- Small for gestational age (SGA)
- Osteogenesis imperfecta
- Chromosomal abnormalities.

Epithelial Pearls

- Small, white, firm lesions
- Location—tip of the prepuce (foreskin) of the penis.

Heart Rate

- Normal newborn heart rate—120–160 beats per minute
- Increases—during and after crying (up to 180 beats per minute)
- Decreases—during sleep (up to 80–100 beats per minute)
- Bradycardia—persistent resting heart rate less than 100 beats per minute (unless term in deep sleep without distress)
- Tachycardia—resting heart rate 180–200 beats per minute, persistent irregular rhythm.

Respiratory Rate

- Normal newborn respiratory rate—40–60 breaths/minute
- Type of breathing—Irregular and shallow
- Periodic breathing—a series of respirations followed by a pause of up to 20 seconds
- Tachypnea—respiratory rate more than 60 breaths/minute
- Bradypnea—respiratory rate less than 25–30 breaths/minute
- Apnea—sudden cessation of breathing that lasts for at least 20 seconds or is accompanied by bradycardia or oxygen desaturation (cyanosis) in a newborn less than 37 weeks of gestational age.

Depressed (Sunken) Fontanelle
- Dehydration

Small Anterior Fontanelle
- Hyperthyroidism
- Microcephaly
- Craniosynostosis-premature closure of one or more sutures of the skull

Chapter 96

APGAR Scoring

Earl Jaspal

Invented by Virginia Apgar in 1952.
A: Appearance (color)
P: Pulse (heart rate)
G: Grimace (reflex irritability)
A: Activity (muscle tone)
R: Respiration (respiratory effort)

APGAR SCORING SYSTEM

Score

Sign	0	1	2
Color	Blue or pale	Acrocyanotic	Completely pink
Heart rate	Absent	Slow (<100 bpm)	≥100 bpm
Reflex irritability	No response	Grimace	Cry or active withdrawal
Muscle tone	Limp	Some flexion	Active motion
Respirations	Absent	Weak cry: hypoventilation	Cry or active withdrawal

- Scoring is done at 1 minute and 5 minutes after birth
- Each component is assigned a value of 0, 1, or 2; the five numbers are then added
- If the newborn does not attain a 5-minute score of at least 7, additional scores are assigned every 5 minutes up to 20 minutes.

Scoring

- Normal—7 to 10
- Intermediate—4 to 6
- Low—0 to 3.

Low Apgar Score

- Associated with risk of long-term neurologic dysfunction
- But is not by itself diagnostic of perinatal asphyxia.

Persistently low Apgar score (below 3 at 10, 15, or 30 minutes)

- Associated with increased risk of neonatal mortality.

Chapter 97

Bag and Mask Ventilation in Newborns

Earl Jaspal

POSITIONING AND THE AIRWAY

- Place the newborn on his or her back with the head in a neutral or slightly extended position, i.e. sniffing position
- Sniffing position or slightly extended position results in optimal airway patency for resuscitation
- Do not hyperextend the neck as this will compress airway
- Placing a towel (shoulder pad) under the shoulder helps in maintaining good position.

MOUTH AND PHARYNGEAL SUCTION

- Do suctioning only if airway is obstructed with meconium, mucous, blood clots or vernix
- Routine suctioning of the nose, mouth or pharynx is not recommended in newborns after birth
- Do pharyngeal suction briefly and with care as prolonged suctioning can delay the onset of spontaneous breathing and cause cyanosis
- Negative suction pressure should not exceed 100 mm Hg
- Use large bore suction catheter—10 or 12 Fg
- Do not pass suction catheter more than 5 cm from the lips in a term infant
- Do not suction deep in the throat as this can cause apnea, bradycardia, laryngeal spasm and trauma to the soft tissues
- Do not repeatedly suction nose as this can cause swelling and obstruct the airway making breathing more difficult.

POSITIVE-PRESSURE VENTILATION

Indications

- Apneic or gasping following initial steps and tactile stimulation
- Heart rate less than 100/minutes after administering the initial steps of resuscitation
- Spontaneously breathing infant—persistent central cyanosis despite free flow oxygen.

Self-inflating Bags

- Following compression, a self-inflating bag re-expands due to its elastic recoil
- It does not depend on a gas source for inflation.

Safety features in self inflating bag:

- Pop off valve—set at 40 cm H_2O
- Pressure gauge (optional)

Advantages of self-inflating bags

- Automatic re-expansion
- Effective operation without a pressurized gas source
- Simple to use
- Portable.

<table>
<tr><td>

Disadvantages of Self-inflating Bags

- Not able to deliver consistent inflating pressures
- Easy to generate unnecessarily high pressures
- Pressure-release valve (usually set at 40 cm H_2O)—inconsistent and can be over-ridden
- Does not provide PEEP
- Cannot be used to deliver free flow oxygen
- Cannot be used to provide CPAP

</td></tr>
</table>

CONTRAINDICATIONS OF BAG AND MASK VENTILATION

- Diaphragmatic hernia
- Nonvigorous baby born through meconium-stained liquor.

Check the Equipment

Self-inflating Bag

- Most appropriate sized bag—240 mL, effectively delivers a tidal volume of 6–8 mL/kg/body weight
- Assemble the device correctly
- Select an appropriately sized face mask
- Attach a reservoir bag or tube (if available)
- If the gas source is attached, set the flow at 10 L/minute
- The open end where the face mask attaches should be obstructed with one hand, squeeze the bag firmly to see that a pressure is achieved and the pressure valve opens
- The bag should reinflate at the end of inflation.

Face Masks

- Appropriate size of face mask must seal around the mouth and nose but not cover the eyes or overlap the chin
- Masks with a cushioned rim are preferable to masks without one
- Size 0 for small infants
- Size 1 for normal weight infant.

Technique of Bag and Mask Ventilation

- Position yourself at head-end or side of baby
- Position the head in neutral or sniffing position
- Mouth should be opened slightly
- Suction the airway, if secretions are present
- Position bag and mask on baby properly
- Ensure good seal—mask should cover the mouth and nose, but not the eyes and it should sit below the mouth on the chin
- If air is heard escaping from the mask, it means the seal is inadequate and the mask should be repositioned
- Ventilate the newborn by squeezing the bag between the thumb and two fingers
- Ventilate at the rate of 40–60 inflations per minute
- Follow this sequence:

Squeeze- two- three- squeeze............... Squeeze- two- three- squeeze..........

- Pressure of initial breath — 30–40 cms H_2O, Later: 15–20 cms H_2O
- Inspiratory time should be about 0.3–0.5 seconds
- Observe for chest movements. Notice the rise and fall of chest with each inflation

- The chest wall movement should be equal to that seen in normal quiet respiration
- If the chest wall does not rise with bag and mask ventilation:
  - Check seal of mask
  - Reposition infant in the neutral position
  - Suction airway
  - Try giving larger breaths with the bag.

How to Assess Effectiveness of Bag and Mask Ventilation?

- Increase in heart rate above 100/minute—primary goal
- Improvement in oxygenation and color
- Rise of chest and upper abdomen with each inflation.

If There is no Improvement or Deterioration as Evidenced by-

- Heart rate does not increase above 100 beats per minute or
- No improvement or worsening in oxygenation or color
- Chest and abdomen does not rise with each inflation.

Causes and Interventions for Ineffective Bag and Mask Ventilation

Cause—inadequate seal
- Intervention—Reapply mask.

Cause—Blocked airway
- Intervention—Reposition the baby
- Clear secretions, if present
- Ventilate with open mouth.

Cause—Insufficient inflation pressure
- Intervention—Increasing inflation pressure.

Cause—Poor oxygen delivery
- Check oxygen delivery system
- Check oxygen supply
- Check oxygen tubing.

If despite above corrective measures

Heart rate remains less than 60/minute
Consider
- Endotracheal intubation
- Provide chest compression in combination with ventilation
  - There should be at least 90 compressions and 30 breaths per minute, with a ratio of 3 compressions with one ventilation (i.e. 3:1 ratio).

Orogastric Catheter

Indication
- Need for bag and mask ventilation for over 2 minutes

Technique
- Use 6–8 Fr size, measure the length, aspirate gastric contents, leave outer end open

Chapter 98

Suctioning in Newborns

Earl Jaspal

Main Indication

- Secretions present in upper airways.

Other Indications

- Restricted air entry
- Increased respiratory effort
- Recurrent apneic episodes
- Excessive mucus
- Poor color
- Blockage of the airway evidenced by:
  - Severe retractions
  - Subcostal and intercostal indrawing
  - Cyanosis.

Equipment Required

- Sterile gloves
- Suction catheter of appropriate size
- Wall suction or suction machine.

Size of Suction Catheter for Oropharyngeal Suctioning

- 10 Fr gauge catheter for term neonates
- 6–8 Fr gauge catheter for preterm and low birth weight babies to avoid mucosal injury.

Procedure

- Ensure hand hygiene. Wash your hands as per hospital protocol
- Wear gloves
- Turns on the wall suction or portable suction machine
- Test the suction equipment by occluding the connection tubing
- Select the appropriate size catheter and attach it to the suction tubing
- Check suction pressure by occluding the tube
- Suction pressure in neonates should be less than 100 mm Hg for neonates when tube is occluded
- Always suction mouth before suctioning the nose
- Remember—M comes before N in English dictionary
- Approximate the depth of insertion of suction catheter:
  - Oropharyngeal suctioning: Measures the distance between the edge of the infant mouth and the tip of infant's ear lobe

- – Nasopharyngeal suctioning: Measures the distance between the tip of the infant's nose and the tip of infant's ear lobe.
- If secretions are present in oral cavity, then turn the newborn head on one side before suctioning so that all secretions collect in mouth
- Apply suction and with a rotatory motion suction the secretions
- Suction for only 5–10 seconds at a time
- Do not push the catheter in and out against the wall of the throat as this may injure the mucous membrane
- Monitor oxygen saturation, heart rate, color of baby throughout the procedure.

Documentation

The following should be documented in neonatal case record sheet:
- Amount of secretions
- Color of the secretion
- Type of secretions
- Respiratory and cardiovascular status of baby before, during and after the procedure
- Steps taken to stabilize the baby, if required.

Complications

- Apnea
- Hypoxia
- Bradycardia
- Arrhythmias
- Damage to delicate oral tissue
- Stimulation of gag reflex causing aspiration
- Cardiac arrest
- Airway collapse
- Tracheobronchial trauma.

Precautions

- Catheter should not be moved so far to the back of the mouth to stimulate the gag reflex
- Apply suction only on withdrawal of catheter, not on insertion
- Suction pressure should be applied continuously while withdrawing the catheter
- Keep the number of suction passes to a minimum.

Things to Remember while Suctioning
- Sterile technique
- Cardiac and respiratory monitoring
- Proper catheter size
- Proper suction pressures
- Adequate oxygenation and ventilation of the patient before, during and after procedure
- Mouth should be suctioned before nose to prevent aspiration of oral contents by reflex when the nose is suctioned
- Duration of suction should be no more than 10 seconds (from insertion to end of withdrawal)

Chapter 99

Oxygen Therapy in Neonates

Earl Jaspal

Oxygen is the most common drug used in neonatal nurseries.

PROPERTIES OF OXYGEN (O$_2$)

- Oxygen is a drug
- Colorless, odorless, tasteless gas
- Makes up 21% of room air
- Is not flammable but does support combustion
- Has dangerous side effects
- Should only be used when prescribed by a treating doctor on treatment chart.
- Ensure oxygen delivery is optimal to avoid hypoxia and prevent hyperoxia
- Transcutaneous oxygen measurement and/or pulse oximetry allow for continuous monitoring of oxygen therapy
- Appropriate use is life saving but inappropriate use has dangers.

INDICATIONS FOR OXYGEN THERAPY

- Hypoxemia—inadequate amount of oxygen in the blood-S_PO_2 less than 90% and/or PaO_2 less than 60 mm Hg
- Any case of respiratory distress:
    - Dyspnea
    - Tachypnea
    - Bradypnea
    - Apnea
    - Use of accessory muscles
    - Intercostal or sternal recession
    - Nasal flaring
    - Cyanosis
    - Lethargy or restlessness
- Excessive myocardial workload.

COMPLICATIONS OF OXYGEN THERAPY

- Retinopathy of prematurity (ROP)
- Bronchopulmonary dysplasia (BPD)
- Drying of nasal and pharyngeal mucosa
- Skin irritation
- Oxygen-induced hypoventilation
- Closure of ductus arteriosus with ductal-dependent anomaly can lead to sudden death
- Absorption atelectasis.

RESUSCITATION

Preterm Infants

- In infants born less than 32 weeks—evidence supports using blended oxygen commencing at 30% rather than 100% O_2 or room air
- Preductal saturation is targeted to 90–95% by 10 minutes
- Use of pulse oximeter during resuscitation and while the infant is on oxygen
- Set alarms limit at 88–96%
- Target range 90–95%.

Term Infants

- It is recommended to start resuscitation at room air for term neonates
- Continuously monitor oxygen saturation using pulse oximeter.

MONITORING

Pulse Oximetry (SpO$_2$)

- Noninvasive monitoring technique that estimates the oxygen saturation
- May be used continuously or intermittently
- Very useful and easy to use
- Maintain normal SpO_2 values between 90 and 95%
- Correlate values with physical assessment findings
- Accuracy is about ± 2%.

Where to Best Site to Place the Oxygen Saturation Probe?

- Best site is on the right hand/wrist
- It provides a preductal reading of oxygen saturation, i.e. the blood going to brain and eyes.

Factors Affecting SpO$_2$ Measurements

- Poor perfusion of baby
- Odema
- Phototherapy
- Patient activity
- Motion artifact
- Vasoconstrictor medications
- Too much light exposure
- Nail polish *(Blue)* when using a finger probe.

Nursing Interventions Related to Pulse Oximetry Monitoring

- Check if the strength of signal in probe is proper
- The red signal/light in probe should be continuous and not blinking
- Attach the probe to baby's hand and then switch on the pulse oximeter
- Place the light and detector opposite to each other
- Set the monitoring alarms at 88% and 96%
- Change the sensor sites every 8th hourly
- Monitor and document SpO_2 values in monitoring sheet
- Notify treating doctor if SpO_2 values are outside specific alarm limits
- Cover the probe site with a sterile cloth while using phototherapy.

Complications of Pulse Oximetery

Burns of the localized area to which probe is attached

Depends on:

- Skin maturation of the newborn
- Tightness with which probe is attached
- Duration of probe attachment

OXYGEN DELIVERY SYSTEMS

Classification

- **Low-flow systems**
    - Contribute partially to the inspired gas that infant breathes
    - Does not provide constant FiO_2
    - Example—simple mask, nasal prongs.
- **High-flow systems**
    - Deliver constant and specific percent of oxygen
    - Oxygen delivered is independent of patient's breathing
    - Example—non-rebreather mask, venturi mask, CPAP, Ventilators.

Simple Mask

- Provide low to medium concentration of oxygen
- Patient exhales through ports on sides of mask
- Should not be used for controlled oxygen levels
- O_2 flow rate—6–8 L
- Can cause skin breakdown.

Oxygen Hood

- Provide a stable concentration, visibility and access to most of the body
- Recommend for acutely ill or unstable infants who require a FiO_2 >0.40
- Current hoods are disposable and lightweight
- Flow rate—
    - Minimum flow rate—3 lit/minute is recommended (in order to prevent CO_2 retention)
    - Flow of 5–10 liters per minute is usually sufficient.
- Monitor temperature and FiO_2 inside the hood
- Too cold of an environment will increase oxygen consumption and cause heat loss
- Too hot of an environment will cause apnea and dehydration
- Proper-sized hood should be used as a hood which does not fit well around the head and shoulders can cause pressure necrosis.

Continuous Assessment Required

Complications of Oxygen Hood/ Headbox use Include:

- Hypoxemia
- Hyperoxemia
- Hypothermia
- Hyperthermia
- Irritation and pressure to neck

You must continuously assess the infant and document the following hourly:
- Inspired oxygen concentration
- Oxygen saturation
- Heart rate
- Respiratory rate and effort
- Baby's temperature
- Position of the oxyhood
- Oxyhood temperature
- Water level in chamber
- Humidification
- Observe the baby's neck for irritation and pressure areas.

Nasal Prongs

- Disposable, plastic device
- Simple and convenient to use

- Two protruding prongs for insertion into the nostrils connected to an oxygen source
- Used for low to medium concentrations of oxygen
- Can be used continuously with activity of the newborn.
- Flow rate for newborns should be lower than or equal to 2 lit/minute
- Prong size should be approximately half the diameter of the nares
- Respiratory rates and depth of breathing influence the amount of oxygen reaching the lungs
- Flow rates more than 4 lit/minute can cause drying and irritation
- FiO_2 is not affected by mouth breathing
- Appropriate size nasal prongs should be used depending on baby's weight and gestational age.

How to Place Simple Nasal Prongs?

- Place nasal prongs along the cheek of the newborn
- Secure the nasal prongs on face with adhesive tape
- Position the tube over the ears and secure behind the baby's head
- Check nasal prong and tubing for patency, kinks or twists at any point
- Check nares for patency, clear with suction as required
- Change the adhesive tape as and when required
- Ensure straps and tubings are away from neck to prevent risk of airway obstruction.

Venturi Mask

- Most reliable and accurate method for delivering a precise O_2 concentration
- Consists of mask with a jet
- Narrowed orifice
- Excess gas leaves by exhalation ports
- O_2 flow rate — 4–10 L/minute
- Can provide FiO_2 of 24–60%
- Can cause skin breakdown.

Retinopathy of Prematurity (ROP) Screening

- Newborns less than 32 weeks gestation at birth or birth weight less than 1250 gm—eye examination is recommended at 4–6 weeks.
- Screening is done for early detection and treatment of ROP
- Newborns less than 36 weeks and have received oxygen—screening depends on individual risk as assessed by the clinician.

Patient Assessment and Documentation

Document hourly:
- Heart rate
- Respiratory rate
- Oxygen saturation
- Work of breathing. (e.g. use of accessory muscles/nasal flaring)
- Oxygen flow rate
- Patency of tubing
- Humidifier settings

Oxygen Safety
- Oxygen should be turned off, when not in use
- Keep the oxygen cylinders safely to avoid injury
- Do not store oxygen cylinders in hot places
- Do not smoke in the vicinity of oxygen equipment
- Do not use any petroleum products or petroleum byproducts while using oxygen

Chapter 100

Preterm and Low Birth Weight Babies

Earl Jaspal

DEFINITIONS

- Gestational age: Defined as time between first day of the last menstrual period and day of delivery in weeks and days
- Chronological age or actual age or postnatal age: Defined as the time actual day of birth in days, weeks, months and years
- Corrected Age: Defined as chronological age minus the number of weeks born before 40 weeks, i.e.

  Corrected age = Chronological age – (40 weeks – weeks gestational age at birth)
- Preterm Infant: Babies born less than 37 weeks of gestational age
- Late preterm: Babies born between 34 and 37 weeks gestational age
- Extremely preterm: Babies born less than 28 weeks of gestational age
- Low Birth Weight (LBW): Birth weight less than 2500 grams
- Very Low Birth Weight (VLBW): Birth weight less than 1500 grams
- Extremely Low Birth Weight (ELBW): Birth weight less than 1000 grams
- Appropriate for gestational age (AGA): Birth weight between 10th and 90th percentile for gestational age
- Small for gestational age (SGA): Birth weight less than 10th percentile for gestational age
- Large for gestational age (LGA): Birth weight more than 90th percentile for gestational age.

Risk Factors for Preterm Birth

- Past obstetrics history
  - Previous spontaneous preterm birth (recurrence rate — 15–50%)
  - Previous 2nd trimester abortion
  - Use of ART.
- Present pregnancy
  - Antepartum hemorrhage
  - Rupture of membranes
  - Cervical/uterine factors
    - Cervical insufficiency
    - Uterine anomalies
    - Fibroids.
- Fetal/intrauterine factors
  - Multifetal gestation
  - Intrauterine fetal death
  - Fetal anonalies
  - Polyhydramnios
  - Maternal hypertension, diabetes, IUGR.

- Infections
  - Chorioamniontis
  - Bateriuria
  - Bacterial vaginosis
  - Gastroenteritis.
- Demographic factors
  - Low socioeconomic status
  - Maternal age less than 18 years or more than 35 years
  - Low level of education
  - Black race.
- Lifestyle issues
  - Cigarette smoking
  - Illicit drug use, stress, physical abuse.
- Inadequate prenatal care
- Low prepregnancy weight
- Poor weight gain in pregnancy
- Iatrogenic.

Characteristics of Preterm Babies

- Hairs
  - The back has abundant growth of fine hairs called lanugo
  - The hairy area turns bald as gestational age increases
  - There is no difficulty in identifying individual hair fibres.
- Breast nodule
  - Measures less than 5 mm and nipple is small or absent.
- Ear cartilage
  - External ear is soft and devoid of ear cartilage and hence on folding the external ear, the recoil is poor.
- External genitalia
  - Males
    - Scrotum is small and does not have rugae
    - Both testes are not descended into the scrotum.
  - Females
    - Labia majora are widely separated, not covering the labia minora, resulting in prominent appearance of clitoris.
- Sole creases—anterior one third of sole reveals a single deep transverse skin crease.
  - There may be multiple superficial creases.
- Skin
  - Shiny
  - Thin
  - Transparent
  - Gelatinous
  - Plethoric.
- Neurologically
  - Less alert
  - Hypotonic
  - Automatic reflexes—Moro's reflex appear at 28–30 weeks of gestation
  - Grasp reflex—appear around 30 weeks of gestation
  - Glabellar tap—blink response to glabellar tap appear at 29 weeks
  - Rooting and coordinated sucking reflexes—appear at 34 weeks of gestation.

- Measurements—small in size
    - Crown heel length is less than 47 cm
    - Head circumference is less than 33 cm.
- Head size
    - Appears large in proportion to the body
    - Sutures are widely separated
    - Fontanelles are smooth and flat.

NEW BALLARD SCORING SYSTEM

- Used for assessment of gestational age
- Helpful for assessment of both preterm and term neonates
- Valid until day 7 of life.

This system includes:

Neuromuscular Maturity

- Posture
- Square window
- Arm recoil
- Popliteal angle
- Scarf sign
- Heel to ear.

Physical Maturity

- Skin
- Lanugo
- Plantar surface
- Breast
- Ear/eye
- Genitals (male)
- Genitals (females).

Complications Associated with Preterm Neonates

- Thermoregulation
    - Hypothermia
    - Hyperthermia.
- Respiratory problems
    - Respiratory distress syndrome (RDS) or Hyaline
    - Membrane disease (HMD) due to surfactant deficiency
    - Apnea of prematurity
    - Bronchopulmonary dysplasia (BPD) or Chronic lung disease (CLD).
- Central nervous system
    - Perinatal depression
    - Intraventricular hemorrhage
    - Periventricular white matter injury.
- Cardiovascular System
    - Patent ductus arteriosus (PDA) may lead to congestive cardiac failure
    - Hypotension.
- Metabolic
    - Hypoglycemia
    - Hypocalcemia.
- Gastrointestinal system
    - Necrotizing Enterocolitis (NEC)
    - Regurgitation
    - Aspiration.

- Hematologic
  - Anemia
  - Hyperbilirubinemia.
- Renal system
  - Low glomerular filtration rate
  - Late metabolic acidosis
  - Inability to handle solute water and acid loads.
- Opthalmologic
  - Retinopathy of prematurity (ROP).
- Immunologic
  - Greater risk of infection due to deficiencies in both humoral and cellular response.
- Nutritional
  - Osteopenia of prematurity
  - Deficiencies of folic acid and vitamin E
  - Anemia.

Long-term Complications

- Cerebral palsy
- Impaired cognitive skills
- Learning disabilities
- Vision problems
- Hearing problems—increased risk of hearing loss
- Dental problems—delayed tooth eruption, tooth discoloration and improperly aligned teeth
- Behavioral and psychological problems—attention-deficit/hyperactivity disorder (ADHD)
- Chronic health issues—Infections, asthma and feeding problems
- Sudden infant death syndrome (SIDS).

Table 1: Energy and nutrient requirement of preterm babies

Name	Requirement
Energy	110–150 kcal/kg
Protein	3.4–4.4 g/kg
Calcium	100–220 mg/kg
Phosphorus	60–140 mg/kg
Iron	2–4 mg/kg
Zinc	1–3 mg/kg
Vitamin A	210–450 mcg/kg
Vitamin D	150–400 IU/kg
Vitamin E	4–8 mg/kg

The etiology, management of the above mentioned complications, fluid therapy and feeding of LBW and preterm babies are been discussed in different chapters in this book.

Chapter 101

Respiratory Distress Syndrome in Newborn

Earl Jaspal

- Also known as hyaline membrane disease
- Most common pulmonary pathology in preterm newborns
- Occurs almost exclusively in premature infants
- Incidence and severity are inversely related to the gestational age.

Pathophysiology

Primary cause—inadequate pulmonary surfactant

Structurally immature and surfactant deficient lung
↓
Decreased compliance of lung
↓
Alveolar collapse
↓
V/Q mismatch
↓
Alveolar hypoventilation   Hypoxemia   Hypercarbia

- V/Q mismatch—ventilation/perfusion mismatch
- Defined as mistmach between the amount of air (ventilation, **V**) and the amount of blood (perfusion, **Q**) in the lungs
- Hypoxemia—Abnormally low concentration of oxygen in the blood
- Hypercarbia—Abnormally elevated carbon dioxide (CO_2) levels in the blood.

Factors which Increase the Risk of RDS

- Prematurity
- Elective cesarean section without labor
- Perinatal Asphyxia
- Baby born to diabetic mother
- Male babies
- Second twin
- Family history of respiratory distress syndrome
- Antepartum hemorrhage
- Erythroblastosis.

Factors which Decrease the Risk of RDS

- Use of antenatal steroids
- Prolonged rupture of membranes
- Intrauterine growth retardation (IUGR)
- Small for gestational age (SGA)

- Pregnancy-induced or chronic maternal hypertension
- Hemolytic disease of the newborn.

Clinical Features

- Tachypnea—respiratory rate of more than 60/minute in a quite resting baby
- Expiratory grunting
- Increase work of breathing in the form of:
  - Subcostal retractions
  - Intercostal retractions
  - Suprasternal retractions
  - Xyphoid retractions.
- Nasal flaring
- Cyanosis.

What is the Natural Course of RDS?

- Symptoms start at or immediately after birth
- Symptoms increase in severity and worsen in the first 48–72 hours
- If not treated, death can occur from inadequate oxygen supply (hypoxia) and respiratory failure
- In those who survive, resolution begins between 2 and 4 days of life.
- There is increased endogenous surfactant production
- This is followed by marked dieresis
- The disease resolves by one week

Composition of Surfactant
- Phospholipids — 70–80%
- Protein — 8–10%,
- Neutral lipids — 10%, primarily cholesterol

Investigations

Fetal Lung Maturity Tests

- Lecithin-to-sphingomyelin(L/S) ratio
  - Ratio is 1:1 until 32–33 weeks gestational age
  - After 33 weeks, lecithin concentration increases while sphingomyelin concentration remains the same
  - Ratio >2 indicates low-risk for RDS.
- Phosphatidylglycerol (PG)
  - Tested by amniocentesis.
  - Concentration of phosphatidylglycerol increases in amniotic fluid several weeks after rise in lecithin
  - Indicates advanced lung maturity
  - Value of >0.3 associated with low-risk for RDS.
- Complete blood count
- Septic screen } to rule out sepsis
- Blood culture

Chest Radiograph

- Helps in making definitive diagnosis of RDS
- According to the chest X-ray findings, RDS graded from grade 1 to grade 4
  - Grade 1—chest X-ray shows very fine granularity
  - Grade 2—there is generalized reticulogranular mottling
  - Grade 3—there are more confluent densities, with air bronchograms extending to second and third bronchial divisions
  - Grade 4—there is complete opacification of lung fields, absence of air bronchograms, also called as "White-out" appearance of lung.

Differential Diagnoses
- Congenital pneumonia
- Aspiration pneumonia
- Transient tachypnea of newborn
- GERD
- Hypoglycemia
- Anemia

Complications

- Neonatal sepsis
- Pulmonary hemorrhage
- Apnea
- Bradycardia
- Bronchopulmonary dysplasia (BPD)
- Necrotizing enterocolitis (NEC)
- Retinopathy of prematurity (ROP)
- Intraventricular hemorrhage (IVH)
- Failure to thrive.

Management

- Use of antenatal steroids
- Proper delivery room management and appropriate neonatal resuscitation
- Surfactant therapy
- Continuous positive airway pressure (CPAP)
- Mechanical ventilation
- Fluid and electrolyte management
- Supportive treatment
- Feeding and nutrition.

Use of Antenatal Steroids

- Two doses of 12 mg betamethasone given intramuscularly 24 hours apart
- **OR** 4 doses of 6 mg dexamethasone given intramuscularly 6 hours apart
- Decreases both incidence and severity of RDS
- Should be ideally given at least 24–48 hours before preterm delivery
- Most effective before 34 weeks.

Delivery Room Management

- Oxygen for resuscitation should be controlled by using an air-oxygen blender
- The lowest concentration of oxygen possible should be used during stabilization
- Monitor oxygen saturation using pulse oximeter
- In infants born less than 32 weeks—evidence supports using blended oxygen commencing at 30% rather than 100% O_2 or room air
- Preductal saturation is targeted to 90–95% by 10 minutes
- Set alarms limit at 88–96%
- Start CPAP as soon as possible, if required.

Surfactant Therapy

- Surfactant is a lipoprotein that decreases the surface tension of distal airways and thus maintains the functional residual capacity (FRC) during expiration
- It increases the lung compliance and hence prevents collapse of alveoli
- Surfactant is produced by type II alveolar cells
- It is a heterogeneous mixture of lipids and proteins in which the predominant component is phospholipid dipalmitoyl phosphatidylcholine (DPCC)
- The production of phosphatiylglycerol is inadequate, if there is damage to type II alveolar cells due to hypoxia, shock, acidosis, hypothermia or antepartum hemorrhage

- The lack of surfactant due to immaturity of lungs leads to hyaline membrane disease (HMD).
- The incidence of HMD is inversely proportional to the gestational age
- Highest incidence is seen in babies born with a gestational age of 26–32 weeks.
- Surfactant replacement therapy reduces mortality and morbidity in babies with RDS
- Surfactant replacement therapy
    - Improves oxygenation
    - Improves lung compliance
    - Resolve atelectases
    - Reduces duration of ventilatory support
    - Decreases pulmonary air leaks (pneumothorax, pulmonary interstitial emphysema)
    - Improves survival.
- Surfactant available as
    - Human
    - Bovine or porcine origin
    - Synthetic preparations.
- Natural surfactants are to be preferred over synthetic surfactants
- Surfactant therapy can be given as
    - Prophylactic therapy
    - Early rescue therapy
    - Late rescue therapy.
- Prophylactic
    - Defined as intubating and administering surfactant within 10–20 minutes after birth, before onset of respiratory distress but definitely after initial resuscitation and stabilization
    - It is preferably given in preterm babies less than 28 weeks gestation.
- Early rescue
    - Surfactant is administered within 2 hours of birth and is preferably given immediately after onset of respiratory distress
    - It is given in preterm babies less than or equal to 34 weeks gestation with respiratory distress.
- Late rescue
    - Defined as surfactant treatment 2 or more hours after birth, administered in preterm babies with established respiratory distress, requiring CPAP or mechanical ventilation.
- Infants receiving prophylactic surfactant have had a lower incidence of
    - Respiratory distress
    - Pneumothorax
    - Pulmonary interstitial emphysema
    - Bronchopulmonary dysplasia
    - Death.
- Therefore, infants who are at a significant risk of RDS should receive prophylactic natural surfactant therapy as soon as they are stable within a few minutes after intubation
- Surfactant is administered intratracheally through an endotracheal tube located in the trachea
- There is no evidence to support the practice of placing the infant in multiple different positions during the administration of surfactant
- Dosage—Bovine-minced surfactant—100 mg/kg or 4 mL/kg; Natural porcine surfactant—200 mg/kg or 2.5 mL/kg

- Single or multiple doses of surfactant depends on clinical condition
- Infants with RDS who have persistent or recurrent oxygen and higher ventilatory requirements within the first 72 hours of life should have repeated doses of surfactant
- Administering more than three doses has not shown to be beneficial
- After surfactant administration, there is rapid improvement in pulmonary function and ventilator settings should be weaned rapidly as follows:
  - For natural surfactants
    - Decrease FiO_2 immediately
    - Reduce inspiratory time
    - Lower PIP according to chest wall movement and blood gases.
  - For synthetic surfactant
    - Decrease FiO_2 cautiously and maintain PEEP.
  - Acute complications
    - Infections
    - Air leak
    - Intracranial haemorrhage
    - Patent ductus arterosis (PDA).
  - Long-term complications
    - Chronic lung disease
    - Neurological impairment
    - Retinopathy of prematurity (ROP).

Other Indications of Surfactant Therapy

- Meconium aspiration syndrome (MAS)
- Persistent pulmonary hypertension of the newborn (PPHN)
- Pulmonary hemorrhage
- Neonatal pneumonia

Causes of Poor Response to Surfactant Therapy

- Wrong dose: Inadequate dosage
- Wrong place: Given into one lung or into esophagus
- Wrong diagnosis: Lung hypoplasia, congenital heart disease, ARDS

Side Effects of Animal-Derived Surfactant

- Transient hypoxia
- Bradycardia
- Acute airway obstruction
- Transient fall in blood pressure and cerebral blood flow
- Slight increased risk of pulmonary hemorrhage
- Potential sensitization to animal proteins.

Noninvasive Ventilation

Nasal Continuous Positive Airway Pressure (CPAP) Ventilation

- First-line treatment of HMD in infants with mild-moderate respiratory distress
- The earlier CPAP is applied, the lesser the need of mechanical ventilation
- Some babies can be managed on CPAP without receiving surfactant treatment
- Early CPAP therapy reduces the incidence of long-term pulmonary morbidity.

Indications

- All newborns less than 30 weeks gestational age at risk for RDS
- Any preterm baby less than 33 weeks gestation with respiratory distress
- Recurrent apneas.

Components of CPAP

- CPAP generator
- Circuit for continuous flow of humidified inspired gases
- Patient interface.

Method of Administering CPAP

- Begin CPAP via nasal prongs or nasopharyngeal tube
- Start at pressure of 5–7 cms H_2O
- FiO_2 of 0.4–0.5
- Pass an orogastric tube.

If oxygenation is inadequate

- Adjust the pressure in increments of 1 to 2 cms of H_2O to a maximum of 8–9 cms H_2O
- Then, increase FiO_2 in increments of 0.05 to a maximum of 0.8.

How to assess improvement by CPAP?

- Decrease in respiratory rate
- Decreased work of breathing
- Reduction in sternal and intercostal recession
- Disappearance of grunting
- Decrease in oxygen requirement to maintain saturation 90–95%
- Improvement in blood gas (if measured).

Weaning off CPAP

- First, decrease FiO_2 by 3–5% (i.e. 0.05) till FiO_2 reaches 0.4
- Now, reduce the CPAP pressure by 1 cm H_2O every 4–6 hours till pressure of 4 cms H_2O is reached
- Now, with FiO_2 of 0.4 and pressure of 4 cms of H_2O—CPAP can be removed
- Transfer baby to head box oxygen
- Adjust oxygen flow rate to maintain oxygen saturation between 90 and 95%.

CPAP Failure

- Worsening of respiratory distress
- Increased work of breathing
- Rapid rise in oxygen requirement
- Rising $PaCO_2$ (>60 mm Hg) and pH lower than 7.25 (arterial)
- Recurrent apnoeic episodes.

Mechanical Ventilation

Types

- Intermittent positive pressure ventilation (IPPV)
- High-frequency oscillatory ventilation (HFOV)
- Mechanical ventilation used to support babies with respiratory failure as this improves survival
- HFOV used in babies with severe respiratory failure on IPPV
- Settings should be adjusted frequently with aim of maintaining optimum lung volume
- Duration should be minimized to reduce its injurious effect on lung.

Supportive Care

Maintain Thermoneutral Environment

- It reduces oxygen and energy requirement of the infant
- Use servo control mode in radiant warmer
- Set the required temperature at 36.5°C.

Monitoring on CPAP

- Temperature
- Heart rate
- Respiratory rate
- Chest retractions
- Oxygen saturation
- Capillary filling time
- Blood gas—if available
- Position of CPAP interface
- Integrity of circuit and equipment

Initial Ventilator Settings in RDS

Preterm baby

- Flow — 6–8 L/minute
- PIP — 18–20 cm H_2O
- PEEP — 5 cm H_2O
- Inspiratory time – 0.3–0.35 seconds
- Rate — 50–60/minute

Fluid and Electrolyte Balance

- Start intravenous fluids at 80 mL/kg/day for preterm babies
- Change IV fluid depending on daily requirement and insensible water losses
- Allow 2.5–4% daily weight loss (15% total) over the first 5 days
- Start small trophic feeds, e.g. 2 mL/kg 3 hourly once the baby is hemodynamically stable.

Antibiotics

- Started after blood culture is drawn
- Start antibiotics until sepsis has been ruled out
- Common regimen—penicillin/ampicillin in combination with an aminoglycoside
- Different neonatal units should have hospital protocols depending on profile of bacterial pathogens.

Treatment of Hypotension

- Volume expansion—10–20 mL/kg 0.9% normal saline
- Dopamine (5–20 µg/kg/min)—if volume expansion fails

If low systemic blood flow and myocardial dysfunction:

- Use Dobutamine (5–20 µg/kg/min) as a first line and epinephrine (0.01–1.0 µg/kg/min) as a second line.

Chapter 102

Transient Tachypnea of the Newborn (TTN)

Earl Jaspal

- Common cause of respiratory distress after birth
- Also called "wet lungs"
- Occurs in near and full-term infants
- Cause—due to delayed alveolar clearance of the lung fluids immediately after birth.

Risk Factors

- Elective cesarean section especially before the onset of labor—most significant
- Large for gestational age (LGA) babies
- Small for gestational age (SGA) babies
- Male gender
- Maternal diabetes
- Maternal asthma.

Clinical Features

- Respiratory distress starts with in first hours of life and persists beyond 4 hours of age
- Tachypnea—respiratory rate ranges from 80 to 120/minute
- Subcostal and intercostal retractions
- Nasal flaring
- Grunting may or may not be there
- Hemodynamically normal
- Neurologically normal
- FiO_2 requirement—≤40% by nasal cannula.

Investigations

- CBC
- CRP
- Septic profile — } to rule out sepsis
- Blood Culture
- Chest X-ray
    - Normal or increased lung volume
    - Mildly cardiomegaly
    - Prominent lung markings
    - Fluid in the interlobar fissures
    - Mild pleural effusions
    - Mild pulmonary edema
    - Chest X-ray findings become normal within 48–72 hours.

Management

- TTN follows a benign course
- It is a self-limiting condition
- Most neonates improve within 2–5 days.

Treatment

- Supportive
- Oxygen therapy to maintain normal PaO_2 levels, given by hood or nasal prongs
- Start feeds as soon as baby can tolerate them
- Antibiotics, if clinical features of sepsis or septic screen positive
- CPAP (continuous positive airway pressure) may be required in some cases, helps in maintaining alveolar surface area as well as absorbing the retained intra-alveolar fluid
- Mechanical ventilation in rare cases.

Prognosis

- Good with no long-term problems.

Chapter 103

Neonatal Jaundice

Earl Jaspal

- Also known as neonatal hyperbilirubinemia or neonatal icterus
- It is defined as yellowish discoloration of skin and sclera
- Most common cause for admission to neonatal unit in first week of life
- It is estimated that approximately 40–50% of all term neonates and 70–80% of all preterm neonates develop jaundice.

Progression of Neonatal Jaundice

- In newborns, jaundice always follow a cephalo-caudal progression, i.e. it first appears at the face and then yellowish discoloration reaches the trunk followed by abdomen, thighs and lastly involves the extremities, i.e. palms and soles
- All babies should be assessed clinically for jaundice at least once a day in postnatal wards by blanching the skin with a fingertip in bright natural day light
- The extent of yellowness of skin can be a useful tool for the assessment of the level of bilirubin.

Factors Affecting the Severity of Neonatal Jaundice

- Inadequate breastfeeding is a common cause especially during first few days of life
- Extravasation of blood, contusion, cephalohematoma
- Dehydration
- Increased weight loss after birth
- Swallowed maternal blood
- Perinatal Asphyxia
- Infant born to a diabetic mother
- GI tract obstruction—increase in enterohepatic circulation
- Acidosis.

Indications for Intervention or Need for Hospital Referral

- Jaundice below lower trunk, corresponding to serum bilirubin of 12–15 mg/dL
- Jaundice within first 24 hours of life
- Rapid rise of serum bilirubin of higher than 0.5 mg/dL/hour
- Yellowish discoloration of palms and soles anytime likely to need exchange transfusion
- Prolonged jaundice of more than 14 days, rule out other conditions, e.g. biliary atresia, neonatal hepatitis
- Clinical symptoms and signs suggestive of other diseases, e.g. sepsis
- Family history of significant hemolytic disease or kernicterus.

Mechanisms of Neonatal Jaundice

- Increased production of bilirubin from heme degradation
- Increased intestinal reabsorption of bilirubin
- Decreased hepatic uptake and conjugation of bilirubin

Kramer's Chart (for Severity of Jaundice)

Area of body and the level of indirect serum bilirubin (mg/dL) corerelates:

- Head and neck — 4–8
- Upper trunk — 5–12
- Lower trunk and thigh — 8–16
- Arms and lower legs 11–18
- Palms and soles — >18

Physiological jaundice is aggravated by:

- Dehydration
- Sepsis
- Perinatal Asphyxia
- Prematurity
- Hemolysis
- Hypoglycemia
- Hypothermia
- Polycythemia
- Breakdown of extravasated blood (e.g. bruising)
- Metabolic disorders including galactosemia, tyrosemia, organic acidemias
- Increased enterohepatic circulation which may be due to gut obstruction

Causes of Pathological Jaundice

- Hemolysis—Rh incompatibility, ABO incompatibility
- G6PD defecieny, puyrate kinase deficiency
- Intrauterine infections— toxoplasmosis, cytomegalovirus, syphilis, rubella
- Crigler Najjar syndrome
- Sepsis
- Hypothyroidism
- Hypoadrenalism
- Hypopituitarism
- Hemolytic anemia
- Hereditary Spherocytosis
- Breast milk jaundice
- Concealed hemorrhage
- Pyloric stenosis or gastrointestinal obstruction

Types of Neonatal Jaundice

Physiological Jaundice

- Usually appears 2–4 days after birth with maximum intensity on 4th–5th day in term and 7th day in preterm newborns
- It usually resolves within 14 days
- Frequently exacerbated by inadequate breastfeeding
- Is not associated with underlying disease and is usually benign
- The serum bilirubin values usually does not exceed 15 mg/dL.

Pathological Jaundice

- Clinical jaundice appearing in the first 24 hours of life
- Increase in the level of total bilirubin by higher than 0.5 mg/dL/hour or 5 mg/dL/day
- Persistance of clinical jaundice more than 2 weeks of age in term babies and more than 3 weeks of age in preterm babies
- Direct serum bilirubin levels of higher than 2 mg/dL.

Investigations

- Total serum bilirubin—direct and indirect fractions
- Mother and baby blood group
- Direct Coomb's test (DCT)
- Complete blood count including hemoglobin
- Reticulocyte count
- Peripheral blood film (PBF)
- G6PD levels
- Blood culture—if infection is suspected.

Measurement of Bilirubin

Noninvasive Method

Transcutaneous bilirubinometry (Tcb)
- It is a handheld, portable and rechargeable instrument but is expensive and sophisticated
- Used to screen babies more than 35 weeks gestation after 24 hours of life
- It has decreased the requirement of blood sampling in postnatal wards
- However, it is unreliable if total serum bilirubin is higher than 14 mg/dL.

Invasive Method

- Estimation of total serum bilirubin on blood samples in laboratory
- It is used to monitor the jaundice in baby before, during and after photo-therapy.

Management of Neonatal Jaundice

Infant Born ≥35 Weeks Gestation

- It is recommended to use American academy of pediatrics charts to treat the jaundice depending on total serum bilirubin levels which are plotted against the age of neonate (in hours)
- There are two age specific normograms, one each for phototherapy and exchange transfusion
- The lines on the normograms indicate three different groups, i.e. infants with lower risk (38 weeks or more and no risk factors), infants at medium

risk (≥38 weeks with risk factors or 35–37 weeks and without risk factors) and infants at higher risk (35–37 weeks and with risk factors).

Infants <35 Weeks

The following levels of total serum bilirubin (Table 1) may be used as a rough guide for starting phototherapy or planning exchange transfusion as there are no consensus guidelines for the same

Table 1: Levels of total serum bilirubin used as a rough guide for phototherapy or exchange transfusion

Weight (grams)	Phototherapy (S. bilirubin- mg/dL)	Exchange transfusion (S. bilirubin- mg/dL)
500–700	5–7	11–14
750–1000	6–8	12–15
1000–1250	8–10	14–18
1250–1500	10–12	16–19
1500–2500	13–15	20–24

Therapeutic Measures

- Phototherapy *(discussed in chapter 104)*
- Exchange transfusion *(discussed in chapter 105).*

Risk Factors

- Isoimmune hemolytic disease
- Sepsis
- Perinatal asphyxia
- G6PD deficiency
- Significant lethargy
- Temperature instability
- Acidosis
- Hypoalbuminemia

Chapter 104

Phototherapy

Earl Jaspal

- Phototherapy reduces bilirubin levels
- It changes bilirubin into more soluble forms to be excreted in the bile or urine
- It is effective in treatment of neonatal jaundice
- Reduction in bilirubin depends on area of skin exposed and irriadance
- Irradiance is the radiant flux received by a surface per unit area
- Blue light in wavelength range of 460–490 nm is most effective for phototherapy
- Blue lights should deliver at least 30 mW/cm^2/nm to the greatest surface area available.

Efficacy of phototherapy is influenced by:

- Wavelength of light
- Irradiance
- Serum bilirubin level
- Cause of jaundice
- Surface area exposed
- Skin thickness
- Day of life
- Birth weight
- Gestational age
- Skin pigmentation

Starting of Phototherapy Depends On

- Level of serum bilirubin
- Day of life or postnatal age
- Gestational age
- Weight
- Cause of jaundice
- Rate of rise of serum bilirubin.

Types of Phototherapy

- Conventional phototherapy
- Compact fluorescent lamp (CFL)
    - Low-setting — 4 blue and 2 white lamps
    - High-setting — 6 blue lamps.
- Light emitting diode (LED) phototherapy
- Fibreoptic pad, e.g. Biliblanket
- Bilibed.

Nursing Care while Giving Phototherapy

- The baby is undressed so that as much of the skin as possible is exposed to the light.
- Supine position is recommended so as to expose the maximum surface area
- Cover the baby's eyes when phototherapy is in use as high intensity light of phototherapy can cause eye injury
- Cover the genitalia or use genital shields
- Ensure the baby is in thermoneutral environment
- Use servo controlled mode of open care warmer while using phototherapy
- Distance between phototherapy and baby bed should be at least 30–45 cm

- High intensity blue light is the treatment of choice for infants with rapidly increasing serum bilirubin
- Monitor serum bilirubin daily or as indicated
- Check irradiance of phototherapy lights regularly
- If irradiance is less than therapeutic level, then replace the lamps of phototherapy
- Monitor the baby's temperature half hourly to detect hyperthermia or hypothermia
- Check the hydration status of baby regularly as prolonged phototherapy can cause dehydration
- Assessment of dehydration by maintaining baby's fluid input and output chart
- Check weight daily and monitor urine output
- Allow mother-baby interaction
- Turn off light during feeding and blood sampling
- Continue breastfeeding during phototherapy
- Observe the baby for sucking, swallowing and attachment of the baby to the mother
- Do not use phototherapy in presence of flammable anesthetics or gases which support combustion
- Asses the skin regularly for localized reddening
- Keep drugs and infusion liquids away from phototherapy
- Do not keep the phototherapy directly under the radiant warmer, as this may block the heat rays from warmer to the baby
- Do not place any objects on the phototherapy unit
- After the phototherapy is started, the color of the baby' skin is a poor marker for assessment of neonatal jaundice
- Hence, always rely on serum bilirubin levels
- Time totalizer is provided in the most phototherapy lamps
- Change the lamps according to manufacture's recommendations
- Stop phototherapy, once two total serum bilirubin values 12 hours apart are below the age specific cut-off
- Look for rebound rise in bilirubin within 24 hours of stopping phototherapy especially in babies with hemolytic disease.

Complications of Phototherapy

- Temperature disturbances—Hypo- or Hyperthermia
- Insensible water loss can lead to dehydration
- Intestinal hypermotility— passage of loose green stools
- Skin rashes
- Bronze baby syndrome— there is bronze discoloration of skin especially in babies with conjugated hyperbilirubinemia
- Photosensitivity— Congenital porphyria or a family history of porphyria is a contraindication to the use of phototherapy

Chapter 105

Exchange Transfusion

Earl Jaspal

INDICATIONS

Blood Volume Requirement
- For term neonates 70–90 mL/kg
- For preterm neonates 85–110 mL/kg

- To treat hyperbilirubinemia when bilirubin reaches toxic levels, such as in Rh incompatibility, ABO incompatibility
- Severe jaundice with risk of kernicterus not responding to phototherapy lights
- Neonatal polycythemia
- Any total serum bilirubin (TSB) higher than 12 mg/dL in first 12 hours
- Cord Hb lower than 10 g/dL and/or Cord TSB higher than 5 mg/dL
- Severe anemia
- Septicemia.

Types of Exchange Transfusion (Depending on Volume)

Size of Aliquot
Depends on the weight of baby
The smaller the baby, smaller is the volume of aliquot
Weight
<1000g – 5mL
1000g–2000g—10 mL
>2000g—15 mL

Double Volume Exchange Transfusion (DVET)

- Removes 85–90% of red cells
- The volume of blood exchanged = 2 × baby's circulating blood volume, i.e. total 140–180 mL/kg in term neonates.

Single Volume Exchange Transfusion

- Removes 60–75% of red cells
- The volume of blood to be exchanged = 1 × baby's circulating blood volume.

Which blood product to use and when?

Documentation in Exchange Transfusion Chart
- Volume in and out
- Time in and out
- Heart rate
- Respiratory rate
- Temperature
- Oxygen saturation
- Color of baby
- Medications administered

- In emergency situations: O Rh negative blood
- If ABO incompatibility: O positive RBCs suspended in AB plasma
- If Rh incompatibility: Rh negative blood of baby's ABO type
- In other babies: ABO type of baby cross-matched with mother's blood.

Prerequisites for Exchange Transfusion

- Ensure that the procedure is explained to the parents in their understandable language and a written consent is obtained
- Place the baby under servo-controlled open care radiant heat source
- Attach multipara monitors and monitor heart rate, temperature, respiratory rate and oxygen saturation throughout the procedure
- Resuscitation equipment and all medicines should be easily accessible
- Baby should be nil by mouth
- Insert a nasogastric/orogastric tube and aspirate stomach contents
- Preparation and documentation of exchange transfusion chart.

Equipment Required

- Protective gowns or plastic aprons
- Protective eye glasses
- Sterile gloves
- Cross-matched blood
- Blood administration set
- Umbilical catheters
- IV cannula No 24
- Exchange transfusion recording sheet
- Sterile drapes; 3-way stopcock/taps
- Syringes assorted sizes as required
- Blood gas syringe
- Tapes
- Suture material
- Resuscitation equipment
- Inj. Calcium gluconate 10%
- Inj. Sodium bicarbonate
- Inj. Frusemide
- Glucose 10%
- Pathology and biochemistry collection tubes
- Alcohol swabs
- Sterile gauze
- Urine drainage bag.

Types of Exchange Transfusion (Depending on Procedure)

Continuous Exchange

- Performed by two operators, one infuses blood and the other simultaneously withdraws it
- It can be done through the following routes:
  - A UVC and UAC
  - A UVC and a peripheral arterial cannula
  - Peripheral cannula and a UAC
  - Peripheral cannula and a peripheral arterial cannula.

Push-Pull Method (Commonly Used)

- Can be done through:
  - A single UVC with tip in IVC or right atrium
  - A single UAC with tip in lower aorta.
- Procedure:
  - The blood is gently withdrawn (out) and the donors blood is slowly injected (in) using push-pull technique
  - The size of aliquot depends on size of the baby
  - During the procedure, the operating person must call out the volume in and out with each infusion and withdrawal (e.g., "six in - six out")
  - A qualified nurse should keep recording the number of cycles with each aliquot and also record HR, RR, color of baby and oxygen saturation every 10 minutes
  - The donor blood bag should be kept moving intermittently to prevent RBC from settling. If any time during the procedure there is dip in baby's oxygen saturation, change in color of baby, respiratory distress or fall in HR less than 100 beats/minute the procedure should be withheld immediately till the baby's condition improves

Blood Samples before Staring the Procedure

- Hemoglobin
- Hematocrit
- Blood gases
- Serum bilirubin
- Potassium
- Blood glucose

Prerequisites for Push-pull Method

- Perform six steps of hand washing. Ensure complete aseptic precautions
- Use fresh CPDA blood
- Make sure that blood has been screened for HIV, Hbs Ag, HCV, malaria and syphilis
- Warm the blood to 37°C
- Preheparinize the umbilical catheter
- Cannulate the umbilical vein or umbilical artery depending on the method used
- Attach the umbilical catheter to two-three ways stopcock/ taps in such a way that its ports are connected to:
  - Umbilical catheter
  - Cross-matched donor blood
  - Sterile container for waste
  - Syringe (used for push-pull technique)

- Inj Calcium gluconate should be given in 1:1 dilution under cardiac monitoring every 50 mL of exchange while using CPDA blood
- After completion, the catheter should be removed gently and umbilical stump should be pressed and dressing should be applied
- The whole procedure takes approximately one hour.

Complications

Cardiac

- Bradycardia
- Hypo- or hypertension
- Arrhythmias
- Arrest and shock
- Volume overload leading to cardiac failure.

Hematological

- Thrombocytopenia
- Neutropenia
- Polycythemia
- Coagulopathy

Metabolic

- Hypocalcemia
- Hypoglycemia
- Hyperkalemia
- Acidosis
- Hypomagnesemia
- Hypernatremia.

Gastrointestinal

- Feed intolerance
- Necrotizing enterocolitis
- Perforation of intestine
- Portal vein thrombosis.

Catheter Related Complications

- Air emboli; thrombosis
- Hemorrhage.

Infection

- Septicemia (bacterial or viral).

Postexchange Care

- Send blood samples for hemoglobin, hematocrit, serum bilirubin, potassium, calcium, blood sugar and blood gases
- Proper dressing over umbilical stump
- Observe for bleeding
- Monitor heart rate, respiratory rate, color of baby, temperature and oxygen saturation every half hourly for 1st four hours
- Continue phototherapy until serum bilirubin level is in normal range

Chapter 106

Thermoregulation

Earl Jaspal

- Thermoregulation is the first and most important aspect of neonatal care
- Temperature regulation is controlled by hypothalamus
- Neutral thermal environment (NTE) is the optimum environmental temperature to ensure the lowest oxygen and energy expenditure
- Cold stress increases metabolism and oxygen consumption.

GRADES OF HYPOTHERMIA

- Normal core body temperature—36.5 to 37.3°C (97.7–99.2°F)
- Cold Stress or Mild hypothermia—36.0 to 36.4°C (96.8–97.6°F).
- Moderate hypothermia 32.0—35.9°C (89.6–96.6°F)
- Severe hypothermia—below 32.0°C (89.6°F).

Methods of Heat Loss

Evaporation
- Heat loss through wet skin.

Convection
- Heat loss from the body surface to the surrounding air via air current

Conduction
- Heat loss through direct contact with a cold surface, e.g. scales, unwarmed mattress.

Radiation
- Transfer of heat to cooler solid objects not in direct contact with the body, e.g. a cold window, wall or incubator wall.

Methods of Heat Production

- Peripheral vasoconstriction
  - Reduces skin blood flow
  - Decreases loss of heat from the body.
- Increased muscle flexion and activity
  - Infants produces muscular warmth through flexion and movement.
- Brown fat metabolism
  - Brown fat is an energy source for infants
  - Storage of brown fat occurs primarily during third trimester of pregnancy
  - Therefore, brown fat may be very limited in preterm babies
  - The more premature the infant, the less brown fat is stored.

Preventive Measures of Heat Loss

Evaporation

- Highest risk immediately after birth and while bathing

Babies at Highest Risk
- Preterm
- Low birth weight
- Small for gestational age (SGA)
- IUGR
- Neonatal sepsis
- Asphyxia
- Respiratory problem
- Cardiac problem

Location of Brown Fat
- Kidneys
- Adrenal glands
- Axilla
- Subscapula
- Mediastinum

- Dry the baby immediately after birth
- Remove wet linens
- Keep prewarmed blankets and linens
- Use plastic wraps or bags for extremely premature and low birth weight babies
- Use heated and humidified oxygen
- Avoid bathing until temperature is stabilized
- Remove wet diapers and pads.

Convection

- Depends on difference in air temperature, speed of movement of the air, and amount of skin exposure
- Warm delivery room
- Warm neonatal nursery and NICU
- Maintain temperature in delivery room and NICU at 25.0°C
- Avoid drafts from vents, doors, windows and fans
- Transport the newborn in prewarmed incubator
- Warm and humidified oxygen
- Use plastic wrap when the baby is under open care radiant warmer
- Using infant servo temperature control mode.

Radiation

- Avoid placing incubators, radiant warmers and bassinets near cold windows, walls, air conditioners.
- Use double-walled incubator or plexiglass heat shield in the incubator
- Wrap the neonate properly
- Placing a knit hat on the infant's head.

Conduction

- Prewarm incubator/radiant warmer before birth
- Placing infant on prewarmed table at the time of delivery
- Avoid placing infants on cold surfaces, such as X-ray plates, scales, examining tables
- Place a cloth between the X-ray plate and the infant
- Prewarm hands, stethoscopes, blankets and other equipment
- Skin-to-skin contact or kangaroo mother care (KMC).

Clinical Presentation

- Cold stress—pale, cool extremities
- Mottling
- Acrocyanosis
- Poor feeding
- Apnea
- Bradycardia
- Tachypnea
- Respiratory distress
- Shallow or irregular respirations
- Central cyanosis
- Irritable
- Lethargic
- Hypotonia
- Hypoglycemia
- Poor cry and activity

- Poor suck
- Abdominal distention
- Increased gastric residuals
- Chronic hypothermia—poor weight gain and possible death.

Treatment of Hypothermia (ACoRN, 2012; WHO, 2003)

Mild Hypothermia

- Skin-to-skin contact, in a warm room (at least 25°C)
- Place cap on newborn head
- Cover mother and newborn with warm blankets.

Moderate Hypothermia

- Under a radiant heater
- In a warmed incubator
- If no equipment is available or if the newborn is clinically stable, skin-to-skin contact with the mother can be used in a warm room (at least 25°C).

Severe Hypothermia

- Using a warm incubator (should be set at 1 to 1.5°C higher than the body temperature) and should be adjusted as the newborn's temperature increases
- If no equipment is available, skin-to-skin contact or a warm room or cot can be used
- Rewarming cold infants should begin immediately in order to avoid complications
- Slow rewarming by providing external heat should be at a rate of 1/2–1°F per hour
- In newborns less than 1000 grams consider 1/2°F per hour since rapid rewarming increases the risk of apnea and intraventricular hemorrhage.

Hyperthermia

- Defined as a body temperature greater than 37.3°C (99.2°F)
- Hyperthermia also has negative consequences for the neonate
- Hyperthermia occurs often due to environmental factors that cause overheating.

Causes of Hyperthermia

- Overheating from incubators, radiant warmers, or ambient environmental temperature
- Maternal fever
- Phototherapy lights, sunlight
- Infection
- CNS disorders (i.e. asphyxia)
- Dehydration
- Excessive bundling or swaddling
- Maternal epidural anesthesia.

Investigations

Septic screen to rule out sepsis.

Treatment

Treat the underlying cause.

Preterm Babies are at a Greater Risk of Heat Loss Due to:

- Large surface area-to-body mass ratio
- Decreased subcutaneous fat
- Poor muscle tone
- Lack of thermogenic brown adipose tissue
- Thin, immature skin leading to increased evaporative water and heat losses
- Poorly developed metabolic mechanism for responding to thermal stress (e.g. no shivering)
- Poor vasomotor response
- Altered skin blood-flow (e.g. peripheral cyanosis)
- Increased handling by health care workers for procedures, IV cannulation, etc.
- Potential birth asphyxia

Signs and Symptoms of Hyperthermia

- Tachycardia
- Tachypnea
- Apnea
- Lethargic
- Hypotonia
- Hypotension
- Poor feeding
- Warm extremities, flushing
- Dehydration
- Skin Temp > Core Temp
- Irritability
- Weak cry
- Seizures
- Coma
- Neurological damage

Chapter 107

Perinatal Asphyxia

- Also known as birth asphyxia
- Defined as the failure to initiate and sustain breathing at birth
- Results from an inadequate intake of oxygen by baby during birth process —before, during, or just after birth
- It causes impaired gas exchange leading to progressive hypoxemia and hypercapnea with significant metabolic acidosis
- Important preventable cause of neonatal morbidity and mortality.

RISK FACTORS

Incidence
Incidence of neonatal encephalopathy due to asphyxia—0.3–1.8%. Incidence of neonatal death—3.2/1000 live births

- Maternal infection
- Hypertensive disease of pregnancy or pre eclampsia
- Premature rupture of membranes
- Intrauterine growth restriction
- Placental abruption
- Fetal anemia
- Unphysiological labor (e.g. induction)
- Prolonged or difficult labor
- Postmaturity
- Malpresentation including vasa previa
- Abnormal fetal positioning
- Fetal anomalies or congenital defects.

Organ System Involvement Due to Asphyxia

Asphyxia Causes
- Peripheral vasoconstriction
- Tissue hypoxia
- Acidosis
- Poor myocardial contractility
- Bradycardia
- Eventually cardiac arrest

Central Nervous System

- Hypoxic-ischemic encephalopathy (HIE)
- Intracranial hemorrhage
- Seizures or convulsions
- Cerebral edema
- Hypotonia.

Cardiovascular System

- Myocardial ischemia
- Hypotension
- Poor contractility
- Congestive cardiac failure (CCF).

Metabolic
- Hypoglycemia
- Hypocalcemia
- Hyponatremia—SIADH
- Acidosis.

Pulmonary System
- Respiratory distress syndrome
- Pulmonary hemorrhage
- Pulmonary hypertension
- Surfactant depletion
- Meconium aspiration syndrome.

Gastrointestinal System
- Necrotizing enterocolitis
- Perforation
- Hepatic dysfunction.

Renal System
- Acute tubular necrosis
- Renal vein thrombosis.

Hematology
- Thermobocytopenia
- Disseminated intravascular coagulation (DIC).

Adrenal Glands
- Adrenal hemorrhage.

Symptoms

Before delivery, symptoms may include:
- Abnormal heart rate or rhythm—periodic deceleration of fetal heart rate in response to uterine contraction.

At birth, symptoms may include:
- Bluish or pale skin color
- Low heart rate or bradycardia
- Poor cry
- Poor muscle tone and reflexes
- Gasping or weak breathing
- Passage of meconium in the amniotic fluid may lead to meconium aspiration syndrome (MAS).

Clinical examination can give clue to the aetiology of asphyxia:
- Meconium staining of amniotic fluid—meconium aspiration syndrome (MAS)
- SGA/IUGR—intrauterine asphyxia
- Caput—prolonged second stage
- Large baby—difficult labor
- Anemia—antepartum hemorrhage
- Depressed baby—drugs, neuromuscular disorder
- Bruises—difficult or traumatic labor.

Grades of Severity of Hypoxic Ischemic Encephalopathy (HIE)

Sarnat and Sarnat Classification

Divided into three grades depending on clinical characteristics and prognostic significance.

Grade 1: Mild HIE characterized by
- Hyperalertness
- Irritability
- Tachycardia
- Dilated pupils
- Jitteriness
- No seizures
- EEG—normal
- Majority of such babies have a normal outcome.

Grade 2: Moderate HIE, characterized by
- Lethargy
- Poor feeding
- Hypotonia
- Proximal weakness
- Low resting heart rate
- Small pupils
- Copious secretions
- Seizures present in 70% of infants
- EEG—abnormal
- Risk of death or significant disability 25–45%.

Grade 3: Severe HIE, characterized by
- Stupor/coma
- Irregular respirations
- Marked hypotonia
- Absent reflexes
- Seizures
- Abnormal EEG—decreased background activity and/or voltage suppression
- Risk of death or significant disability more than 90%.

Investigations

- Complete blood count
- Septic screen
- Hematocrit
- Blood gases
- Blood culture
- Serum electrolytes
- Serum and ionized calcium
- Blood glucose
- Chest X-ray
- EEG
- CT scan/MRI
- Echocardiogram (ECHO).

Management

General principles of supportive therapy in babies with suspected perinatal asphyxia at risk of HIE.

Resuscitation

Delivery room treatment

Appropriate and timely resuscitation to prevent hypoxia, hypercarbia and acidosis. Maintain TABC, i.e.

- Temperature—maintain temperature
- Airway—establish a patent airway by suctioning, if necessary by endotracheal intubation
- Breathing—initiate breathing by tactile stimulation or positive pressure ventilation (PPV) with a bag and mask or through endotracheal tube
- Circulation—maintain circulation with chest compression and medications, if needed.

Measure cord blood gases, if possible as it is the most effective way to assess the baby's condition just before birth.

Admission to a nursery

Babies who require more than simple resuscitation should receive monitoring and admission in neonatal nursery.

Correction of Hypoglycemia

- Do blood sugar estimation
- If hypoglycemia—take corrective measures (refer chapter on hypoglycemia).

Thermoregulatiom

- Avoid hyperthermia
- Maintain thermoneutral environment
- Shift the baby under radiant warmer
- Maintain core temperature between 36 and 37°C
- Maintain skin temperature between 36 and 36.5°C
- Chances of hypothermia are maximum in the first few minutes after birth.

Therapeutic Hypothermia

- Aims to lower temperature of vulnerable brain structures especially basal ganglia, to a temperature of 33–34°C
- Most effective in term and late preterm newborns with moderate to severe hypoxic ischemic encephalopathy, if identified before 6 hours of age
- Should be given in a level III NICU.

Fluids and Electrolytes

- Insert an intravenous cannula and start intravenous fluid
- Fluid restriction essential, if risk of inappropriate antidiuretic hormone secretion and renal failure
- Monitor urine output
- In babies with anuria/oliguria, restrict fluids to 30–40 mL/kg/day until adequate urine output established
- Monitor fluid balance, serum electrolytes and creatinine.

Sepsis

- Draw sample for septic screen and blood culture before starting antibiotics
- Start antibiotics depending on hospital policy.

Monitoring
- Heart Rate
- Respiratory rate
- Capillary refill time
- Blood pressure
- Temperature
- Oxygen saturation
- Urine output
- Blood Sugar
- Blood gases
- Hematocrit

Neurological Management

Treatment of Seizures

Phenobarbitone

- Drug of choice
- Initial Dose: 20 mg/kg IV slowly over 30 minutes
- Repeat dose: If seizures persist after completion of this loading dose, repeat dose of phenobarbitone 10 mg/kg every 20–30 minutes till a total dose of 40 mg/kg
- Maintenance dose: 3–4 mg/kg/day in 1–2 divided doses, started 12 hours after the loading dose
- Rate of infusion of phenobarbitone — 1 mg/kg/minute
- Note—respiratory depression can occur from higher doses of phenobarbitone
- Preparations:
    - 200 mg/mL—1 mL ampoule
    - For slow IV bolus, dilute 1:10 with 0.9% saline and give at a maximum rate of 1 mg/kg/minute.

Phenytoin sodium

- Indication: If maximal dose of phenobarbitone (40 mg/kg) fails to resolve seizures
- Dose is 20 mg/kg slow IV infusion over 30 minutes
- Caution: It should only be mixed with saline and not with dextrose as it precipitates in dextrose
- Repeat dose of 10 mg/kg may be tried in refractory seizures
- Maintenance dose is 5–8 mg/kg/d in two divided doses, started 12 hours after the loading dose
- Discontinue before discharge
- Cardiac rate and rhythm should be monitored during the infusion
- Preparations: 50 mg/mL

In refractory seizures, use the drip of

- Midazolam
- Lorazepam or diazepam
- Newer anticonvulants—lamotrigene, clobazam, gabapentin may be used.

Duration of Anticonvulsant Therapy

- Neonatal period:
    - If neurological examination normal—discontinue therapy before discharge
    - If neurological examination is persistently abnormal—consider etiology, obtain EEG
    - In such cases—continue phenobarbitone, discontinue phenytoin and reevaluate after 1 month.
- One month after discharge:
    - If neurological examination is normal—discontinue phenobarbitone
    - If neurological examination is persistently abnormal—obtain EEG
    - If no seizure activity on EEG—discontinue phenobarbitone.
- No role of prophylactic anticonvulant therapy.

Respiratory Management

- Attach a pulse oxymeter and monitor oxygen saturation
- Maintain oxygen saturation between 90 and 95%
- Monitor for hypoxia, acidosis and hypercarbia
- Maintain normocarbia (pCO_2 35–45)
- Avoid hypoxia and hypocarbia
- Intubation and ventilation, if there are
    - Ineffective spontaneous breaths
    - Respiratory failure
    - Not able to maintain oxygen saturation despite oxygen.

Treatment of Hypovolemia

- If capillary filling time (CFT) of more than 3 seconds
- Give 10 mL/kg of normal saline over 5–10 minutes
- Hypotension is a common consequence of myocardial ischemia
- Maintain a mean blood pressure of more than 35 mm of Hg in term babies
- Maintain cardiac output by using inotropes like dopamine or dobutamine
- Start dopamine at 5 microgram/kg/min and escalate rapidly to 10 microgram/kg/min
- In case of inadequate perfusion, further add dobutamine at 5 microgram/kg/min and escalate to 20 microgram/kg/min
- Suspect septic shock in presence of intrapartum risk factors for sepsis and positive septic screen.

DIC- Bleeding or Petecchiae

- Investigations—Platelet count, coagulation profile (PT, APTT)
- Treatment
    - Injection vitamin K
    - Fresh frozen plasma (FFP) transfusion
    - If thrombocytopenia—platelet transfusion.

Feeding

- Starting of feeds depends on severity of asphyxia and association of respiratory distress, hypotension, encephalopathy, and renal impairment
- Feed intolerance is common in asphyxia, may lead to necrotizing enterocolitis (NEC)
- Preferred milk—mother/s expressed breast milk.

Predictors of Poor Outcome

- Refractory seizures
- Neurological defect at the end of first week
- HIE stage 3 at the time of discharge.

Chapter 108

Meconium Aspiration Syndrome

Earl Jaspal

- Meconium is formed as early as 12–16 weeks gestational age
- Frequency of meconium staining of the amniotic fluid increases with increasing gestational age
- Prevalence increases to 10% after 38 weeks and 30% at 42 weeks gestation
- Incidence of meconium staining of the amniotic fluid (MSAF) ranges from 5–25% of childbirths
- Of the infants presenting with MSAF, 3–8% of infants will develop meconium aspiration syndrome (MAS)
- Mortality associated with MAS and pulmonary hypertension can be as high as 20%
- Appropriate intrapartum care with early detection and management of fetal hypoxia is important in minimizing the risk from meconium staining of amniotic fluid.

CONSTITUENTS OF MECONIUM

MAS occurs most frequently in term, or post-term newborn infants who have passed meconium in utero.

- 75–80%—water
- Remaining 25%:
    - Gastric secretions
    - Bile salts
    - Mucus
    - Blood
    - Lanugo
    - Squamous cells
    - Free fatty acids
    - Vernix
    - Pancreatic enzymes.

Pathophysiology of Meconium Aspiration Syndrome (MAS)

- History of fetal distress and meconium in the liquor
- Intrauterine distress leads to gasping in utero
- This results in amniotic fluid and particulate matter to be inhaled into large airways, which then causes obstruction at delivery
- The meconium causes a ball-valve effect in the airways, resulting in areas of collapse and areas of overexpansion due to trapping of gas
- Air leaks are common
- Chemical inflammation from the meconium leads to a pneumonitis
- Meconium inhibits endogenous surfactant. Secondary persistent pulmonary hypertension of the newborn (PPHN) occurs as a result of atelectasis, hypoventilation, and intrapulmonary shunting.

Signs and Symptoms of MAS

- Typically, a postmature or mature newborn with long fingernails and dry skin
- Skin, nails and umbilical cord are often stained greenish yellow
- Baby is depressed at birth
- Tachypnea
- Grunting
- Retractions—intercostal and subcostal indawing
- Nasal flaring
- Cyanosis
- Barrel chest appearance due to gas trapping and alveolar over distension
- On auscultation—rales and rhonchi may be heard
- Affected newborns develop progressive respiratory failure with significant hypoxemia during the first 48–72 hours of life.

POSTDELIVERY MANAGEMENT OF MAS

Neonatal Management

- Assess the infant immediately after birth
- Decide whether the newborn is vigorous or depressed at birth

Vigorous Infant	Depressed Infant
Heart rate more than 100 beats/min	Heart rate less than 100 beats/min
Spontaneous respiratory efforts	Absent or depressed respiratory efforts
Good muscle tone	Decreased muscle tone

If the infant is vigorous
- Remove secretions from mouth and nose using suction catheter or bulb syringe or mucus trap. The suction pressure should be adjusted on the suction machine so that when the suction catheter is blocked the negative pressure is 100 mm Hg
- Follow routine steps of resuscitation
- No role of routine intubation and tracheal suctioning in a vigorous infant.

If the infant is depressed
- According to American Academy of Pediatrics (AAP) guidelines, in a depressed baby born through meconium-stained amniotic fluid, direct suctioning of trachea is to be done soon after delivery before many respirations have occurred.

Procedure

- Immediately perform direct laryngoscopy, using a large bore suction catheder of 12 F or 14 F and suction any meconium that is in mouth and posterior pharynx
- Then intubate the infant's trachea, and attach a suction source directly to the endotracheal tube as it is slowly withdrawn from the trachea
- Repeat, if necessary until little meconium is recovered or the heart is less than 60 beats/minute. Do not intubate and suction more than three times. Then proceed with routine resuscitation.

Treatment of Established MAS

The main aim of treatment is supportive until the alveolar macrophages clear debris and lung function returns to normal.

Therapies instituted for MAS include:

- Oxygen therapy
- Continuous positive airway pressure (CPAP)
- Intermittent positive pressure
- High-frequency oscillatory ventilation
- Antibiotics
- Pulmonary vasodilators
- Surfactant therapy
- Blood volume and blood pressure monitoring
- Steroid administration
- Extracorporeal membrane oxygenation.

General Measures

Maintain Thermoneutral Environment

- Nurse the baby in a thermoneutral environment of 36.0–37.0°C.

Airway Clearing

- No role of oral or nasal suction for neonates while the head is on the perineum.

Provide Respiratory Support

- Aim of ventilation is to optimize oxygenation while minimizing air-trapping.

Continuous Positive Airway Pressure (CPAP)/Bubble CPAP

- Effective if air trapping is not a major problem.

Convential Mechanical Ventilation

Recommended settings on ventilator

- Low inspiratory pressure
- Short inspiratory time
- Long expiratory time
- Rapid rates
- Low PEEP.

High-frequency ventilation (HFV)

- Provides effective gas exchange at low tidal volumes
- Start the infant on a MAP equal to that on the conventional ventilator and gradually increase it.

Advantages of HFV

- Improve oxygenation
- Improve CO_2 removal
- Less barotraumas
- Increased mobilization of airway secretions
- Quicker attainment of respiratory alkalosis.

Provide Cardiovascular Support, Avoid Hypotension

- Monitor blood pressure and capillary filling time (CFT) closely
- Systemic arterial blood pressure should be greater that pulmonary arterial blood pressure
- Maintain mean blood pressure 55–60 mm Hg
- If hypotensive, treat aggressively with proper fluid management
- Start inotropic support—Dopamine, and adrenaline infusions as required.

Minimal Handling

- Keep handling to minimum
- Agitation can cause hypoxia and acidosis in these infants.

Antibiotics

- No role of routine use of antibiotics
- Use antibiotics only when indicated depending on clinical condition and septic screen.

Maintain Nutrition

Provide parenteral nutrition until feeding is established.

Surfactant Therapy

- Indicated in severe meconium aspiration syndrome
- Meconium inactivates endogenous surfactant
- It is more effective, if given earlier
- Dosage—100–200 mg/kg of phospholipid
- Repeat dose 6 to 8 hourly till oxygenation improves.

Advantages

- Improves gas exchange
- Improved oxygenation
- Decreased incidence of air leaks
- Reduced the severity of respiratory failure
- Decrease need for extracorporeal membrane oxygenation (ECMO).

Note: Surfactant therapy does not reduce mortality in infants with MAS.

Inhaled Nitric Oxide (INO)

- Potent pulmonary vasodilator
- Decreases pulmonary arterial pressure
- Effective therapy in treatment of persistent pulmonary hypertension of newborn (PPHN) which accompanies MAS
- Recommended dosage of INO is 20 parts per million (PPM)
- Ensure adequate ventilation before starting iNO.

Bronchoalveolar Lavage (BAL)

- No role of saline or surfactant lavage.

Extracorporeal Membranous Oxygenation (ECMO)

- Effective in reducing both mortality and severe disability in neonates with MAS.

Steroids

- No role of corticosteroids use in management of MAS.

Chapter 109

Hypoglycemia in Newborns

Earl Jaspal

DEFINITION

- Blood glucose levels of less than 40 mg/dL or plasma glucose levels of lower than 45 mg/dL in both term and preterm infants
- Most common metabolic problem in newborn period
- Glucose is an essential nutrient for the brain
- Abnormally low level, prolonged or recurrent hypoglycemia can lead to long-term neurological injury.

Risk Factors

- Prematurity
- Low birth weight babies (<2500 gm)
- Small for gestational age babies
- Intrauterine growth retardation
- Infant of a diabetic mother (IDM)
- Macrosomic infant
- Neonatal sepsis
- Perinatal asphyxia
- Cold stress or hypothermia
- Polycythemia
- Erythroblastosis fetalis
- Respiratory distress syndrome
- Hypothyroidism
- Adrenocortical deficiency
- Congenital heart disease
- Maternal intake of terbutaline, propranolol, or oral hypoglycemic agents
- Inborn errors of metabolism—glycogen storage disease, galactosemia, beta oxidation defects
- During exchange transfusion.

Symptoms

- Jitteriness
- Irritability
- High-pitched cry
- Seizures
- Hypothermia
- Temperature instability
- Poor suck
- Refusal to feed
- Apnea

- Irregular rapid breathing
- Hypotonia
- Cyanosis
- Coma.

Indications of Blood Glucose Measurement

- All high-risk babies
- Babies receiving intravenous fluid in neonatal intensive care
- Babies having symptoms of hypoglycemia
- Babies with neonatal convulsions.

Measurement of Blood Glucose

Testing Method

- Bedside glucose testing reagent strips.

Advantages

- Inexpensive
- Practical
- Easy to use.

Disadvantages

- Inaccurate values
- Not reliable—significant difference from true blood glucose levels
- Always confirm suspected hypoglycemia with laboratory levels of blood glucose
- Laboratory blood glucose sample should be processed immediately and urgently.

Screening of At-Risk Neonates

- Screen all high-risk neonates
- Measure blood sugar by glucometer at ages 1, 2, 4, 6, 9 and 12 hours
- If blood glucose is stable, then monitor blood sugar every 6th hourly.

Prevention

- Encourage early feeds via breastfeeding usually within 30–60 minutes of birth
- Maintain thermoneutral environment
- Screen all high-risk newborns and observe for signs of hypoglycemia
- Feed frequently either 2nd or 3rd hourly
- If newborn is nil by mouth then start intravenous fluids as soon as possible.

Treatment

Nonsymptomatic Infants

- All hypoglycemic babies should be monitored
- Maintain a thermoneutral environment.

If Blood Glucose Levels between 20 and 40 mg/dL and Asymptomatic

- Feed immediately
- Check the blood glucose levels 30 minutes after the feed.

- If blood sugar greater than 40 mg/dL, continue 2nd hourly feeds
- Monitor blood glucose levels every 6th hourly for the first 48 hours of life
- These babies can stay with the mother in the postnatal ward
- Record and document all the readings on the neonatal blood glucose observation chart
- If blood glucose remains less than 40 mg/dL despite feedings, begin intravenous fluid therapy
- Continue feeding during IV fluid therapy
- If blood glucose levels are less than 20 mg/dL and asymptomatic
- Insert an intravenous cannula and start intravenous fluids as per protocol for treatment of symptomatic babies.

Symptomatic Infant

- Immediate bolus—2 mL/kg intravenous bolus of 10% dextrose over 1–2 minutes
- Start continuous glucose infusion at the rate of 6–8 mg/kg/min
- Check blood sugar levels after 30 minutes and then 6th hourly, if euglycemia is achieved
- Target glucose levels should be higher than 45 mg/dL and should be maintained higher than or equal to 50 mg/dL with IV glucose infusions
- If blood sugar remains below 40 mg/dL, then titrate and increase the glucose infusion rate by 2 mg/kg/minute up to a maximum of 12 mg/kg/minute
- Intravenous infusion of solutions with more than 12.5% glucose are best given through an umbilical venous catheter or central line to avoid complications
- Encourage frequent breastfeedings
- Monitor glucose concentrations before feeding and as IV is weaned until values stabilize off intravenous fluids
- Careful documentation of all the blood sugar readings on the neonatal blood glucose observation chart.

Weaning from High Glucose Concentrations

- Once glucose concentrations have stabilized for 24 hours, start weaning
- Continue to monitor blood glucose 4th to 6th hourly while IV dextrose is being gradually reduced.
- Rapid reductions in glucose infusion can cause rebound hypoglycaemia.
- If blood sugar is 45 mg/dL or more on two consecutive measurements, start decreasing glucose infusion @ 2 mg/kg/min 6th hourly
- Wean IV glucose as serum glucose normalizes and increase feeds simultaneously
- Stop IV fluids when oral feeding reaches at least 2/3 of daily requirement
- Feed the baby every 2nd hourly
- Cease blood sugar monitoring when three consecutive blood sugar values are more than 45 mg/dL on full feeds.

Persistent or Severe Hypoglycemia

- Babies requiring more than 10 mg/kg/minute of glucose or lasting longer than 1 week
- Requires further investigation and management for example, with glucagon, diazoxide, steroids or surgery.

Treatment Options

- If increases of glucose intake further than 12—15 mg/kg/minute are necessary, commence glucagon infusion—2 mg/kg in 48 mL 5% dextrose at 1 mL/hour
- In a symptomatic infant where i.v. access cannot be gained give glucagon 0.1–0.2 mg/kg intramuscular
- If glucagon fails to control blood glucose further glucose may be given using 20% or 25% solutions
- Rarely steroids may be needed. They are essential in adrenal and pituitary insufficiency
- Give hydrocortisone max. 5–10 mg/kg/day po, i.v. or i.m. 12 hourly
- If hyperinsulinemia has been diagnosed then diazoxide may be used
- Give diazoxide 1.5–6.5 mg/kg 8 hourly p.o.

HYPERGLYCEMIA

Definition

- Serum glucose higher than 125 mg/dL in term infants and higher than 150 mg/dL in preterm infants.

Etiology

- Excess glucose administration (>8 mg/kg/min)
- Transient neonatal diabetes mellitus
- Hyperosmolar formula
- Sepsis
- Hypoxia
- Medications
- Stress.

Clinical Features

- Nonspecific symptoms may be related to the cause
- Osmotic diuresis
- Dehydration
- Weight loss
- IVH
- Increased mortality.

Monitoring

- Serum glucose q 1 hour until lower than 150 mg/dL then q 4 hours until normoglycemic.

Treatment

- If serum glucose higher than 150 mg/dL
- Reduce glucose infusion rate (GIR) 2 mg/kg/minute by decreasing total fluids.
- If total fluids cannot be decreased, decrease glucose concentration
- IV human regular insulin administration (0.1 unit/kg IV), if reducing the GIR is not effective or is not possible
- Continuous insulin infusion starting at 0.01 units/kg/hour, increase gradually to 0.05-0.1 units/kg/hour may sometimes be indicated.

Chapter 110

Hypocalcemia in Newborns

Earl Jaspal

DEFINITION

Defined as total serum calcium level - less than 7.0 mg/dL in preterm babies
less than 8.0 mg/dL in term babies.
Or ionized calcium concentration of less than 4.0 mg/dL in preterm babies or less than 4.8 mg/dL in term babies.

Types of Neonatal Hypocalcemia

a. Early neonatal hypocalcemia
b. Late neonatal hypocalcemia

Early Neonatal Hypocalcemia

Defined as hypocalcemia that occurs in the first three days of life.
- Mostly seen in premature babies
- Etiology:
    - Premature and Low birth weight babies
    - Perinatal Asphyxia
    - Small for gestational age (SGA)
    - Intrauterine growth retardation (IUGR)
    - Infant born to diabetic mother
    - Maternal hyperparathyroidism.
- Symptoms—usually asymptomatic
- Usually occur in first 12–24 hours
- Spontaneously resolves by 5–10 days.

Late Neonatal Hypocalcemia

Defined as hypocalcemia that occurs between the fifth and tenth days of life.
- Usually symptomatic
- Rarely seen in breast-fed babies
- Etiology:
    - High phosphate formula feeding
    - Cow's milk feeding
    - Neonatal hypoparathyroidism
        - Transient — idiopathic, maternal hyperparathyroidism
        - Congenital — idiopathic, congenital hypermagnesimia.
    - Vitamin D deficiency
    - Hypomagnesemia
    - Congenital hypoparathyroidism
    - Renal disease

Symptoms of Hypocalcemia

- Usually asymptomatic
- Irritiability
- Muscle twitches
- Jitteriness
- Seizures
- Hypotonia
- Tachycardia
- Tachypnea
- Apnea
- Poor feeding
- Lethargy
- Tremors

- Hypoalbuminemia
- Exchange transfusion.

Investigations

- Total or ionized serum Ca level—blood serum levels of total and ionized serum calcium
  - Total serum calcium level of less than 7.0 mg/dL in preterm babies or less than 8.0 mg/dl in term babies.
  - Ionized calcium concentration of less than 4.0 mg/dL in preterm babies or less than 4.8 mg/dl in term babies
- Electrocardiogram (ECG) shows prolongation of the corrected QT interval (QT_c)
- Serum magnesium levels—lower than 1.5 mg/dL indicate hypomagnesemia, which can accompany hypocalcemia
- Alkaline phosphatase levels— more than 225 IU/L and can be an early sign of rickets
- To rule out causes of hypocalcemia
  - Serum albumin
  - Phosphorus
  - Magnesium
  - Vitamin D_3 levels
  - Renal function
  - Paratharmone levels (PTH)
  - Urinary calcium.

Treatment

- Early onset: IV 10% Ca gluconate
- Late onset: Oral calcitriol or Ca
- Early-onset hypocalcemia usually resolves in a few days
- Preterm hypocalcemic infants who are asymptomatic
  - Require no specific treatment
  - Hypocalcemia usually resolves within 3 days.
- Asymptomatic newborns: Serum calcium levels higher than 7 mg/dL or ionized Ca higher than 3.5 mg/dL rarely require treatment.
- Asymptomatic hypocalcemia as diagnosed by screening—
  - Give 80 mg/kg/day of elemental calcium or 8 mL/kg/day of 10% calcium gluconate.
- Infants with increased risk of hypocalcemia:
  - Give 4 mL/kg/day of 10% calcium gluconate or 40 mg/kg/day of elemental calcium
  - If baby is on oral feeds, add oral calcium every 6th hourly
  - Therapy should continue for 3 days
  - If serum calcium level is less than 6.5 mg/dL
    - Start continuous calcium infusion
    - Starting dose—45 mg/kg/day or 5 mL/kg/day of 10% calcium gluconate.
- Symptomatic hypocalcaemia
  - Injection 10% Ca gluconate—2 mL/kg/dose diluted with 1:1 of 5% dextrose by slow IV infusion over 10-15 minutes under cardiac monitoring.

- Maintenance dose:
  - Continue maintenance IV infusion of calcium gluconate at the rate of 0.5–1.0 mmol/kg/day or 8 mL/kg/day of 10% calcium gluconate or 80 mg/kg/day of elemental calcium for 48 hours.
- Monitor ionized calcium levels every 12–24 hours
- If plasma calcium levels are normal and infant is asymptomatic:
  - Decrease calcium gluconate infusion by 50%, i.e. 4 mL/kg/day of 10% calcium gluconate or 40 mg/kg/day of elemental calcium for the next 24 hours and stop the infusion after another 24 hours.
- Change to oral calcium therapy on the last day
- Continue oral calcium at dose of 1 mmol/kg/day of elemental calcium in divided doses.

<table>
<tr><td>

Contraindications to Calcium Therapy

- Hypercalcemia
- Severe renal disease
- Severe hypercalcuria

</td></tr>
</table>

Care to be Taken while Giving IV Calcium Therapy

- Monitor heart rate
  - Too rapid infusion causes
    - Bradycardia
    - Arrhythmias
    - Cardiac asystole.
- Check IV cannula site, if cannula is not properly inserted
  - Infiltration of calcium gluconate causes
    - Skin redness
    - Local tissue damage
    - Necrosis
    - Calcium deposition.
- Never give intramuscularly calcium gluconate injection.

Strength Available of Injection Calcium Gluconate

- 10% = 100 mg/mL (9 mg [0.45 mEq] of elemental calcium per milliliter).

Symptomatic Hypocalcemia not Responding to Calcium

- Cause—may be hypomagnesemia
- Diagnosis—Serum magnesium levels less than 1.2 mg/dL
- Treatment of hypomagnesemia—
  - 0.1–0.2 mL/kg of 50% $MgSO_4$ per kg deep I/M.
- Dose may be repeated after 12 hours deep intramuscular
- Maintenance dose
  - Oral administration of $MgSO_4$ 50% — 0.2 mg/kg/day orally for 3 days.

Chapter 111

Intrauterine Growth Retardation

Earl Jaspal

- Incidence affects 3–10% of pregnancies
- Neonatal mortality is 8 to 10 times higher in growth retarded infants
- Neonatal morbidity occurs in 50% of surviving infants.

DEFINITIONS

- Intrauterine growth restriction (IUGR)—a rate of fetal growth that is less than normal for the growth potential of a specific infant
- IUGR infants have marked increased risk of neonatal mortality and morbidity and long-term sequel.
- Appropriate for gestational age (AGA): Birth weight between 10th and 90th percentile for gestational age
- Small for gestational age (SGA): Birth weight less than 10th percentile for gestational age.
- Large for gestational age (LGA): Birth weight more than 90th percentile for gestational age.

INTRAUTERINE GROWTH RESTRICTION (IUGR)

Symmetrical IUGR

- Constitutes 20–30% of IUGR
- Occurs due to an insult during early pregnancy
- There is a proportionate decrease in length, weight and head circumference for gestational age
- All parameters are less than 10th percentile on growth chart
- Decreased growth potential
- Lower risk for transitional problem
- Example—genetics, chromosomal, TORCH infections.

Asymmetrical or Head Sparing IUGR

- Constitutes 70–80% of IUGR
- Related to under nutrition or hypoxia in late pregnancy
- Weight and length is decreased less than 10th percentile for gestational age
- Head circumference remains normal, i.e. appropriate for gestational age
- Higher risk for transitional problem
- Growth arrest
- Example—maternal malnutrition, placental dysfunction.

Intrinsic *(Fetal)* Causes

Genetic
- Chromosomal (7–20%)
- Single gene defects
- Deletion disorders
- Inborn error of metabolism
- Constitutional
- Congenital abnormalities.

Infections
- TORCH
- Syphilis
- Malaria
- Viruses.

Toxic
- Substance abuse
- Cigarette smoking
- Therapeutic irradiation
- Cocaine
- Hydantoin
- Radiation.

Extrinsic *(Maternal/Placental)* Causes

- Maternal age— less than 16 year or more than 35 year
- Maternal illness
  - Cardiac—cyanotic heart disease
  - Anemia
  - Chronic renal disease
  - Hemoglobinopathies
  - Malnutrition.
- Uteroplacental insufficiency
  - Pre eclampsia
  - Chronic hypertension
  - Infection
  - Vascular disease
  - Placental infarcts
  - Abuptio placenta
  - Vlamentous insertion of umbilical cord.
- Multiple gestation
- Demographic
  - Low socioeconomic status
  - Race.
- Behavioral
  - Stress.
- Teenage preganacy
- In utero constraint
  - Tumor
  - Mass.

Common Morbidities Associated with IUGR

- Perinatal asphyxia
- Hypothermia
- Hypoglycemia requiring intravenous (IV) therapy
- Polycythemia
- Neonatal sepsis
- Necrotizing enterocolitis (NEC)
- Severe growth restriction
- Congenital anomalies
- Hemorrhage.

Ponderal Index (PI)

Ponderal index (PI) is a ratio of body weight to length expressed as

$$PI = [\text{weight (in grams)} \times 100] \div [\text{length (in cm)}]^3$$

Typical values are 20 to 25.

Postnatal Assessment

- Growth parameters: document weight, length and head circumfrence
- Assess gestational age by using new Ballard score
- Plot growth parameters on growth chart.

Physical Appearance of IUGR Infants

- Heads are disproportionately large for their trunks and extremities
- Facial appearance has been likened to that of a "wizened old man"
- Widened skull sutures
- Large fontanelles
- Soft tissue wasting
- Dry, peeling skin
- Long nails
- Plethoric
- Thin umbilical cord
- Neurological—hyper alert or jittery
- Exaggerated moro's reflex
- Scaphoid abdomen
- Advanced sole creases
- Shortened crown—heel length.

Hypothermia

Higher risk in IUGR infants due to:
- Prematurity
- Increased surface area:body mass ratio
- Diminished glucose supply
- Diminished fat for insulation and energy
- Impaired lipid metabolism.

Management
- Warm delivery room
- Drying the baby after birth with prewarmed towels
- Skin-to-skin contact
- Early initiation of breastfeeding
- Radiant warmer/incubator care.

Ponderal Index
Used to distinguish the types of IUGR:
Asymmetrical IUGR
- Restriction late in gestation
- Only the weight affected
- Low ponderal index
Symmetrical IUGR
- Restriction early in gestation
- Weight and length affected
- Normal ponderal index

Investigations
- Septic profile
- Hematocrit
- Platelet count
- Blood glucose
- Serum Calcium
- Blood culture and sensitivity

Hypoglycemia

Higher risk due to:

- Reduced glycogen stores
- Hyperinsulinemia—increased insulin levels
- Reduced fat stores
- Increased brain:body mass ratio
- Immaturity of hepatic enzymes
- Reduced expression of glucose 6 phosphatase
- Reduced ketogenesis.

Polycythemia

Results from:

- Chronic hypoxia
- Increased EPO levels
- Increased red cell mass.

Necrotizing Enterocolitis

Results from:

- Absent end-diastolic flow
- Reversed end-diastolic flow
- Chronic hypoxia.

Management

- Be cautious in feeding these babies.

Perinatal Asphyxia

- Hypoxia during labor with compromised placental flow
- Increased risk of in utero passage of meconium.

Outcome of IUGR Infants

- Babies with symmetrical IUGR have poor outcome compared to asymmetrical IUGR
- Symmetrical IUGR associated with:
  - Cerebral palsy
  - Learning deficits
  - Behavioral problems
- Asymmetrical IUGR associated with:
  - Increased fat mass
  - Central adiposity
  - Insulin resistance
- Perinatal mortality for IUGR infants—5–20 times greater than for AGA
- Neurological morbidity—5–10 times higher than for AGA infants
- Preterm IUGR has high incidence of abnormalities
- Congenital infection has poor outcome—neurological sequel in more than 50% cases
- IUGR has higher rate of learning disability
- IUGR with chromosomal disease—100% incidence of handicap

Chapter 112

Convulsions/Seizures in Newborns

Earl Jaspal

- Seizures occur more frequently in the neonatal period (the first 28 days of life) than at any other time
- Incidence in newborns
  - 1.5–3.5 per 1000 live term births
  - 10–130 per 1000 live preterm births.
- Seizures are very common and occur in up to 70% of preterm infants with intraventricular hemorrhage or periventricular leukomalacia.

CAUSES OF NEONATAL SEIZURES

- Hypoxic-ischemic encephalopathy (HIE)—most common
- Intracranial hemorrhage
  - Intraventricular hemorrhage
  - Intracerebral hemorrhage
  - Subdural hemorrhage.
- Metabolic disorders
  - Hypoglycemia
  - Hypocalcemia
  - Hypomagnesemia
  - Hypo- and hypernatremia.
- Central nervous system infection
  - Bacterial meningitis
  - Viral meningitis
  - Encephalitis.
- Intrauterine (TORCH) infections
- Inborn errors of metabolism
- Drug withdrawal syndromes
- Kernicterus
- Benign idiopathic neonatal convulsions
- Congenital CNS malformations
- Idiopathic.

Clinical Signs of Subtle Seizures

- Staring look
- Blinking of eyes
- Horizontal deviation of eyes
- Chewing movements
- Sucking movements
- Lip smacking
- Repetitive mouth and tongue movements
- Boxing movements
- Pedaling movements
- Swimming movements
- Tachycardia
- Apnea

TYPES OF NEONATAL SEIZURES

Subtle Seizures

- More common in term babies
- Occur in babies with HIE and intraventricular hemorrhage.

Clonic Type

- Occurs in 50% cases
- More common in term babies

<table>
<tr><td>

How to differentiate jitteriness from convulsions?

Jitteriness:

- No associated eye movements
- No autonomic changes, i.e. there is no tachycardia, increase blood pressure, apnea, salivation or pupillary change
- Movements start by stimulus or may be spontaneous
- Movements stop by holding the limb
- Predominant movement in jitteriness are tremors which are rhythmic and of equal rate amplitude

</td><td>

- Rhythmic jerking movements
- Consciousness may be preserved
- May be focal, multifocal or generalized depending upon underlying lesion
- Focal clonic seizures—good prognosis.

Tonic Type

- Occurs in 20% cases
- More common in preterm babies
- Most common in the first 24 hours of life following hypoxic—ischemic insult
- May be focal or generalized, i.e. involving one limb or the entire body
- Presents as sustained extension of the upper and lower limbs or sustained flexion of upper with extension of lower limbs.

Myoclonic

- Rare in newborn period
- Present as rapid isolated jerks
- May be focal or generalized
- Poor prognosis.

</td></tr>
</table>

INVESTIGATIONS

- Septic screen, including blood cultures
- Lumbar puncture—CSF analysis
- Blood glucose
- Serum total and ionized calcium
- Serum magnesium
- Serum sodium
- Serum urea and creatinine
- Serum electrolytes
- Metabolic screening
- Blood ammonia and lactate
- TORCH
- Ultrasound cranium to rule out intracranial hemorrhage
- MRI to confirm the cause of seizures
- Electroencephalography (EEG) to predict the risk of electrographic seizures and prognosis.

MANAGEMENT

- Require urgent treatment to prevent brain injury
- Maintain TABC, i.e. Temperature (T), Airway (A), Breathing (B), Circulation (C).

Correct Metabolic Disturbances (If Documented)

- Hypoglycemia: 2 mL/kg IV bolus of 10% dextrose followed by continuous intravenous infusion at the rate of 6–8 mg/kg/minute
- Hypocalcemia: 2 mg/kg/dose of 10% calcium gluconate IV in 1:1 dilution with 5% dextrose over 10–15 minutes under cardiac monitoring
- Hypomagnesemia: 0.1–0.2 mL/kg of 50% $MgSO_4$ deep I/M.

Anticonvulsant Therapy

Start only after adequate ventilation and perfusion have been established.

Phenobarbitone

- Drug of choice.
- Initial Dose: 20 mg/kg IV slowly over 30 minutes
- Repeat dose: If seizures persist after completion of this loading dose, repeat dose of phenobarbitone 10 mg/kg every 20–30 minutes till a total dose of 40 mg/kg
- Maintenance dose: 3–4 mg/kg/day in 1–2 divided doses, started 12 hours after the loading dose
- Note—respiratory depression at higher doses of phenobarbitone
- Preparations:
    - 200 mg/mL–1 mL ampoule
    - For slow IV bolus, dilute 1:10 with 0.9% saline and give at a maximum rate of 1 mg/kg/minute.

Phenytoin Sodium

- Indication: If maximal dose of phenobarbitone (40 mg/kg) fails to resolve seizures
- Dose is 20 mg/kg slow IV infusion over 30 minutes
- Caution: It should only be mixed with saline and not with dextrose as it precipitates in dextrose
- Repeat dose of 10 mg/kg may be tried in refractory seizures
- Maintenance dose is 5–8 mg/kg/d in 2 divided doses, started 12 hours after the loading dose
- Discontinue before discharge
- Cardiac rate and rhythm should be monitored during the infusion
- Preparations: 50 mg/mL.

Duration of Anticonvulsant Therapy

- Neonatal period:
    - If neurological examination is normal before discharge—discontinue therapy
    - If neurological examination is persistently abnormal—consider etiology, obtain EEG
    - In such cases—continue phenobarbitone, discontinue phenytoin and reevaluate after 1 month.
- One month after discharge:
    - If neurological examination is normal—discontinue phenobarbitone
    - If neurological examination is persistently abnormal—obtain EEG
    - If no seizure activity on EEG—discontinue phenobarbitone.

Midazolam

Indication
- Babies who continue to have seizures after phenobarbitone and/or phenytoin.

Dose and administration
- 0.15 mg/kg IV over minimum of 5 minutes.

Continuous Infusion:
- 60–400 micrograms/kg/hour.

Reconstitution and dilution
- Dilute 1 mg/kg of midazolam up to a total of 50 mL with 0.9% sodium chloride, 5% glucose or 10% glucose:

    1 mL/hour = 20 micrograms/kg/hour.

Complications of Neonatal Seizures

- Cerebral palsy
- Hydrocephalus
- Epilepsy
- Learning disability
- Mental retardation
- Feeding difficulties

DOCUMENTATION

Document each episode of seizure in neonatal case record sheet. This should include:

- Date of seizure
- Time of seizure
- Duration of each seizure
- Type of seizure (subtle, tonic, clonic, myoclonic and focal or generalized)
- Any abnormal eye movements
- Associated autonomic system changes, e.g. apnea, hypotension, hypertension
- Any provoking stimulus, e.g. handling, noise
- Treatment given
- Dose and route of the drug
- Response to treatment.

PROGNOSIS

- Depends on underlying etiology
- Hypocalcemic seizures—excellent prognosis
- Symptomatic hypoglycemia and meningitis—50% chance of sequelae
- Hypoxic ischemic encephalopathy—prognosis depends on the grade of HIE
- CNS malformations—poor prognosis.

Chapter 113

Neonatal Sepsis

Earl Jaspal

- Bacterial sepsis is a major problem in the newborn unit
- Neonatal sepsis is associated with significant morbidity and mortality
- Most common organisms causing neonatal sepsis both in hospital and community in India
  - *Klebsiella pneumonia*
  - *Staphylococcus aureus*
  - *E. coli.*

TYPES

- Early-onset sepsis (EOS)
- Late-onset sepsis (LOS).

Early Onset Sepsis (EOS)

- Sepsis occurring in the first 72 hours of life
- Etiology result from vertical transmission of bacteria from mother to neonate during intrapartum period
- Manifests with pneumonia and/or septicemia
- Oganisms predominantly acquired from the birth canal
- High-risk of mortality—10–30%.

Late Onset Sepsis (LOS)

- Sepsis occurring beyond 72 hours of life
- Etiology results from horizontal transmission of pathogens from environment or hands of the care giver
- Manifests as septicemia, pneumonia or meningitis
- Rate of infection is inversely related to birth weight and gestational age
- Infants less than 1000 gms are at highest risk
- Pathogens causing late-onset neonatal sepsis:
  - Coagulase negative staphylococci (CONS)
  - Methicillin resistant Staphylococcus aureus (MRSA)
  - Methicillin sensitive Staphylococcus aureus (MSSA)
  - Gram-negative species
  - Candida albicans.
- Mortality rate—5%.

Risk Factors for Late Onset Sepsis

- Prolonged hospital stay
- Presence of foreign bodies, e.g. intravenous catheters, endotracheal tubes

Risk Factors for Early Onset Sepsis

- Clinical chorioamnionitis
- Maternal intrapartum fever (>38.0°C),
- Prematuity
- Low birth weight
- Rupture of membranes (ROM) >18 hours before delivery
- More than three vaginal examinatons
- Maternal GBS colonization
- Previous infant with GBS infection
- Inadequate intrapartum antibiotic prophylaxis

- Prematurity
- Low birth weight
- Mechanial ventilation
- Total parental nutrition (TPN)
- Cross infection by staff and parents.

Clinical Features

Generally nonspecific:
- Hyperthermia or hypothermia and/or temperature instability
- Respiratory distress
  - Increased respiratory rate
  - Chest indrawing
  - Grunting
  - Cyanosis.
- Apnea
- Bradycardia or tachycardia
- Lethargy
- Irritability
- Seizures
- Poor feeding/refusal to feed
- Hypoglycemia or hyperglycemia
- Abdominal distension
- Feed intolerance—vomiting, altered and excessive gastric aspirates
- Unexplained jaundice
- Signs of shock—CFT more than 3 seconds, poor perfusion, hypotension
- Altered muscle tone—hypotonia
- Absent reflexes
- Thrombocytopenia or abnormal coagulation
- Signs of local infection—eyes, skin and umbilicus
- Need for mechanical ventilation.

Investigations

- Complete blood count
- Septic screen—components
  - Total leukocyte count
  - Absolute neutrophil count
  - Micro-ESR
  - Immature to total neutrophil (I:Tratio)
  - C-reactive protein (CRP).
- Positive septic screen—if two or more of above mentioned parameters are abnormal
- Total leukocyte count (TLC):
  - Less than 5,000/mm^3
  - Reliable indicator of infection but is less sensitive and nonspecific, if considered individually.
- Absolute neutrophil count (ANC)—low counts
  - Use Manroe chart for term neonates and Mouzinho's chart for VLBW babies.
- Immature to total neutrophil ratio
  - I:T ratio ≥0.2 considered to be significant in terms of infection.
- Micro-erythrocyte sedimentation rate
  - More than 15 mm in 1st hour.

- C-reactive protein (CRP):
  - CRP level begins to increase 4–6 hours after an inflammatory trigger
  - Peaks between 36–50 hours
  - Normal concentration of CRP in neonates—1 mg/dL or lower
  - CRP more than 1 mg/dL—marker for established neonatal bacterial infection
  - Serial CRP values taken 24–48 hour after the onset of symptoms—better sensitivity and specificity
  - Levels decrease rapidly with resolution of inflammation
  - Lacks specificity—CRP can be increased in noninfectious etiology by about 10 times of its normal concentration.
- Blood culture
  - Gold standard
  - Minimum volume for culture—1.0 mL of blood when a single pediatric blood culture bottle is used
  - Collect blood culture before administering the first dose of antibiotics
  - Take strict aspectic precautions while taking blood culture.
- Chest radiograph
  - If clinical signs of respiratory disease are present.
- Lumbar puncture (LP)
  - Consider lumbar puncture in all neonates with late onset sepsis
  - If an lumbar puncture was not done at presentation, an LP should be considered if:
    - CRP greater than 10 mg/l
    - Positive blood culture
    - Low white cell count
    - Poor response to antibiotic treatment
    - If there is a strong clinical suspicion of infection or signs/symptoms suggestive of meningitis.

TREATMENT

Supportive Care

General

- Maintain thermoneutral environment
- Place the baby under radiant warmer/incubator
- Monitor vital signs—heart rate, respiratory rate, CFT, blood pressure, oxygen saturation.

Respiratory

- Manage respiratory distress
- Treat hypoxia, hypercapnea and apnea
- Depending on clinical condition give respiratory support
  - Oxygen therapy
  - Noninvasive ventilation—continuous positive airway pressure (CPAP)
  - Invasive ventilation—mechanical ventilation.

Cardiovascular

- Measure capillary filling time and blood pressure
- If poor perfusion or hypotension
  - Consider volume expansion by normal saline
  - Inotropic support dopamine or dobutamine, if required

Antibiotics

- Initial choice of antibiotics depends on the individual hospital policy, pathogens and susceptibility pattern of the organisms in that unit
- Antibiotic can then be rationalized or upgraded on the basis of culture and sensitivity results and clinical condition.

First Line Therapy

- Standard therapy (Injection ampicillin or penicillin G and an aminoglycoside (gentamycin/ amikacin) by intravenous or intramuscular route
- Discontinue antibiotics in asymptomatic baby with negative cultures after 48 hours
- Continue more than 48 hours, if there is a high-index of suspicion for sepsis or a positive blood or CSF culture
- Once the organism and antibiotic sensitivity is identified by culture and sensitivity report, select the appropriate drugs.

Dosage and frequency of administration of antibiotics depends on—
- Gestational age
- Postnatal age
- Birth weight
- Hepatic and renal function.

Second Line Therapy

- Considered, if no clinical improvement after 48–72 hours
- Should cover both gram-positive and gram-negative organisms
- Cloxacillin/ciprofloxacin and amikacin/netilmycin may be used
- In suspected septic shock due to gram-negative organism, use vancomycin, gentamycin/amikacin
- In suspected meningitis, use cefotaxime
- In necrotizing enterocolitis, use amoxicillin, gentamicin/amikacin, metronidazole.

Third Line Therapy

- Injection meropenam and vancomycin or
- Inj piperacillin tazobactum and netilmycin
- If Methicillin resistant Staphylococcus aureus (MRSA) is suspected use vancomycin
- Change antibiotics depending on blood and CSF culture and sensitivity patterns.

Duration of Antimicrobial Therapy

Blood Culture Negative, Septic Screen Negative, Clinically Asymptomatic

Stop antibiotics after 48 hours if:
- Baby is asymptomatic with no clinical signs of possible infection
- Septic screen is negative
- CRP less than 10 mg/l on both tests
- Blood culture is negative.

Blood Culture Negative, Septic Screen Positive, Baby Clinically Symptomatic

- Duration of antimicrobial therapy—7–10 days

Blood Culture Positive Sepsis without Meningitis

- Blood-culture-positive sepsis—antibiotics for 10–14 days
- Choice of antibiotics depends on sensitivity pattern
- Stop antibiotics by 7–10 days if:
  - Gestational age more than 32 weeks
  - Birth weight more than1500 grams
  - Asymptomatic within 5 days of appropriate therapy
  - Ensure a proper follow-up for these neonates.

Antimicrobial Choice and Duration of Therapy for Neonatal Meningitis

- Third generation cephalosporins have excellent central nervous system penetration
- In suspected gram-negative meningitis, use cefotaxime
- Decision of antibiotic based on:
  - Activity of antibiotic against the causative pathogen
  - Relative penetration into cerebrospinal fluid (CSF) in presence of meningeal inflammation.
- Treatment of early-onset neonatal meningitis:
  - Combination of ampicillin and cefotaxime or ampicillin and aminoglycoside.
- Treatment of late-onset meningitis:
  - Combination of vancomycin plus a third-generation cephalosporin
  - Change antibiotics depending on blood and/or CSF culture and susceptibility results.
- Duration of antibiotics for neonatal meningitis—21 days.

Fungal Sepsis

- Considered, if infants deteriorate whilst receiving antibiotics
- Generally seen in VLBW infants in neonatal intensive care unit (NICU)
- Use amphotericin B as empirical treatment
- Fluconazole should be reserved for prophylaxis
- Duration of treatment depends upon the site of infection
- Treatment usually ranges from 3 to 6 weeks.

Risk Factors for Fungal Sepsis

- Gestational age less than 28 weeks
- Presence of central lines
- Endotracheal tube
- Thrombocytopenia ($<100,000/mm^3$)
- Exposure to broad spectrum cephalosporins or carbapenem
- Multiple courses of IV antibiotics
- Extensive areas of skin breakdown

Chapter **114**

Apnea of Prematurity

Earl Jaspal

DEFINITION

- Defined as a sudden cessation of breathing that lasts for at least 20 seconds or is accompanied by bradycardia or oxygen desaturation (cyanosis) in a newborn less than 37 weeks of gestational age
- Commonly occurs in premature babies
- Incidence is inversely proportional to gestational age
- Most common at lower gestational age and usually ceases by term
- Universal in babies less than 26 weeks of gestation and very common in babies of less than 34 weeks of gestation
- Usually resolves by 37 weeks postmenstrual age but occasionally persists for several weeks post-term
- Usually occurs in the first 2 days of life and at most within 7 days of life
- Occurrence beyond the first week is very uncommon
- It usually relates to immature respiratory control systems in the mid-brain and brainstem which must mature ex utero.

Conditions Causing or Accentuating Apnea

Systemic Illness

- Sepsis
- Shock (e.g. NEC)
- Hypoxemia.

CVS Disorders

- Congenital cyanotic heart disease
- Patent ductus arteriosus
- Congestive cardiac failure (CCF).

Central Nervous System Disturbances

- Asphyxia
- Seizures
- Intracranial hemorrhage
- Malformations.

Pulmonary Causes

- Respiratory distress syndrome (RDS)
- Pneumonia
- Pneumothorax

- Pulmonary hemorrhage
- Atelectasis
- Chronic lung disease.

Thermal Disturbance

- Hypothermia
- Hyperthermia.

Metabolic Disturbances

- Hypoglycemia
- Hypocalcemia
- Hyponatemia
- Inborn errors of metabolism.

Anatomical Narrowing of Airways

- Micrognathia
- Tracheomalacia
- Macroglossia
- Choanal atresia.

Drugs

- Opiates
- Sedation.

TYPES OF APNEA

Central Apnea

- Defined as cessation of both breathing efforts and airflow to lungs for more than 20 seconds.
- Associated desaturation will be detected by a saturation monitor.

Obstructive Apnea

- Defined as upper airway collapse causing cessation of airflow to the lungs in presence of breathing efforts
- Clinically diagnosed by desaturation on pulse oximeter with or without associated color change and bradycardia.

Mixed Apneas

- Most common
- Start as obstructive apnea and progress to central apnea or vice versa.

Investigations

To rule out secondary causes of apnea
- Complete blood cell count with differential count
- Hematocrit
- Septic screen
- Blood culture
- Blood glucose
- Serum and ionic calcium
- Serum electrolytes

- Blood gases
- Chest X-ray
- Echocardiography
- Head ultrasound.

TREATMENT

- Pharmacological treatment
- Nonpharmacological treatment

Pharmacological Treatment

Most commonly used agents
- Aminophylline/Theophylline
- Caffeine citrate

Main effect of xanthine is to increase the output of the respiratory center, which determines an increase in ventilation.

Aminophylline/ Theophylline

- Loading dose—4–8 mg/kg/dose IV
- Maintainence dose—1.5–2 mg/kg/dose IV 8th hourly
- Therapeutic levels—7–12 mcg/mL
- Toxic levels more than 20 mcg/mL
- Lower therapeutic to toxic ratio
- No role of prophylactic aminophylline
- Continue till 34 weeks corrected gestational age
- Stopped after apnea free period for 7 days.

Side effects

- Sinus tachycardia
- Ventricular tachycardia
- Agitation/irritability
- Feed intolerance
- Seizures/jitterness
- Hyperglycemia
- Electrolye abnormalities
- Diuresis
- Gastrointestinal bleeding.

Caffeine Citrate

- Drug of Choice
- Therapeutic levels—5–25 mcg/mL
- Toxic levels— higher than 40 mcg/mL
- The earlier the caffeine is started, the more beneficial effects it has
- Caffeine has been proven safe and effective in large multcenter randomized controlled trials.

When to start treatment?

- Infants <34 weeks of gestation with symptomatic apnea of prematurity
- Infants <30 weeks of gestation at birth who are on respiratory support
- Recurrent episodes of apnea requiring tactile stimulation and bag and mask ventilation to terminate the event.

Dosage

- Loading dose—20 mg/kg caffeine citrate
- Maintenance dose—5 mg/kg/day once a day
- If apneas persist, increase maintenance dose to 10 mg/kg/day
- Maintenance dose is given after 24 hours of loading dose.

Advantages of Caffeine

- Reduction in episodes of apneas
- Less side effects
- Once a day dosage schedule as it has a long half-life
- Plasma half-life—40 to 230 hours (mean -103)
- Wider therapeutic to toxic ratio
- Reliable enteral absorption
- Decreased need for mechanical ventilation
- Decreased oxygen requirement
- Reduced incidence of chronic lung disease and patent ductus arteriosus (PDA).

Side effects

- Nausea
- Vomiting
- Tachycardia
- Hypertonia
- Sweating
- Metabolic disturbances
- Pulmonary edema
- Cardiac failure.

Strength Available

- Injection: 20 mg/mL as caffeine citrate (10 mg/mL as caffeine base)
- Oral: 20 mg/mL as caffeine citrate (10 mg/mL as caffeine base)

When to stop caffeine?

- Postconceptual age—32–34 weeks
- Baby is off respiratory support and with minimal symptoms
- No significant apnea/bradycardia events for one week
- As caffeine has very long half-life, it can be stopped abruptly.

When to stop monitoring?

- Gestational age—34 weeks
- Apnea free for 8 days
- If caffeine has been given, must be off caffeine for 8 days and apnea free
- Minimum of 5 days off Ventilation/CPAP, if it has been used
- If vitals are stable and symptoms of apnea have resolved, baby can be discharged.

Doxapram

- Indication—If apnea persists despite caffeine/aminophyllin and CPAP
- It is a potent stimulator of breath
- Mechanism of action is not well known
- Its use in the newborn has been studied in limited and uncontrolled case series.

Side Effects of Doxapram

Has a serious adverse effect

- Jaundice
- Respiratory distress
- Convulsions
- Vomiting
- Diarrhea
- Irritability
- Hypertension
- Tachycardia
- Increased gastric residuals
- Abdominal distention
- Hyperglycemia,
- Glycosuria

Dosage

- Continuous infusion intravenous started at 0.5 mg/kg/hour
- Can be increased to maximum of 2.5 mg/kg/hour
- Infusion rate should be decreased when apnea control is achieved.

Nonpharmalogical Treatment

Maintain TABC, i.e.
   T- Temperature
   A- Airway
   B- Breathing
   C- Circulation

Positioning

Randomized study shown that nursing a preterm infant prone does not reduce rate of apnea when compared with side sleeping.

Continuous Positive Airway Pressure

- Indication—if apnea persists despite caffeine or aminophylline.
- Continuous positive airways pressure via nasal prongs reduces the severity of the apnea
- CPAP—start at 2–4 cm of H_2O.

Mechanical Ventilation

- Indication—Apnea and bradycardia not be controlled by drug therapy or nasal CPAP
- Low-pressures should be used at the rate necessary to prevent apnea.

Anemia

Transfusion is indicated, if:
- Symptomatic baby on oxygen or on respiratory support
- Not feeding well
- Low-hematocrit—less than lower than 21–25%
- Low-reticulocyte count.

   However, in many studies blood transfusion has not been shown to be effective in reducing apnea in anemic infant.

L Carnitine

- No effect on apnea rate with L-carnitine supplementation.

Creatine

- No effect on apnea rate with creatine supplementation.

Chapter 115

Fluid and Electrolyte Management in Newborns

Earl Jaspal

FLUID AND ELECTROLYTE MANAGEMENT

- Newborns fluids and electrolytes requirements are unique
- There is an excess of extracellular water (ECW) at birth and this decreases over the first few days of life
- Term babies normally lose up to 5% of their body weight
- Preterm babies may lose up to 10–15% of their body weight

Insensible water loss (IWL)—highest in very low birth weight and very premature babies due to:
- High surface area to body mass ratio
- Immature, water-permeable skin.

Factors that increase IWL:
- Immature skin
- Prematurity
- Hyperthermia/fever
- Radiant warmers
- Phototherapy
- Skin defects/breakdown
- Tachypnea
- Nonhumidified oxygen/environment.

Factors that decrease IWL:
- Mature skin
- Humidity
- Heat shields
- Humidified oxygen/environment.

Energy Requirements

Depends on:
- Gestational age
- Postnatal age
- Weight
- Route of intake (less calories if parenteral)
- Growth rate
- Activity level
- Thermal environment
- Medical problems.

Initial Fluid Administration

How to Start and Increase Intravenous Fluids?

Starting Points:
- Birth weight <1000 gm = 80 mL/kg/day
- Birth weight 1000–1500 gm = 80 mL/kg/day
- Birth weight >1500 gm = 60 mL/kg/day

Advancement Example: Baby weight <1000g
- Start 1st Day of life—80 mL/kg/day
- 2nd Day of life—100 mL/kg/day
- 3rd day of life—120 mL/kg/day
- 4th day of life—130 mL/kg/day
- 5th day of life—140 mL/kg/day
- 6th day of life—150 mL/kg/day
- 7th day of life—160 mL/kg/day

Advancement Example: Baby weight 1000g–1500g
- Start 1st Day of life—80 mL/kg/day
- 2nd Day of life—95 mL/kg/day
- 3rd day of life—110 mL/kg/day
- 4th day of life—120 mL/kg/day
- 5th day of life—130 mL/kg/day
- 6th day of life—140 mL/kg/day
- 7th day of life—150 mL/kg/day

Advancement Example: Baby weight more than 1500g
- Start 1st Day of life—60 mL/kg/day
- 2nd Day of life—75 mL/kg/day
- 3rd day of life—90 mL/kg/day
- 4th day of life—105 mL/kg/day
- 5th day of life—120 mL/kg/day
- 6th day of life—135 mL/kg/day
- 7th day of life—150 mL/kg/day

- Use birth weight for calculation of IV fluids
- For the first 24 hours, IV fluid is 10% dextrose solution
- Maintain a glucose infusion of 4–6 mg/kg/min
- Add calcium to IV fluids on day 1 of life in infants who are
  - Preterm
  - IUGR/SGA
  - Asphyxiated
  - Septic
  - Postoperative
  - Infants of a diabetic mother.
- Maintenance dose of Calcium—4 mL/kg/day of calcium gluconate
- No sodium or potassium should be added to fluids in first 24 hours
- Daily weight and urine output should be recorded and documented properly
- Daily increment of fluid depends on
  - Weight change
  - Urine output
  - Serum sodium.
- Do not increase fluids if there is
  - Inadequate urine output

- Baby has gained weight
- Serum sodium less than 135.
- Monitor daily weight, vital signs, urine output and blood urea nitrogen
- Add sodium and potassium to IV fluids after 48 hours
- After 48 hours of life:
  - Maintenance for sodium (Na+): 2–4 mEq/kg/day
  - Maintenance for potassium (K+): 1–3 mEq/kg/day.
- At 1 week of life:
  - Requirement of sodium: 3–5 mEq/kg/day
  - Requirement of potassium: 2–3 mEq/kg/day
- Monitor urine output:
  - Polyria—urine output >5 mL/kg/hour
  - Oliguria—urine output <1 mL/kg/hour
  - Anuria—urine output <0.5 mL/kg/hour
- Common Fluid Problems
  - Hypervolemia/volume overload
  - Hypovolemia/dehydration.

Conditions Requiring Fluid Restriction

- Respiratory distress syndrome (RDS): Excessive fluid can lead to fluid overload and increased risk of BPD
- Bronchopulmonary dysplasia (BPD): Excessive fluid can worsen, therefore, treated with diuretics to reduce pulmonary edema
- Patent ductus arteriosus (PDA): Volume overload can open ductus and worsen respiratory status
- Hypoxic ischemic encephalopathy (HIE): Associated with acute tubular necrosis (ATN) and/or SIADH and can lead to subsequent volume overload.

ELECTROLYTE ABNORMALITIES

Sodium Abnormalities

Hyponatremia

- Definition: Serum sodium—less than 130 mEq/L.
- Causes:
  - Water overload (most common cause in the first week in the preterm infant)
    - Excessive maternal fluid intake during labor/delivery can lead to neonatal hyponatremia
    - Excessive administration of fluid
    - Syndrome of inappropriate secretion of antidiuretic hormone (SIADH) with low urine output and high urine specific gravity
    - Acute renal failure in the oliguric phase before fluid restriction with decrease urine output and usually a low urine specific gravity.
  - Sodium deficiency:
    - Inadequate sodium intake
    - Diuretic therapy, especially loop diuretics (e.g. furosemide)
    - Renal sodium losses, especially in preterm babies
    - Excessive sodium loss: Diarrhea, gastric losses, 17OH progesterone deficiency.
- Signs/symptoms:
  - Lethargy

- Seizures
- Coma.
- Treatment:
  - Restrict intravenous fluids
  - Give additional sodium.
- Total body deficit of Na^+ can be calculated by:
  Na^+ deficit (mEq) = (desired $[Na^+]$ - current $[Na^+]$) × 0.8 × body weight (kg)
  (0.8 × body weight is the volume of distribution for Na^+)

Hypernatremia

- Definition: Serum sodium—more than 150 mEq/L.
- Causes:
  - Excessive water loss
    - Very preterm insensible water loss
    - Diarrhea
    - Polyuria.
  - Excess sodium intake
    - Relatively common with sodium bicarbonate infusions
    - Medications and infusions may contain large quantities of sodium.
- Signs/symptoms:
  - Lethargy
  - Seizures
  - Coma.
- Treatment:
  - Increase fluid intake
  - Decrease sodium intake.

Note: Always correct hypernatremia slowly. Rapid correction of hypernatremia can cause seizures and permanent neurodevelopmental sequelae.

Potassium Abnormalities

Hypokalemia

- Definition: Serum potassium—less than 3.5 mEq/L.
- Causes:
  - Inadequate intake of potassium
  - Metabolic alkalosis—secondary to overventilation, loss of acid from gastric secretions, bicarbonate treatment
  - Increased potassium losses—diuretics, renal causes, diarrhea.
- Signs/symptoms:
  - Lethargy
  - Ileus
  - Arrhythmias
  - Altered renal function.
- Investigations:
  - EKG changes—flat T waves, prolonged QT interval, U waves.
- Treatment:
  - Correct metabolic alkalosis
  - Increase potassium in daily maintenance intravenous fluids.

Note: Always correct hypokalemia slowly by IV route; Do not give potassium by bolus infusion or rapid push as it can cause arrhythmias.

Hyperkalemia

- Definition: Serum potassium—more than 6 mEq/L.

- Causes:
  - Iatrogenic—excessive administration of potassium in IV fluid
  - Severe acidosis
  - Acute renal failure
  - Congenital adrenal hyperplasia (CAH)
  - RBC breakdown
  - Laboratory error or hemolysis of blood sample.
- Signs/symptoms:
  - Arrhythmias
  - Ventricular fibrillation.
- Investigations:
  - EKG changes—peaked T waves, wide QRS, bradycardia/tachycardia, Ventricular tachycardia, Ventricular fibrillation.
- Treatment options:
  - Discontinue all potassium containing solutions
  - Calcium gluconate—200 mg/kg IV over several minutes to reach high-normal calcium range
  - Sodium bicarbonate to correct acidosis
  - Increase rate of glucose infusion
  - Insulin infusion
  - Injection furosemide
  - Kayexalate—cation exchange rasin
  - Dialysis
  - Exchange transfusion.

Calcium Abnormalities

Hypocalcemia

- Defined as total serum calcium level—less than 7.0 mg/dL in preterm babies less than 8.0 mg/dL in term babies.
- Or ionized calcium concentration of less than 4.0 mg/dL in preterm babies or less than 4.8 mg/dL in term babies.

Causes, clinical features and management discussed in chapter on Hypocalcemia

Hypercalcemia

- Definition: Serum calcium—more than 11mg/dL or ionized calcium (iCa) more than 5
- Usually associated with preterm fortifiers (HMF)
- Rare in neonates.

Magnesium Abnormalities

Hypermagnesemia

- Definition: Serum magnesium more than 2.3 meq/L.
- Causes: Maternal treatment with magnesium
- Signs/symptoms:
  - Respiratory depression
  - Apnea
  - Hypotonia
  - Decreased GI motility.
- Treatment: Self-limited, resolves within a few days.

Chapter 116

Feeding in Low Birth Weight Babies

Earl Jaspal

- Low birth weight babies—birth weight of less than 2.5 kg, irrespective of the period of their gestation
- Includes both preterm and small for gestation (SGA) babies
- India—25-35 percent of babies are low birth weight
- Low birth weight (LBW): Babies born with birth weight between 1,500 and 2,499 gm
- Very low birth weight (VLBW): Babies born with birth weight less than 1,500 gm.
- Extremely low birth weight (ELBW): Babies born with birth weight less than 1,000 gm

What Should be the Choice of Milk for LBW Babies?

- Mother's expressed breast milk is highly recommended.

Duration of Exclusive Breastfeeding

- Exclusively breastfed up to 6 months of age.

How to and When to Start Feeding?

- Babies more than 34 weeks—if able to breast feed, start as soon as possible after birth.
- Babies between 32 and 34 weeks—not able to breast feed, start feeding with cup and spoon or palladai
- Babies between 30 and 32 weeks or birth weight 1250-1500 gm—gavage feeding either nasogastric or orogastric
- Babies between 28 and 30 weeks or birth weight 1000-1250 gm—intragastric tube feeding either nasogastric or orogastric
- Babies less than 28 weeks or birth weight 500-1000 gm—start IV fluids.

Feeding guidelines—based on birth weight and gestational age:

Birth Weight 500–1000 gm or Gestational Age <28 Weeks

- Start with intravenous fluids as per protocol
- Feeds can be started once baby is clinically stable
- Feeds can be started as early as day 1 of life
- Start trophic enteral feeds at 5–10 mL/kg/day or 1–2 mL q 6 hours
- Preferred milk—mother's expressed breast milk
- If baby tolerates initial trophic feeds for 2-3 days—increase feeds by 10 mL/kg/day
- When feeds reach 100-120 mL/kg/day—add human milk fortifier.

Birth Weight: 1000–1250 gm or Gestational Age 28–30 Weeks

- Gavage feeding through an orogastric or nasogastric tube
- Choice of milk—mother's expressed breast milk
- Start with 10–20 mL/kg/day feeds in divided volumes every 2nd or 3rd hourly
- Increase feeds by 15–20 mL/kg/day, if baby tolerates.

Birth Weight: 1200–1500 gm or Gestational Age 30–32 Weeks

- Gavage feeding through an orogastric or nasogastric tube
- Choice of milk—mother's expressed breast milk
- Start with 10–20 mL/kg/day feeds in divided volumes every 2nd or 3rd hourly
- Increase feeds by 15–20 mL/kg/day, if baby tolerates
- Gradually shift to cup and spoon feeds/ palladai feeding as gestational age advances
- Once full feedings of 20 cal/oz are tolerated, advance to 24 cal/oz, if desired or add human milk fortifier.

Birth Weight: 1500–2000 gm

Gestational age—more than 34 weeks
Birth weight—more than 1600 gm   } **Try Breastfeeds**
Hemodynamically stable
Neurologically intact

For babies between 32 and 34 weeks and hemodynamcally unstable:
- Try spoon feeding/palladai feeding or use gavage feeding through an orogastric or nasogastric tube depending on the condition of the baby
- Start feeds by 15–20 mL/kg/day
- Increase feeds by 20–30 mL/day, if baby tolerates.

Absolute Contraindications to Feeding
- Congenital gut malformation
- Necrotising enterocolitis (NEC)
- Any evidence of bowel obstruction

Birth Weight: 2000–2500 gm or Gestational Age >34 Weeks

If hemodynamically stable and neurologically normal—begin breastfeeding.

FEEDING METHODS

Nasogastric / Orogastric Feeding

- Orogastric tube feeding is preferred over nasogastric feeding.

Equipment

- Infant feeding tube—6FG or 8FG with markings
- Disposable gloves
- 10 mL syringe
- Adhesive tape—micropore or transpore
- Tegaderm.

Monitoring during Insertion of Feeding Tube
- Heart rate
- Respiratory distress
- Vomiting
- Color change
- Resistance

Procedure

- Wash your hands following all 6 steps of hand washing
- Wearing disposable gloves before the procedure
- Baby is placed in supine position with the head in midline
- Measure the distance from either nostril for nasogastric or mouth for orogastric to the tragus (lobe of the ear) to the half-way point between the xiphisternum and the umbilicus

- Check position by aspirating with 10 mL syringe
- Once correct position of tube is ensured, properly fix the tube with adhesive tape
- To prevent epidermal stripping, apply tegaderm to skin of face before applying adhesive tape
- Document date, time and depth of insertion in the treatment chart.

How to Give Tube Feeding?

- Ask mother to give expressed breast milk in a cup with lid or katori with lid
- Ensure the cup/katori has been sterilized properly
- Label the cup/katori with type of milk, date and time
- Visually check position of tube before each feed and aspirate to confirm position.
- Do not give feeds without confirming tube position
- Take a 10 mL syringe, remove the plunger and connect the syringe to the feeding tube
- Pinch the end of tube before connecting to the syringe
- Put the prescribed volume of milk in the syringe following all aseptic precautions
- Allow milk to flow down the tube by gravity
- Do not apply pressure with the plunger
- Hold the tube higher because the higher the tube is held, the faster the milk will flow
- Document the type of milk, amount of feed, date and time of feed in the treatment chart.

> **What are the signs of feed intolerance?**
> - Vomiting
> - Abdominal distension
> - Large gastric aspirates
> - Altered gastric aspirates- especially hemorrhagic aspirates

Complications

- Displacement of gastric tube into trachea or esophagus leading to aspiration and pneumonia
- Malposition of gastric tube while coughing or retching
- Vasovagal response on passage of tube resulting in apnea, bradycardia and cyanosis
- Nasal trauma
- Pharyngeal trauma
- Esophageal trauma
- Trauma to skin below the fixation
- Gastroesophageal reflux.

When to Withhold Feeds?

- If the gastric aspirates are more than 5 mL/kg and more than 50% of the previous feed, do not give the current feed
- If these aspirates continues in next feeds then decrease the feed amount to the last tolerated feed
- Look for signs of feed intolerance.

Feeding with Cup and Spoon or Palladai

- Wash your hands following all 6 steps of hand washing
- Cup and spoon or palladai should be properly sterilized
- Hold the baby sitting little upright
- Hold the cup to the baby's lower lip
- Touch the edge of cup/spoon/palladai to outer part of baby's upper lip
- Let the baby become alert and let him open his mouth

- Keep the cup at the baby's lips allowing the baby take milk slowly into mouth with his tongue
- Let the baby swallow the milk as babies tend to keep some amount of milk in mouth before swallowing
- Monitor the baby during feeds
- Once the baby is full and had enough milk, baby will close his mouth
- Burp the baby properly after feeds
- Cup and spoon or palladai feeding should be given by a trained staff.

Supplements

- Vitamin D supplements—400 i.u–1000 i.u/day for 6 months of age
- Calcium and phosphorus supplementation—120–140 mg/kg/day and 60–90 mg/kg/day, respectively daily during the first months of life
- Iron supplementation—2–4 mg/kg/day, start at 2 weeks and continue up to 6 months of age.

Criteria of Discharge of Preterm and Low Birth Weight Infants

- All medical problems have been treated
- Sustained weight gain has been achieved
- Baby is able to maintain his/her temperature
- Baby is sucking all feeds
- Mother is confident in feeding and taking care of the baby
- Proper kangaroo mother care (KMC) technique is being practiced
- Appropriate vaccinations have been delivered
- Proper follow-up services have been established

Chapter 117

Intravenous Cannulation in Neonates

Earl Jaspal

INTRAVENOUS CANNULATION

Most common procedure in neonatal nurseries and neonatal intensive care units.

How to differentiate between artery and vein?

- An Artery has bright red blood
- On palpation, artery pulsates while vein does not
- When an artery is flushed, it blanches

Equipment

- Clean trolley
- Sterile dressing pack—sterile gauze, sterile drape/towel
- Skin cleansing agent
- Gloves
- Sterile cotton balls
- IV Cannula—24g or 26g depending on gestational age
- 0.9% Normal Saline—10 mL ampules
- Transparent sterile adhesive dressing—tegaderm
- Luer lock extension set—single or double lumen
- Disposable syringes—5 ml
- Adhesive tapes
- Baby board splint.

What are the preferred sites for I.V cannulation?

- Dorsal venous plexus on the hand
- Cephalic vein on the radial border of the wrist
- Accessory cephalic and cubital veins in the antecubital fossa
- Dorsal venous plexus of the foot

How to Select a Site for I.V. Cannulation?

Ideal site for vein/area:
- Vein that is relatively straight
- Vein that has not been infiltrated previously
- Area that is not bruised
- Joint of the extremity can be immobilized.

Cannulas Available for Neonates

- 24 gauge—commonly used in neonates
- 26 gauge—suitable for extremely small veins

Size	Color code	Catheter length (mm)	Water flow rate (mL/min)
24 G	Yellow	19	23
26 G	Purple	19	17

Procedure

- Take all aseptic precautions
- Follow all steps of hand washing, dry hands and wear gloves
- Inform the parents about the procedure and take a written consent
- Ensure aseptic nontouch technique is followed

- Place the infant properly on a firm surface and use comfort measures
- Prepare the IV cannula, tapes, board splint, tegaderm and prefilled syringe containing 0.9% normal saline
- Locate the infant's vein for cannulation
- Clean the selected site with appropriate antiseptic solution
- Clean the skin thoroughly in a circular motion for at least 30 seconds
- Allow to air dry. Do not re-palpate the area
- Stabilize the vein by stretching the skin and holding it taut
- Hold I.V cannula at sides so as to allow view of flashback chamber
- Insert cannula into the skin at an angle of 10–30 degrees in the direction of the venous blood flow with bevel facing upwards and introducer facing downwards
- Puncture the selected vein, observe for blood flashback in cannula hub
- When a blood flashback is seen, withdraw the stylet slowly while inserting the cannula further into the vein
- Gently flush the vein with 0.9% normal saline to ensure patency
- If swelling or resistance occurs, remove cannula and apply pressure to site to prevent hematoma formation
- If the cannula flushes properly, stabilize and secure the cannula with transparent sterile adhesive dressing
- Use board splint to support the limb, shape the splint to the limb and immobilize the joint above the insertion site
- Attach the intravenous fluid to the cannula with luer lock plug
- Secure the cannula with the correct strapping
- Dispose sharp and nonsharp materials in a proper manner
- Wash hands after procedure
- Document the date, time and vein used for cannula insertion in neonatal case record sheet.

Documentation
- Date of insertion
- Time of insertion
- Site of insertion
- Signs of infiltration
- Any manipulation done

Taping Peripheral IV Cannula

- Apply transparent sterile adhesive dressing over the tip of the cannula to observe the signs of infiltration
- Tapes should secure the limb proximal and distal to the cannula
- Do not apply tape too tightly as it may interfere with circulation of extremity
- Do not apply tape on the nail beds as it will interfere with assessment of peripheral circulation
- Do not tape over pre-existing tapes
- If retaping is required, then remove the existing tapes first
- Make tabs at ends of each tape so that tapes can be easily removed
- Do not use scissors to remove tapes
- Make sure baby is comfortable after taping
- Tape in a way that is developmentally appropriate for the baby
- For extremely premature babies use little adhesive tape directly to skin due to the fragility of skin.

Care of IV Cannula Site

- Inspect intravenous cannula site every 4th hourly for:
    - Redness
    - Swelling
    - Pain
    - Leakage
    - Position
    - Secure placement

Signs and Symptoms of Infiltration
- Pain
- Swelling
- Erythema—superficial reddening of the skin
- Leakage at the site of insertion
- Blistering
- Lack of blood return

- Check infusion pump for:
  - Correct infusion rate
  - Pumping action
  - Pressure limits
  - Occlusion
  - Alarms
  - Air in circuit.

Removal of Peripheral Intravenous Cannula

Objectives
- To prevent cannula related sepsis
- To ensure minimal handling and discomfort to the baby
- To safely remove the intravenous cannula.

Removal of IV Cannula

- Take all aseptic precautions including hand hygiene
- Remove adhesive tape gently and carefully
- Gently remove transparent adhesive dressing or tegaderm
- Slowly and carefully withdraw the cannula and apply pressure with sterile gauze to site of removal
- Observe the site for bleeding
- Do not apply dressing or adhesive tape over the bleeding site
- Press with sterile gauze until the bleeding stops
- Document the removal of cannula and date and time in the case record sheet.

Complications of IV Cannulation

- Infections—local and/or systemic
- Phlebitis—inflammation of a vein
- Hematoma—collection of blood
- Bleeding—if disconnected
- Air embolism
- Thrombus
- Accidental insertion into an artery
- Extravasation with blistering or tissue necrosis.

Blood Sugar Estimation in Newborns

Earl Jaspal

Blood sugar estimation is done to detect hypoglycemia and/or hyperglycemia
- Hypoglycemia—blood glucose levels less than 45 mg/dL
- Hyperglycemia—blood glucose higher than 125 mg/dL in term infants and higher than 150 mg/dL in preterm infants.

Risk Factors for Hypoglycemia

- Small for gestational age (birth weight <10th centile)
- Large for gestational age (birth weight >90th centile)
- Birth weight less than 2.5 kg or greater than more than 4.5 kg
- Baby born to a diabetic mother
- Any baby thought to be at risk of hypoglycemia for clinical reasons (e.g. not feeding well).

Risk Factors for Hyperglycemia

- Infants born less than 35 weeks gestation
- Septicemia
- Infants on intravenous fluids
- Infants on total parentral nutrition (TPN)
- Infants with glycosuria.

Measurement of Blood Glucose Levels

- Laboratory methods
- Rapid estimation by glucometer.

Advantages of glucometers
- Simple
- Easy to use
- Less quantity of blood required (~5 microL)
- Quick reading
- Little training required to operate
- Effective in primary, secondary and tertiary set ups.

Procedure

- Inform parents about the procedure and obtain informed written consent
- Prepare the glucometer before sampling
- Ensure hand hygiene. Follow all steps of hand washing
- Put on disposable gloves
- Make sure that the heel is warm
- Rub with hands if heel is cold

Lab Methods Include

a. Glucose oxidase method—most commonly used
b. Folin Wu method
c. O-toluidine method
d. Nelson Somaygi method

Equipment Required

- Sterile disposable lancet (tip length ≤ 2.4 mm)
- Disposable gloves
- Sterile cotton wool balls or gauze swabs
- Glucometer
- Test strips
- Sharps disposal box

- Additional warming is not recommended as it does not improve collection or reduce pain
- Ensure proper grip of newborn's heel—Place the fore finger at arch of foot and thumb to be placed below sampling site at ankle
- Select the site for sampling
- Ideal site—sampling should be done from medial and lateral limits of a warm well perfused heel
- Aim—obtain blood from the capillaries located at junction of lower dermis and upper subcutaneous tissue estimated at a depth of 0.35–1.5 mm from the skin
- Avoid previous used puncture sites
- Clean the site with a sterile cotton ball or gauze swab. Allow to dry thoroughly
- If 70% isopropyl alcohol is used, make sure alcohol has completely dried off before sampling
- Alcohol on the skin may adversely affect the test results
- Do not use povidine iodine or betadine
- Use a sterile lancet, and puncture the heel at a 90 degree angle
- Never use a lancet longer than 2.5 mm
- Application of gentle pressure and holding the foot downwards will encourage a good blood flow
- Wipe the first drop of blood away as it may be diluted by interstitial fluid
- Obtain a fresh drop of blood on the test strip that is attached to the glucometer
- If blood does not flow freely, another puncture should be performed at a different site
- On completion of sampling, press a cotton ball onto sampling site until the bleeding stops
- Ensure bleeding has stopped and baby is comfortable
- Do not apply adhesive tape at sampling site
- Wait for result to be displayed on glucometer
- Read the result and document in neonatal case record sheet
- Reconnect the monitors if they were removed for sampling
- Dispose all the sharps according to protocol.

Index